#3

OLIVER E. BYRD, Ed.D., M.D.

Professor of Health Education, Stanford University

HEALTH

THIRD EDITION

Philadelphia   London

W. B. SAUNDERS COMPANY

Preface

MANY changes, starting with *Health* as a new title, have been made in this revision of the *Textbook of College Hygiene*. These changes have been brought about by new research and new facts in the field of health, by further studies of the health problems and interests of college students and by suggestions for modifications by college and university teachers who have adopted previous editions of the textbook for their classes.

Seven new chapters have been added, with the following titles: *Reasons for Health, Stress and Tension, Physical Fitness, Safety in Sports, Malaria, Radiation and Health* and *Civil Defense*. By condensation and fusion of previous chapters it has been possible to present the new, revised edition within a total of thirty chapters.

Factual material in the text has been

brought up to date with an abundance of new topics, such as drownproofing, nalline, griseofulvin, suntan chemicals, food additives, the Rh-factor, live vaccine for poliomyelitis, atherosclerosis, mouth-to-mouth resuscitation, germ warfare, stress, and other subjects currently discussed in the medical and public health literature.

The basis for the selection of topics has remained the same, but some chapters have been enlarged. More than 100,000 consecutive calls at the Stanford University student health service have been analyzed for the discovery of the leading health problems of college students. In addition to information from this source the existing or potential health problems of about 5,000 undergraduates were explored by means of a *Personal Health Inventory* which the author had previously developed as a health history for use in schools and colleges. Studies of student health interests have been broadened through the use of an expanded checklist of 500 health problems which the author prepared from the reading of approximately 25,000 scientific articles on health which appeared in medical, public health, and allied professional journals over a period of 15 years. A fundamental concept in the preparation of this checklist was that no health problem

of trivial nature would appear in these technical journals; hence the student would have an opportunity to express an interest in only significant problems.

Topics selected on the basis of information from the foregoing explorations of the health needs and interests of college students were supplemented by a careful consideration of personal, community, and other health problems identified through the extensive readings indicated in the previous paragraph. For example, *Malaria* was added as a separate chapter because of the importance attached to this disease on a global scale by the World Health Organization, even though its conquest has been achieved within the United States. Chapters on *Radiation and Health* and on *Civil Defense* were added because of the significance of these topics in the current world situation.

References for further reading have been expanded at the end of many chapters into a deeper-level reading list for advanced, gifted, or pre-medical students. Recommended films have been increased in number. Questions for stimulation of discussion have again been provided.

As in previous editions the emphasis on the functional approach has been maintained.

OLIVER E. BYRD

Contents

2

3

4

5

6

NUTRITION AND HEALTH 58

7

OVERWEIGHT AND UNDERWEIGHT 76

8

COFFEE, TEA AND COLA DRINKS 89

9

10

11

12

13

14

15

16

17

18

19

20

21

22

23

24

25

26

27

28

29

30

1

REASONS FOR HEALTH

THERE are many reasons why people should learn about health. The reasons why college students should learn about health range from its significance in world affairs to the strictly personal needs of the late adolescent.

College students represent the intellectual cream of the nation's population in an early stage of development and maturation. The college students of today will play major roles tomorrow in the leadership of communities, states and nations. It would be unfortunate if such leaders were ignorant of the powerful impact of health and disease upon world affairs.

Medical history gives us many illustrations of the importance of health and disease in the rise and fall of nations and civilizations. The lessons of the past are accentuated in the portents of the future. For the first time in man's history, there exists the potential in nuclear, bacteriological and chemical warfare for virtual extermination of the world's population. Survival, as never before, may be a matter of understanding and preparing for the prevention or elimination of the multiple hazards that can impair or destroy life itself.

CHALLENGE OF OUR TIMES

"The challenge of our own time is to decipher the nature and the biochemical substrate of diseases and its natural history—the biological cycles of the pathogenic agents, the enigmas of genetics, and the secrets of ecology—and thus be able to anticipate the biological destiny of man and to make of therapeutics a subtle diagnostic key with which to unlock the last door opening to the threshold of life."

Felix Marti-Ibañez, 1960

At the strictly personal level, the college student needs to learn about the kinds of health problems that will confront him or his family on an increasing scale for the rest of his life. He needs to know about the significance of vitality in industry, in military service and in all kinds of endeavor. He needs to know that there is a special obligation to protect our gifted persons and to sustain them at a high level of vitality for as long as we can. He needs to know that his own personal health experience will probably include illnesses and accidents that may make profound changes in his life. He needs to know that the habits he is developing today will have an important relation to both his present and future health. He needs to know that knowledge of disease is important in international travel and that a shrinking world may expose populations to new and exotic diseases.

These and many other things in the field of health should be known to the intelligent, educated person. A thorough knowledge of the values of good health and the hazards of disease and accidents should be the possession of every cultured individual.

The Shrinking World

The world is changing as it has never changed before.

The population of the world is rapidly reaching an explosive point. The health problems that may be created by a dense packing of the earth's surface with human beings may be overwhelming. Epidemics such as humanity has never before seen may burst forth, and some of them may emerge from the laboratories of bacteriological warfare. Within a few centuries the capacity of the world to produce food to provide for all nations on a sustained basis may be challenged.

Transportation and communication have made such spectacular advances that remote and exotic diseases may suddenly comprise a threat to all the world.

The pestilence and famines of the past may be repeated in the future on grander scales in all countries.

HEALTH AND WORLD AFFAIRS

"I have been deeply impressed with the vital importance of better health to raising standards of living for the underdeveloped regions and underprivileged peoples of the world."

Nelson A. Rockefeller, 1960

The leaders of the present and those of the future who do not have an adequate understanding of the significance of health in future population problems will be poorly qualified to meet them.

Indeed, a thorough knowledge of world health problems on the part of an individual may ultimately mean his personal survival as well as that of his family, his community and even his nation.

An example of how health problems in other parts of the world differ from those in the United States can be found in the continent of Africa. The World Health Organization recently called attention to these major health problems in Africa: bilharziasis (snail fever), leprosy, malaria,

malnutrition, mental illness, onchocercia-
sis (river blindness), plague, sleeping sickness, small pox, tuberculosis, yaws and yellow fever. Although some of the diseases
are indigenous to Africa, they are a hazard
to a person from any other part of the
world who travels in that continent, and
some could be brought to the United
States by air transportation of persons who
are in the incubation period (before the
appearance of symptoms).

Other parts of the world have other
problems. It can be expected that diseases
from other nations may make their appearance in this country, and it is entirely
possible that under certain circumstances
these appearances could be on an epidemic scale.

In July 1960 President Dwight Eisenhower signed the Health for Peace Act in
which Congress expressed its desire to
give financial support to the conquest of
disease in foreign countries.

The Health for Peace Act symbolizes
the growing importance of international
health in world affairs and makes possible
an expression of good will and sympathy
on the part of the United States that may
contribute to better understanding among
the peoples of the world.

Part of a man's education should be the
understanding of the international significance of health.

> "Massive success in international health coopera-
> tion could well serve as a model for other efforts
> to build a cooperative world characterized by
> peace, freedom and justice."
> *Milton S. Eisenhower, Ph.D., 1959*

The Challenge of Vitality

There is an ever-present challenge to
the intellect of mankind to create a higher
level of individual, national and world vitality than is now in existence.

Meeting the challenge to create in the
minds of men a state of supreme mental
health would afford perhaps the greatest
potential for enlightened world leadership.
So great is the world's need for stable,
well-balanced, far-sighted leaders with an
abundance of vitality that it would be
tragic if the history of the world were repeated in respect to the deranged and
mentally ill despots of the past.

> ### HIGH-LEVEL WELLNESS
> "... our eyes have been so long turned in a dif-
> ferent direction, concentrating fixedly on disease
> and death. When we take time to turn our gaze
> in the opposite direction, focusing it intently on
> the condition termed good health, we see that
> wellness ... is a complex state, made up of over-
> lapping levels of wellness ... the state of being
> well ... is a fascinating and everchanging pano-
> rama of life itself, inviting exploration of its every
> dimension."
> *Dr. Halbert L. Dunn, M.D., Ph.D., 1959*

Health and vitality of both a physical
and mental nature is an urgent necessity
for all future leaders. The world can no
longer afford the catastrophic results of
leadership by fatigued, ill, declining and
even unbalanced persons.

Good health and vitality are necessary
for effective, able and long-sustained leadership. Perhaps some day the peoples of
the world will develop an effective screening program for the elimination of the
physically and mentally unfit from positions of power and prominence. If this
ever occurs, we should expect to see a
more stable and mature approach to world
problems. We need to have good leaders
at high levels of vitality and health, and
their replacements should meet similar
standards.

High levels of vitality and mental health
have many foundations. A superior genetic
inheritance, sound, well balanced nutrition, protection from contagious diseases,
avoidance of many harmful substances,

freedom from disabling accidents, the wise use of medical care, thorough understanding of human relations and many other physical and mental factors are related to vitality and emotional health.

SOCIAL PATHOLOGY

"A sizeable body of information has been accumulated which suggests . . . a positive correlation between physical illness and various aspects of social pathology."

Zdenek Hrubec, Sc.D., 1959

An example of a devitalized population is the one in which malaria exists on a widespread scale. It has often been said that for every death from malaria there are 100 cases of the disease in the community. It is well known by health authorities that malaria causes a serious decline in health and vitality even when it does not destroy life. A devitalized population suffering from malaria on a massive scale is often not aware of its lack of vitality. People who live in a world of perpetual semi-sickness and low vitality are not apt to understand the need for improvement unless somewhere and somehow the horizon is lifted so that they can see the promise of better things.

Emotional Health and Human Relationships

There is much to be learned in the field of mental health.

Although we do not understand all of the causes of mental illness we do know a great deal about emotional health for normal people.

A full understanding of human relationships will make a person happier and far more effective in his relations with other people, including his own family. A knowledge of basic emotional needs and of how to adjust every-day situations can prob-

ably do more than any other single thing for the promotion of human happiness.

It is also helpful for the college student to know about the kinds of emotional problems that are commonplace among his peers. The emotional problems experienced by one group of college students are indicated in the associated table.

It is also wise for a person to learn about some of the major symptoms of mental illness. To recognize that a person is mentally ill may save much distress in human relationships and may eventually lead to the securing of proper medical and psychiatric care for the afflicted person. Such symptoms are described in a later chapter.

EMOTIONAL PROBLEMS OF A GROUP OF 187
UNIVERSITY STUDENTS

Rank	Focal Point of Problem	Number of Students
1.	Occupation	32
2.	Insecurity, sense of inferiority, lack of confidence, self-consciousness	24
3.	Love and marriage problems	17
4.	Mother or father conflict	14
5.	Grades in college	9
6.	Confusion in sex adjustments	6
7.	Religion	5
8.	Financial	5
9.	General outlook on life	5
10.	Social adjustment	4
11.	Worry	4
12.	Procrastination	4
13.	Present world situation; possibility of war	4
14.	Learning how to study	3
15.	Poor health of parents	2
16.	Disappointment in athletics	2

Personal Health Experiences

The great majority of college students have already had a number of health experiences of significance. On a restricted scale the health problems of the total pop-

ACCIDENT AND SURGICAL EXPERIENCE OF A
CLASS OF 92 UNIVERSITY STUDENTS

Surgical Experience	
No surgery	28
Surgery	64
Tonsillectomy	48
Appendectomy	13
Hernia	3
Aural (ear)	2
Eye	2
Oral	2
Malignancy—leg	1
Infected hand	1
Herniated disk	1
Moles	1
Deviated septum	1
Nasal Polyps	1
Submucous resection	1
Bone biopsy	1

Accidents (40% of class)		
Cuts, bruises, etc.		12
Broken arms		9
Broken legs		5
Broken clavicles		4
Broken noses		4
Broken ankles		3
Broken patellas		2
Broken wrist		1
Broken rib		1
Broken toe		1
Broken foot		1
Dislocated knee		3
Dislocated shoulder		1
Ruptured tendons		2
"Torn" ligaments		5
Ankle	3	
Spine	1	
Knee	1	
Head injury		1
Optic nerve severed		1
Sacroiliac subluxation		1
Burn		1
Temporary paralysis		1
Sprains		6

ACCIDENT AND SURGICAL EXPERIENCE OF A CLASS
OF 92 UNIVERSITY STUDENTS (*Continued*)

Accident Sources	
Falls	16°
Athletics	13
Skiing	9
Automobile	6
Horses	3
Dogbite	2
Roller skating	2

One Case Each

Shotgun, ice skating, tobogganing, bolt, arm through window, jumping rope, pick in head, pedestrian hit by auto.

ulation are represented by those of the current college generation.

Analysis of the personal health experiences of a group of college students can be expected to reveal that about 40 per cent have had a serious accident, that about 60 per cent have had some kind of surgery during their lives and that as many as 20 per cent or more have family health backgrounds that provide a special hazard.

The accident and surgical experience of 92 students in a single college class is summarized in the associated tables.

As many as 30 per cent of the students on the average college campus can be expected to have lost some member of their immediate families by death. An additional 5 per cent can be expected to have some member of the family living with a serious health problem such as heart disease, cancer, ulcers, arthritis, diabetes, mental disorder, gallbladder disease or other disorder. The family health experience of death or disease is certain to affect the college student in a highly personal way sooner or later.

The person who goes through life without a single medical or surgical experience is indeed rare. Most college students have already had one or more illnesses, broken bones, automobile accidents, surgical operations, athletic injuries and emotional problems of varying intensity. If you have not yet had a serious illness, the chances are that you will have one.

Personal and family health experiences ought to alert the intelligent student to the fact that he cannot and will not escape the impact of life-and-death problems.

Safeguarding the Gifted

The gifted, by virtue of their unusual talents, have a special place in society. The premature loss of special talents by illness or death represents a deficit for society the magnitude of which is difficult or impossible to measure.

The child with great natural talents who dies before maturity never has the opportunity to contribute to society those things he might have achieved had he lived. The mature, gifted adult who functions at a low level of vitality may make great contributions to the civilization of which he is a part, yet even greater things might come from such genius if it were coupled with vitality. The premature loss of genius by death may have a profound impact upon a society, which, perhaps, can never be recognized.

In an age of great emphasis upon science it does not make sense to ignore information that may protect our leadership genius. Civilizations rise and fall on the collective contributions of its gifted people.

Health and Legal Affairs

It is important for the well informed person to be aware of the legal implications of health, disease and injury.

There are laws in industry of compensation for injured workers. There are legal regulations covering many health benefits of various groups in our society. There are legal requirements pertaining to the health of the school child. There are laws governing the medical care of indigents and old persons. There are legislative enactments pertaining to the medical and surgical correction of physical defects in persons under the age of twenty-one.

Courts often award heavy damages for injury to life or limb because of accidents. Similar awards have been made in the case of the transmission of communicable disease. Other damages have been ruled because of negligence on the part of an individual or group in the protection of others.

There are many public health laws that protect the people of a community, such as regulations for the control of air pollution, water pollution and other hazards. There are many legal rights that the individual must forfeit if his actions constitute a health threat to others, such as may be involved in the spread of tuberculosis and other diseases. In short, there are many laws pertaining to the health of the individual and the community about which the educated person should be informed.

Knowledge in Emergencies

In a critical health emergency a knowledge of what to do, and what not to do, may save your own life or that of another.

The educated person should know what to do in any emergency that threatens life. He should know how to conduct himself so that he does not cause further injury to a person who is already suffering from disease or accident. He should know his ethical, moral and legal obligations when confronted with a health emergency. He should have an adequate knowledge of first aid and he should have faith in his knowledge.

The educated person should know that there are only two critical health emergencies, severe bleeding and cessation of breathing. In all other situations a greater amount of time is available for doing the right thing. In these two emergencies a knowledge of what to do, and prompt action based on this knowledge, can and will save lives.

Knowledge is power in an emergency. The intelligent, educated person can and should exercise this power. It may save the life of someone in his family. It may result in the gift of life to a total stranger. It may mean the saving of a talented person that society can ill afford to lose.

Fitness for Work

Many intelligent people believe that a high level of physical fitness is valuable only for physical performance in sports, military service or physical labor. Nothing could be further from the truth. A high level of physical vitality enables anyone in any field to work with greater intensity and for a longer period of time. Fitness is an advantage in any line of effort.

The laboratory worker who becomes physically fatigued is a less efficient worker. The research person who is tired is no longer as brilliant an investigator as when his vitality was at a high level. The speaker who is physically fatigued may lose much of the sparkle and vitality of his presentation. The judgment of the business executive is apt to be less acute as he declines in vigor.

There never has been and never will be any sharp cleavage between mind and body. Mental and emotional stress have been shown to produce actual physiologic and anatomic changes in the human body. Physical fatigue definitely impairs the functioning of the intellect. The products of mankind reflect the sum total of both physical vitality and intellectual capacity. It can never be otherwise.

MOTIVE FOR LIVING

". . . sustained growth and vigor depend, to a large degree, on some positive motive for living. Without motive, a person of 35 might be old . . ."
Medicine at Work, 1957

To many people it will be a novel concept that a person might follow training rules for top performance in his work just as an athlete trains for a high level of physical performance. The training rules are different, but they can pay dividends in executive ability, laboratory research, salesmanship or in any other kind of work.

Military Conflict

Wars of the future can be expected to involve nuclear fission and radioactive fallout, new and deadly gases, destructive chemicals and contagious diseases on a scale never before seen by mankind.

Survival in future military conflict may be strictly a matter of two factors: (1) luck and (2) knowledge.

It would be foolish for the educated person to leave out of his cultural preparation a knowledge of those things that may permit him to survive under the annihilating conditions of modern warfare. A full knowledge of how to protect yourself from radioactive materials, from contagious diseases, and from nerve gas and other chemicals can make a substantial difference in the welfare of you and your family.

Military conflict always places a high premium upon physical fitness. A thorough knowledge of the multiple factors involved in the creation of a high level of physical fitness may some day make the difference between survival and death.

An intelligent appraisal of the kinds of hazards that will be encountered in any war of the future does not mean that a student must conclude that war is inevitable. For a man to subscribe heavily to life insurance when his children are young does not mean that he anticipates dying early. It does mean that he is preparing for the contingency or possibility that his untimely death may plunge his family into financial distress.

Knowledge of the hazards of war con-

MORE DIFFICULT THAN MEDICINE

"Politics has a depth and complexity encountered in no other human pursuit. Einstein perceived this and succinctly summed it up when he was asked why it was that men who can develop wonder drugs and stamp out epidemics, cannot understand politics. The wise old man answered that politics is more difficult than medicine."
Elliot Lee Richardson, 1959

stitute a strong incentive to resolve all international conflicts by mediation and compromise.

For war or peace, let us learn about the hazards to life and health of modern warfare.

Travel and Health

Foreign lands are no longer inaccessible from the United States. It has become commonplace for college students and others to travel to many different parts of the world. It is likely that this mobility of population will increase during the generations to come.

Travel abroad is governed by certain international health regulations and by certain global health problems.

The person who leaves the United States for travel must carry with him an international certificate of vaccination proving immunization against smallpox, yellow fever and cholera. In addition to this requirement the traveler must meet the vaccination requirements that are established by specific foreign countries. Upon his return to the United States he must meet our own immunization requirements or he will not be admitted to this country.

GEOGRAPHY OF DISEASE

"The pattern of disease on our planet today dates back hundreds of millions of years. . . . Disease is inseparable from its environment, and . . . the vital factors of geography."

Jacques M. May, 1953

In certain areas of the world the traveler will be confronted with diseases about which he knows little unless he has deliberately prepared himself in the field of health for travel in such areas. Certain immunizations will be recommended for the traveler's own protection in certain parts of the world, even though these are not required by international regulations.

To protect himself against devitalizing disease, the foreign traveler must be well informed in the field of health. He must make the maximum use of immunization procedures. He must conform to certain international health standards. If his family accompanies him he must give serious thought to the protection of young children; failure to do so may result in needless illness or loss of life.

Even within the United States the well-informed person will recognize that he should not go by air when he has an ear infection; that he should recognize poison oak or poison ivy when he is in the wilds; that mosquitoes and ticks and other insects may spread serious diseases in certain sections of the country; that animals may spread disease and that there are many health hazards of which a person should become aware when he leaves his own community.

Emerging Health Habits

The college student is at a period of life where health habits are emerging that may become fixed throughout a lifetime. Many of the alcoholics in this country began drinking heavily in college or during the college age period; those who smoke tobacco usually have the habit well established by the time they leave college; driving patterns on streets and highways are emerging for good or bad.

Faulty eating habits may have developed long before the student entered college, but for many students college life represents the first years away from home, and eating patterns will depend upon self-direction and independence in the choice or rejection of foods.

Some indication of the health habits of a typical group of college students may be achieved by an analysis of a group of 200 students in which it was shown that 20 per cent were smoking between one-half and one package or more of cigarettes daily;

approximately 38 per cent were not meeting the nutrition standards of the National Research Council; 12 per cent were drinking alcohol daily (mostly beer); and approximately 10 per cent were taking medicines such as thyroxin, antihistamines, aspirin, sleeping pills, reducing pills, and certain antibiotics on prescription (for the prevention of the recurrence of rheumatic fever).

It is likely that health habits established during college days may persist throughout the major part of a lifetime. The thinking student may well contemplate the establishment of desirable health habits of exercise, rest, nutrition, and control over the use of alcohol and tobacco. Decisions and habits now may well have a deciding influence upon his present and future health.

Quackery in Health

In our society there are many charlatans who profess to cure the sick and promote human vitality. These unscrupulous persons defraud the public with false claims of cures for cancer, arthritis and other perplexing medical problems. They operate vigorously in the field of nutrition and in other areas of human health where good or bad results are often difficult to measure.

These health quacks often cause fatal delays for people suffering from illnesses that could be cured with proper medical or surgical attention. Besides defrauding the American public of millions of dollars annually these confidence men in the field of health actually cause needless loss of life in some instances.

> **HEALTH BELIEFS**
> "Anthropologists and physicians have remarked on the tenacity with which certain beliefs . . . regarding the causation of disease are held by some of the world's more primitive peoples."
> **M. Margaret Clark, Ph.D., 1959**

The intelligent, educated person should be able to distinguish between the signs of charlatanism and the dignity of sound medical advice.

Health Plans for the Future

The intelligent, educated person can plan ahead more effectively than the less intelligent and less educated person.

Health plans for the future should take into consideration as broad a preventive program as possible. They can be built around the following factors: (1) health education, and (2) health insurance and life insurance.

Plans for the future call for an intelligent understanding of the many health problems that can impair or shatter the health of the individual or his family. This knowledge can only be gained through health education, although information on health problems may come from many directions and many fields of study.

Full use should be made of all the preventive measures that science has evolved for the protection of health. For example, effective use should be made of immunizations in the protection of adults as well as children.

Plans ought to be made for the securing of good medical care when preventive measures fail. These medical care plans should include all the major professional services that may be needed in the treatment of the sick or the injured, and they should also provide for sufficient family income during the period of illness so that a family is protected against economic distress. To plan ahead is one of the marks of intelligence and maturity.

Questions

1. What do you consider adequate preparation in planning for the health protection of a family of four?

2. What is the significance of health in world affairs?

3. If five young scientists were lost in an airplane crash at an average age of thirty-five years, how could you estimate the loss to society?

4. What special justification is there for a gifted person to learn about health?

5. Is the money spent by a community in the correction of physical handicaps in young people a financial advantage?

6. Why is health assuming greater significance in the world?

For Further Reading

1. Clark, M. Margaret: *Health in the Mexican-American Culture*. Berkeley, California, University of California Press, 1960.

2. Cook, James: *Remedies and Rackets: The Truth About Patent Medicines Today*. New York, W. W. Norton and Company, 1959.

3. Roth, A.: *The Teen Age Years: A Medical Guide for Young People and Parents*. New York, Doubleday and Company, 1960.

4. Rule, Colter: *A Traveler's Guide to Good Health*. Garden City, New York, Doubleday and Company, 1960.

For Advanced Reading

Gallagher, J. Roswell: *Medical Care of the Adolescent*. New York, Appleton-Century-Crofts, Inc., 1960.

2

EMOTIONAL HEALTH

VERY often some remarkably simple change in the way of living can result in substantial improvement in the mental or emotional health of the person who is basically stable. Even thirty minutes' additional rest in the period of twenty-four hours may make a person less irritable, friendlier, and therefore easier to get along with. This is especially apt to be so if the additional rest is secured in the form of one or two periods of physical relaxation or sleep during the daytime.

Eating a better breakfast or an earlier dinner may help greatly in preventing fatigue and irritability. This is especially true in those persons who tend to have low blood sugar levels. A great many tensions in the normal person can be traced directly to fatigue and undernourishment. A good starting point for mental health is to see that you get adequate rest and good food.

11

Mental health for the person in good physical health with reasonably adequate health habits is largely a problem in human relations.

To understand other people and to know that they have precisely the same emotional needs that you have is probably the most fundamental step toward both the maintenance of good mental health in yourself and the creation of sound emotional development in others.

When people understand which emotional needs are fundamental and when they realize the destructive psychologic effects of deficiencies in emotional experiences upon the personalities, it can be expected that the normal person will have a greater opportunity for a stable and emotionally rich life.

The Need for a Sense of Security

For emotional stability a person must have a reasonable sense of security.

When worries, tensions, fears and anxieties plague a person, it should be obvious that his emotional stability will be affected. Research has shown that anxiety, for example, may have profound influences on both the physical and mental status of the individual.

One of the harmful effects of anxiety lies in its impairment of the power to reason. One psychiatrist who studied, for a period of several years, a large group of patients suffering from anxiety found that in almost all cases it was more difficult for these persons to solve problems whenever they were in a state of acute anxiety. Perhaps even more significant was his discovery that about 10 per cent of the patients suffered from *utter and complete destruction of the power to reason.* About one person in ten in this group of patients was unable to do any effective reasoning at all while suffering from acute anxiety, although during a period of calm these same patients could work all the problems in reasoning given to them by the psychiatrist.

Such research is very important, for it tells us that the patient who is insecure and anxious cannot think as well as the person who feels secure and serene.

A sense of insecurity and anxiety can be spread from one person to another. In one interesting experiment a group of psychiatrists listened to recordings made of patients suffering from acute anxiety. After the records had been played the psychiatrists themselves were in a state of anxiety. Other studies as well as practical experience tell us that anxiety is a communicable disease. In fact, some psychiatrists believe that it should be classified among the communicable diseases by public health authorities.

A group of psychiatrists in making studies of anxiety found that it was primarily spread from one person to another through sound. So far as practical human situations are concerned this means that anxiety will be spread from one person to another mostly through speech. To establish a sense of security in someone else, attention should be given to the quality of the voice. The person who learns voice modulation may be making a considerable contribution to the reduction of family tensions and quarrels. Almost everyone knows that when a person elevates his voice in anger, there is apt to be instant transmission of tension to another. Most likely that person's voice then climbs higher, and tension is transmitted back again to the other person. Such shuffling of anxiety builds tensions and makes it difficult or impossible to settle any quarrel through the use of reason.

The Need To Be Loved

The need for affection is basic and universal among all people of all races and at all ages.

Most people need to develop the capacity for expressing affection. With small children it is a relatively simple procedure to embrace them or tell them frankly that you love them. At the college level the problem is more complicated. Affection from friends takes the form of liking rather than outright love. In other words, we need to have the feeling that we have friends who like us. To be deprived of friends is to be deprived of a mature form of affection.

It is easy to make friends. All you have to do is be nice to people, be considerate of them, recognize their good qualities, overlook their bad habits, be modest about your own accomplishments, and smile and be cheerful when you are with others.

Many people have a genuine liking for their friends, but fail to let them know about it. Often one member of a family may have a deep and genuine love for the other members of the family, but may fail to indicate this in any way whatsoever.

This is a mistake. Since people have a basic emotional need for the regard of others, we should let them know about it when we do like them.

People who are shy or have a deep reserve may find it most difficult to come out of their shells to express an emotion. It can be done, however, for there are hundreds and even thousands of different ways of expressing regard or affection for others.

A friendly smile, a word of approbation, a pat on the back, a friendly wink, an expression of courteous attention, depriving oneself of a privilege in favor of another are all ways of saying, "I like you" or "I love you."

The important thing for people to remember when they have a difficult time showing any emotion is that the other person needs that expression of liking or regard in order to achieve a normal and wholesome level of mental health. In other words, when you express yourself, you are actually serving others rather than exposing yourself. People who are reluctant to express their inner feelings are not only depriving themselves of many friends, but

are also overlooking opportunities for contributing to the welfare of others. This is a mistake that you ought not to make.

The Need for Independence

The psychologic structure of the human being is such that he is happiest when he has independence.

Independence, however, must be coupled with respect and consideration for others. The most effective kind of independence is that which supports the emotional need of the individual without taking from others their instinctive right to be independent.

Independence should not be granted indiscriminately. It should be gauged to the capacity and maturity of the individual. It should be associated with a sense of responsibility. Independence without a sense of responsibility is essentially a form of license. When responsibility is associated with independence, the latter is freedom rather than license.

Independence, then, carries with it responsibilities for the intelligent use of that freedom. Until people are mature enough to understand that the achievement of independence must be linked with the development of social responsibilities for the good of all, there will be evidence that the capacity for independence has not yet been adequately developed.

To shelter a child from harmful influences is a responsibility of parenthood. To extend this protection into a long-lasting overprotection is psychologic disservice to the individual. The parent who overprotects a child or young adult for fear that the individual will make a mistake is actually destroying, or at least hindering, development of the capacity to do the right thing.

Every parent should have a deliberate program to yield independence to his or her children. In the long run it pays dividends of happiness for all members of the family.

The Need To Be Successful

For emotional satisfaction all people need to feel that they have accomplished something worthwhile.

In looking for the success that we need for our emotional development, however, many people make a serious error. The mistake is to look only for a major success. Great triumphs are for the gifted few or the fortunate ones who achieve results of significance by force of circumstances.

Sometimes it is necessary for us to broaden our sense of values to recognize our achievements. Success should not be counted solely in terms of business leadership, professional competence or financial independence. In a spiritual and psychologic sense the person who contributes to the happiness of others in the family, who brings up children to an understanding maturity, or who enriches the emotional lives of others through kindness, consideration, tolerance and understanding, may have achieved a far greater success than others who have concentrated on the material things. If we add up intangible achievements, we can draw spiritual and emotional satisfaction from them. Even the smaller successes of daily life should be recognized and cumulated deliberately as a contribution to the meeting of our emotional needs.

Knowing that success or accomplishment is essential to our own emotional life, we should not be reluctant to recognize and praise success in others. Whenever we acknowledge an accomplishment by someone else we are contributing to the mental health of that person.

The Need for Recognition

When we are recognized by others, we have psychologic evidence of our importance to them. This is good for our mental health, for recognition is apt to be an indication of regard, respect, and friendship that helps to establish in us a sense of value.

If there is any doubt in your mind that recognition includes an emotional component, think back to the last time you passed an acquaintance to whom you nodded or spoke, but from whom you received only indifference or rejection in return. Most likely your own emotions boiled up to a distressing point of resentment. Chances are that you still harbor a sense of resentment against the person even though the experience may have taken place months or years ago. Emotional reactions of this type are not easily forgotten.

Recognition, of course, can take many different forms. It is not solely a matter of saying "Hello" to a person or calling him by name. Some of the finest kinds of recognition may be carried out in the absence of the person being recognized. For example, praising the work of one person to a group, even if the person involved is not at that particular meeting or assembly, may give great emotional satisfaction to the person commended when he hears about it.

If you seek the opinion of another, especially if you respect the advice you may secure, you are giving recognition. If you exhibit the work of another, even without comment of any kind, you are expressing recognition. If, in a conversation, you defer to the comment or wisdom of another, you are giving recognition.

Such things are intangible, but they are apt to bring emotional satisfaction to both the giver and the receiver.

The Need for Self-Respect

A mature person, aware of life's responsibilities, should not see himself as an utterly insignificant part of family and community affairs. The ego is a powerful force in emotional life and must be sustained at a normal level.

Self-respect rests mainly upon an independent spirit, a sense of having accomplished something worthwhile, and recognition by others of the useful things you have done.

Your worthwhile achievements, however, may not always be apparent to others. They may be unknown even to you.

The housewife and mother who does a good job of bringing up children who are honest, truthful, capable of self-direction, creative because they have been encouraged, confident and poised and many other desirable qualities, has been a major success in life even though she, as well as others, may not realize this fact for years—if at all. Self-respect, based on knowledge of accomplishment in such a situation, can invigorate and sustain a person's mental health.

Self-respect is recognized by others even though they may not know what that self-respect is grounded upon.

To live well with one's self is to assure a calm and orderly progress through life.

The Need To Be Taken as We Are

Personalities cannot be changed overnight, but they *can* be changed. This is apparent in our everyday living and in the adjustments we make to other people. There is a limit, however, to our capacity for change.

If adjustment to others is always one-way, then this giving in and modifying of our own way of living and thinking must eventually lead to a disturbing surrender of independence and self-direction.

There is a fundamental emotional need for acceptance as we are. In other words, each of us has a basic personality structure beneath which no changes can be made without unhappiness and disturbance of our mental health. Knowing this, we should be willing to accept others even though there may be uncongenial elements in their personalities.

Knowing that each person has a funda-mental need for acceptance should make it easier for us to get along with those who have ugly personalities as well as those who have attractive ones. There is no perfection anywhere in the world; hence we must expect that all people will have faults. That person who has the greatest number of faults will also have the greatest amount of rejection by other people. As a consequence, his emotional need for acceptance will be greater than average.

If we know that the person with an unattractive personality has a greater than average need for acceptance, this may make it easier for us to give that acceptance. In giving, we help in the reconstruction of the mental health of that person and we also enrich our own sense of accomplishment and self-respect.

Authority and Mental Health

Authority may be good or bad, depending upon its quality. Harsh, unjust authority becomes tyranny which those with independence and spirit may revolt against. Authority which is just and fair and clarifies the rules under which we live, so that everyone has a better understanding of his relation to others, is the kind of leadership that aids mental health.

Many people draw great strength from religion because to them it represents the highest kind of authority. When this authority has also prescribed a reasonable code of ethics or set of rules of conduct for human affairs which is adapted to the needs of the individual, mental health is apt to flourish.

We have a fundamental need for guidance in human affairs that will keep us out of confusion. To be confused is to be uncertain and insecure, to lack confidence in one's self, to court failure and to have little self-respect. A major function of the right kind of authority is to dispel confusion and uncertainty. When this is done in a wholesome manner, it is a distinct contribution to the emotional health of the individual.

Those in positions of leadership who understand the need of others for authority are responsible for seeing that their leadership is democratic, just and fair.

Mental Health Is Based on Giving as Well as Receiving

To give is a richer experience than to receive. That person who has not discovered the deep value of generosity has yet to understand one of life's richest rewards. So it is with mental health. He who contributes to the emotional welfare of others will draw strength, security and understanding by so doing.

A most important move toward one's own mental health is learning the fundamental emotional needs of all human beings and then setting out to make contributions to others with those needs in mind. Such contributions cost nothing to the giver. They bring intangible rewards, but mental health is composed more of intangibles than material things.

That person who expresses kindness and affection, security, recognition and respect to others is most apt to receive the same in return. To meet the basic emotional needs of others is to provide the basis for one's own mental health.

Some Common Emotional Problems

All normal people have emotional problems, and everyone has a breaking point. Anyone, if troubles pile unceasingly upon him, can have a nervous collapse. Even a sheep dog, placid lamb or guinea pig can have a breakdown if the conditions are bad enough and last long enough.

Many normal people, however, do not have emotional problems of any particular intensity at any given time. Today, for example, you may not feel that you have a problem in mental hygiene. Tomorrow you may feel differently, for conflicts and other difficulties may arise between now and then. In the meantime there is no use getting agitated about trivial emotional problems. It makes sense, however, to *know* what kinds of emotional problems *normal people have* and to be aware in advance that you will probably have similar problems at various times throughout life.

Types of Problems

The worries and difficulties that beset normal college students, ranked in order of greatest frequency, are about as follows. Uncertainty as to future occupation or employment is apt to lead the list in frequency, but not in severity. Next most common are mental problems centered around a feeling of insecurity, a sense of inferiority, lack of confidence, and self-consciousness. In fact, it is from this group of emotional problems that the greatest intensity of difficulties will be found.

Next in line, so far as frequency is concerned, are problems of love and marriage and mother or father conflict. Grades in college are a source of worry to some students.

The highest proportion of severe problems is apt to occur among those students who experience confusion in sex adjustments. Religion, too, may create emotional problems for some students as well as resolve problems for others.

Financial difficulties and social adjustments will worry only a minority of college students.

In a small group there will be a variety of mental health problems centered around physical illness (such as eczema), fainting spells, overeating, death of some person in the family, and so on. Emotional problems may also be related to miscellaneous fac-

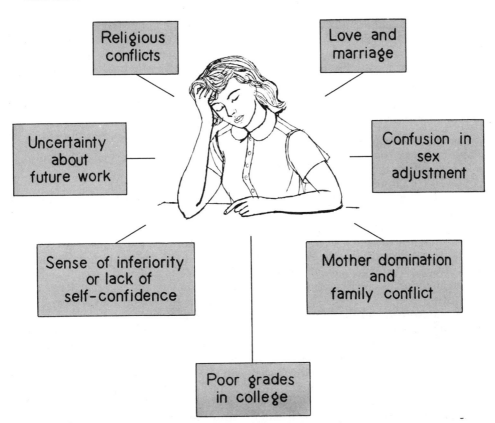

Religious conflicts

Love and marriage

Uncertainty about future work

Confusion in sex adjustment

Sense of inferiority or lack of self-confidence

Mother domination and family conflict

Poor grades in college

Figure 1. Emotional problems of college students.

tors such as gambling, trouble with in-laws, disappointment in athletics, and many other items.

Remember, if you are experiencing a mental health problem such as any of the foregoing, you are confronted with an emotional difficulty typical of those experienced by normal college students.

Mental Health and Occupation

Circumstances may be more important than your training so far as *getting* a job is concerned. Once the job has been obtained, however, it will most likely be your performance that decides the issue of future promotion and satisfaction rather than any specific training for the particular job that you may have experienced. In fact, it is unlikely that you will be trained in college in the specific details of your future work. College should be a maturing experience rather than a trade school which qualifies you in a particular occupation. *Personal qualities rather than knowledge of facts will probably be more important in your work progress in the long run.*

You should know also that many people train for special occupations and then work in a totally different field.

For the professions, of course, the problem is different. An engineer must have had training in engineering; a doctor must have had training in medicine; a lawyer must have had preparation in law; and so on. Even so, there are many persons trained as lawyers who end up in politics, business or other fields. Many business students change to the professions even when they have had to undergo late preparation in the new field.

Do not be dismayed, for your problems are like those of most other people in respect to preparation for work.

Lack of Confidence

The emotional problems that have the greatest intensity as well as next to greatest frequency in normal college students are: a sense of inferiority, lack of self-confidence, feelings of insecurity, and self-consciousness.

From the academic viewpoint, college students have already demonstrated their superiority. Only a minority of high school graduates enter college; college students are definitely of a superior group, at least academically.

The widespread lack of self-confidence that exists among normal college students appears to indicate that even if they are superior, they do not recognize it.

It is important for any individual college student who feels a sense of inferiority to know that a substantial number of his classmates have precisely the same feeling about themselves. Even students who occupy leadership positions often doubt their own abilities and feel self-conscious when speaking to their fellow students, though they may give no inkling of this.

Rather than worry about his self-consciousness, the student should look upon it as a normal phenomenon for his particular age group. In fact, if the question were discussed widely among college students, it would be apparent that all have about the same hesitations, doubts and misgivings.

Sometimes a sense of inferiority can be traced directly to a failure to achieve emancipation from an overdominant parent. If this be the case, the student should realize that college itself affords a first major experience in the achievement of independence. Time, rather than psychologic devices, may bring the confidence and security that a person needs for his own emotional satisfaction. Knowing that feelings of inferiority are common among others, however, will decrease the severity of the problem for many college students. This can be a first step toward overcoming feelings of inferiority.

Mother or Father Conflict

Domination of normal college students by one or both parents is often a source of severe emotional conflict. Resolving such a conflict requires a thorough understanding of the psychologic mechanisms involved.

Mother domination is apt to be more commonplace than father domination. There is a logical and sensible reason for this; to understand that there is makes the problem easier and may lead to its ultimate solution.

When a child is born he is completely helpless or very nearly so. In other words, every one of us starts life almost completely dependent upon an adult. This adult almost without exception is the mother. From the start of your life, then, your mother has been in the psychologic position of dominating your activities, a responsibility she could not avoid without being charged with neglect. It is also a position from which she draws great psychologic satisfaction, because taking care of a baby or young child is a service. To serve others is to gain emotional satisfaction.

In the early years of life the mother is compelled to make decisions for her child. To let the child make decisions at too early an age may result in severe damage or loss of life. For example, to permit a two-year-old child to cross the street unguided through heavy traffic may lead to the death of the child. Some adult control is obviously needed.

On the other hand, to continue making decisions for a child long past the time he is able to make them for himself is to do him a severe injustice. If freedom of decision is granted too soon, great psychologic and physical harm may be done, but if freedom of decision is postponed too long, the harm may be as great.

It takes almost genius in human understanding to be able to judge accurately just when independence in respect to the responsibilities of life should be granted to a young person. Many mothers do not have that genius, but they do have love for the child involved, and it is this affection that may cause them great distress. Emotional problems accumulate for the child, too, if the power of self-decision is not encouraged and promoted gradually under parental direction.

It is a wise parent who plans deliberately to release emotional controls and to stimulate and promote the power of self-decision and the growth of independence in his or her children. Such parents should be treasured and respected, for they are all too uncommon. The college student is more apt to have one or both parents who learn by blunder, confusion and slow experience that a child cannot grow into an adult until independence has been achieved.

Religion

Many people are apt to draw strength and security from religion. Belief and faith in an ultimate authority makes possible an interpretation of life that makes the latter full of meaning.

Most religions have a code of ethics aimed at making people live together in greater peace and security.

One of the basic emotional needs of all human beings is for an authority that clarifies the rules of human conduct. Working in ignorance of or confusion about the regulations that govern social affairs fosters poor emotional health. Religion, by the provision of a supreme authority, meets a fundamental emotional need.

For the troubled individual religion may provide a means of sharing and distributing psychologic burdens.

On the other hand, religion can be, and is at times, a source of serious problems of mental health. At the college level a fairly common emotional problem is created when young people of opposite religious faiths fall in love. Merely falling in love with a member of another church does not in itself automatically create a problem in mental health. However, when the parents of the two young people are so devout in their attachments to their own churches that they cannot accept marriage of their children to those of other denominations, then the seed of emotional conflict has been sown.

Since love is apt to be based upon personality rather than upon religious beliefs, it should be obvious that people of various faiths and denominations can become enamoured of each other. When trouble arises, it is almost invariably caused by the family rather than by the individuals who have fallen in love.

Problems of religious adjustment should be explored not solely in terms of those who are contemplating marriage, since many times no conflict exists at this point. But when children are born, a problem may arise concerning the faith which these children are to be encouraged to adopt. Prospective marriage partners should discuss such a problem in detail before entering into wedlock. They should also discuss with their families the wisdom of marriage between members of conflicting faiths. If possible, religious leaders should be consulted, for when they are tolerant many family dissensions on the issue can be resolved.

Love and Marriage

Emotional problems of love and marriage are often frequent and severe. Not to be loved creates emotional problems, but to be loved also creates emotional difficulties because love is a highly emotional experience, as everyone knows.

The lovers' quarrel is so commonplace as to be normal and expected. The violent emotional upheavals involved in such a quarrel actually serve a useful purpose. If people are genuinely fond of each other, they will survive the handicap of many quarrels. On the other hand, if there is no genuine affection, the lovers' quarrel is apt to end in dissolution of the affection. In the absence of true love who is to say that this is not a good result?

The emotional problems of unrequited love are not easy to solve. Fortunately, most people are so constructed that they can fall in love again with someone else.

Some college students have emotional problems associated with love because, although they are determined to get married eventually, they feel that to do so while each is still in college would be unwise for financial or other reasons. This is not necessarily so.

When young people are so in love that the intensity of their emotional attachment begins to give them difficulties, it would be well to discuss it with members of the family. In many cases, families will not only approve marriage while the students are still in college, but may be able to help financially until the college training has been completed. Even when such financial assistance is not possible, family approval will mean much to many young people.

In general, elopements are not advisable. Studies have shown that there is a higher percentage of divorces among those who have eloped than among those who have married under standard conditions.

Confusion in Sex Adjustments

Some of the most severe emotional problems of college students are in the field of sex adjustment. Invariably these problems are associated with sex conduct which is at variance with that of the average college student.

As a group, college students conform to social standards of sex behavior more completely than almost any other adult group. The Kinsey Report has shown that there is less deviation from socially accepted sex

behavior by college students than by those who do not go to college. Venereal disease studies have shown consistently that the college group has a lower rate of infection with venereal disorders than any other group studied. Most college students conform to the social standards most acceptable to the total adult population.

It is among those who disrupt this general pattern that emotional problems based upon confusion in sex adjustment are apt to arise.

Since perfection does not exist among human beings, it is expected that college students will make mistakes. Some of these mistakes will be biological, others will be mental or social.

In most colleges today, counsellors, religious advisers and physicians are available for consultation. The student who is confused on sex matters would be well advised to seek guidance and help from these three major sources. Often, by open discussion, a particular problem may be solved when older and wiser people are consulted.

Grades in College

Many students worry about their grades in college. With relatively few, however, is it a problem of major concern, unless there is some danger of flunking out of school, or of losing a scholarship or some other advantage that depends upon superior academic performance.

Some top students worry about the possibility of even a slight deviation from superior grades. Often such concern is not impelled by the importance of the grades themselves, but of the psychologic satisfaction they bring to these superior students. Many students try for better grades because they have found themselves inferior in sports, social activities, student government or other situations and attempt to make up for these deficiencies by a superior scholastic performance.

Most college students achieve a balanced outlook on the matter. They come to realize that even in preparing for the professions qualities other than scholarship are important in qualifying for admission to graduate school in such fields as medicine, law and engineering.

So far as future work is concerned, the college student should realize that many successful business men who employ young people will want the well rounded person rather than one who has obtained superior grades at the expense of all else that college has to offer. The dean of at least one large school of business has reported that many employers are requesting recommendations for students who have not achieved the top grades. Obviously, these requests must rest upon reason or experience suggesting that qualities other than scholarship are needed for success on the job.

As a matter of fact, it is likely that once the college student has finished his academic training and has left the college or university with the degree he sought, no more than one to half a dozen people will ever look at his academic transcript during the rest of his life. Grades are not as important as some people think they are.

On the other hand, it is obvious that if a student wishes to remain in college he must do satisfactory academic work. If he wishes to be admitted to a graduate school that requires top grades he must attain these grades. He should therefore strive for a reasonable balance of scholarship together with other enriching experience that the thoughtful and discriminating student can derive from college.

Questions

1. Why is a feeling of inferiority so common among superior college students?

2. When does a feeling of being "down" become depression of such intensity as to justify psychiatric help?

3. Is there ever a person who does not have some of the symptoms that mentally ill patients have?

4. What is the most effective way of securing independence from parents without rejecting them or making them feel that you do not love them?

5. How can a person with an unattractive personality become more appealing to others?

6. When does independence become license rather than liberty?

7. How can a person contribute to his own emotional health while contributing to the mental health of others?

For Further Reading

1. Bertine, Eleanor: *Human Relationships.* New York, Longmans, Green and Company, 1958.

2. Jahoda, Marie: *Current Concepts of Positive Mental Health.* New York, Basic Books, 1958.

3. Liebman, Samuel: *Emotional Forces in the Family.* Philadelphia, J. B. Lippincott Company, 1959.

4. Pressey, S. L., and Kuhlen, R. G.: *Psychological Development Through the Life Span.* New York, Harper and Brothers, 1957.

5. Roth, A.: *The Teen-Age Years: A Medical Guide for Young People and Their Parents.* New York, Doubleday and Company, 1960.

6. Valentine, C. W.: *The Normal Child and Some of His Abnormalities.* Baltimore, Penguin Books, 1956.

7. Wilkes, Edward T.: *Family Guide to Teenage Health.* New York, Ronald Press, 1958.

3

MENTAL ILLNESS

MENTAL illness is a serious problem the world over.

The human brain can get sick in people of any language or nationality.

The difficulty is that we do not know the cause of a great deal of mental illness. We do have some information and our knowledge of mental disease is growing. We are, perhaps, on the threshold of a major breakthrough in research on the reasons why people become mentally ill. In the meantime we are still greatly hampered by lack of knowledge. We do know, however, that there is no single unified cause of mental illness.

Many different factors may be a source of mental disease. Emotional disturbances can be prevented and their treatment consistently successful only when specific causes are known, treated or counter-balanced in advance.

There is always a close association between physical and mental health. So frequently are mind and body confused in illness that the psychiatrist takes great pains to rule out physical or organic causes of mental illness before he decides that the problem is strictly psychologic. Even when it is concluded that the disease is psychogenic, it is likely that the health of the body may have been impaired by mental illness. Some physicians have stated that about 75 per cent of the patients who come to a doctor's office have emotional as well as physical problems.

An illness of the mind can come primarily from physical causes, from psychologic causes or a combination of both. Once the illness has been established it is almost inevitable that both mind and body will be involved.

Mental Illness of Unknown Origin

Unfortunately, the origin of all types of mental illness is unknown. For example, in the case of schizophrenia, also known as dementia praecox, the ultimate cause has not yet been determined. Since schizophrenia is the leading type of mental illness for which patients are put in hospitals and institutions, it is pathetic that we must treat this illness without knowing its fundamental cause. Apparently the seeds of this disorder are present at birth or in early childhood. It has long been observed

that the onset of this particular illness occurs usually before the age of thirty. If a person has survived that long without suffering schizophrenia, it is unlikely that he will ever suffer from it.

It has not been proved, however, that schizophrenia is hereditary. Nevertheless, indications of the disease are found at an early age when a careful, retrospective study is made of those who acquire it. At the Judge Baker Guidance Center in Boston, for example, a study was made of two groups of children. The early years of the lives of fifteen children with schizophrenia were compared to a similar period in the lives of fifteen children who did not have this disease. The study showed that those with schizophrenia had early feeding difficulties, severely disturbed or retarded speech, poor school adjustment or achievement, a high incidence of bizarre behavior and extremely poor social relations with other children.

It is possible that eventually a disturbed biochemistry of the brain may prove to be the cause of the most severe types of mental illness not obviously caused by injury or other factor. This is discussed more fully in a later section of this chapter.

Physical Causes of Mental Illness

There are many physical causes of mental disease. Among these are communicable diseases, nutritional deficiencies, accidents involving the brain, nervous system or other parts of the body, severe anemia, the use of certain drugs, alcohol, glandular disturbances, allergies, poor heredity and a great variety of other factors.

Physical defects can also produce emotional problems in an indirect way. For example, facial defects, protruding ears or harelip may cause children to become exceedingly self-conscious due to ridicule from other children. Sensitivity to such defects may become greatly exaggerated during the teen-age period. Adjustment to members of the opposite sex may be made more difficult by such disorders, which may lead to acute emotional problems.

As discussed in another chapter, nutritional deficiencies may sometimes cause a serious impairment of the stability of the mind and emotions. A deficiency of vitamin B complex is perhaps more closely linked to nervous disorders than most other food elements.

The emergence of accidents as a leading public health problem has brought an increase in the number of injuries to the brain and central nervous system. Severe head injuries always carry the possibility of permanent damage which may change the personality to a distressing extent.

Most mental illness is not hereditary in origin, although it is estimated by some authorities that about 80 per cent of the severe depressive type of mental illness is transmitted from parent to child.

It has been shown in recent years that many different infections may create an inflammation of the brain that results in behavior disorders and personality changes. Whooping cough, measles, influenza, poliomyelitis, pneumonia, diphtheria, scarlet fever, chickenpox, meningitis and other toxic conditions have all been proved to have caused brain inflammation in children or adults at one time or another. This encephalitis is, of course, not an ordinary symptom of these disorders, but can result as a complication.

In one study it was found that about 80 per cent of the children who suffer from this complication have a characteristic personality makeup in which restlessness, impulsiveness, unpredictability of behavior and lack of inhibition are the dominant personality traits.

Recent studies have shown that inflammation of the brain may also occur as an allergic reaction to certain foods, and that this may cause a gross disturbance to the personality. It is expected that such cen-

tral nervous system inflammation may result from other allergic conditions.

The excessive consumption of alcohol over a long period of time may damage the brain as well as other parts of the body, sometimes in a direct manner. Usually, however, it is the nutritional deficiency that causes damage rather than any direct action of the alcohol. On the other hand, there is actual destruction of parts of the central nervous system when a person consumes wood alcohol.

In severe anemia there may be such a deprivation of oxygen to the brain that this organ is damaged. The brain may also be damaged from a deficiency of oxygen in carbon monoxide poisoning. Sometimes such poisonings are accidental, but they may occur in attempted suicide.

Almost any physical cause of illness may have complicating effects upon the mental health of the individual. In the great majority of cases, however, these physical ailments do not cause severe personality disturbances. It is only in the unusual or complicated case that such results sometimes occur.

Body Chemistry and Mental Health

It may be that the ultimate explanation of a serious mental illness such as schizophrenia is chemical changes within the brain. Although no research has definitely identified specific chemical changes as the cause of serious mental illness a number of studies have linked them together.

In a certain army camp, at the close of World War II, ten soldiers exhibited psychoneurotic symptoms that caused them to be temporarily classified as mentally ill. Blood studies on this group, however, showed that all suffered from low blood chloride levels. Because the men had been involved in tank maneuvers in a desert area and had lost a great deal of water and salt through perspiration, army medical officers suspected that a severe salt deficiency might explain their symptoms.

The symptoms of deficiency were both physical and psychologic. There was loss of appetite, frequent nausea, occasional vomiting, abdominal cramps, headaches, dizziness, tremor, nervousness, apprehension, restlessness, insomnia, depression, personality changes and even anxiety. When blood chloride levels were restored to normal, there was rapid improvement of all the psychoneurotic symptoms. Physical symptoms of the illness also disappeared, and the patients became normal.

It is not yet possible to make a diagnosis of schizophrenia on a biochemical basis although it has been determined that there are certain blood changes in people with this mental illness. For example, blood glutathione levels are diminished in the schizophrenic person.

Certain chemical substances produce auditory and visual hallucinations with loss of insight when they are given to volunteer human subjects. Most notable among these substances are LSD and JB-336. The giving of LSD to normal people results in temporary effects very similar to those of schizophrenia. In fact, in some psychiatric hospitals nurses and doctors are given LSD temporarily so that they get a momentary impression of what the schizophrenic patient suffers.

One of the substances extracted from the blood of a schizophrenic is taraxein which is thought to be a protein. When this substance is injected into the blood of normal volunteers, effects come within five to ten minutes and subside in about two hours. In the interval a normal patient experiences many of the same phenomena that harass the schizophrenic.

Chemical research at the National Institute of Health has shown that reserpine, one of the tranquilizing drugs that often improves mental health, will remove certain chemicals from the brain and other parts of the body. All of this research suggests that schizophrenia is a mental illness involving biochemical changes in the brain. It is not likely that this most serious of the mental illnesses results from any purely psychogenic stress.

The significance of the chemistry of the body in mental health is also suggested in certain types of mental retardation in children. Some families, apparently through genetic mechanisms, pass on a certain biochemical structure that results in mental retardation. The link between biochemistry of the brain and levels of human intelligence has never been fully understood. After two years of investigations at the National Institute of Mental Illness, research personnel have been unable to identify any significant biochemical abnormalities among schizophrenics other than the changes already noted.

Symptoms of Mental Illness

Situations that create feelings of anxiety, guilt, depression, confusion, fantasy, obsession and suspicion are usually complicated by the personality structure of the individual showing such symptoms.

Anxiety or fear indicates insecurity which may be based primarily upon an environmental situation or primarily upon an apprehensive nervous system. Often it is the interplay between the two that creates anxiety. However, it is possible, as has been shown in certain cases, that this expression of mental illness may come predominantly from the mind because of real or imagined hazards.

A feeling of guilt may arise solely within the mind because the individual is not aware that normal people sometimes have unwholesome feelings or impulses. To feel guilty about such phenomena is often to create an unjustified emotional problem. Sometimes, of course, a feeling of guilt may develop because of a genuine reason for such a reaction. When a guilt reaction is severe, there is serious danger of depression or even suicide. In such instances psychiatric help should be sought.

Depression and anxiety represent the most frequent type of emotional reaction. Depression may come from physiologic changes in the body chemistry or from what goes on in the mind. The loss of a loved one precipitates a feeling of depression, and sometimes one wonders whether life is worth living.

Everyone feels depression at one time or another, but it is not usually severe. It is normal for a person to fluctuate in his emotions to some extent, but when these variations in mood become more extensive or more frequent mental illness may be involved. Medical and psychiatric treatment for depression can be quite effective, and if the condition is severe enough, help should be sought in that direction.

Confusion, suspicion and fantasy are symptoms of mental illness that should not be neglected. There is always the possibility that such symptoms may come from a disturbed biochemistry of the brain or from other physical changes. The physician may be unable to find any organic cause of such mental illness, however.

Suspicious reactions reflect a danger to other people because the mentally ill person is apt to defend himself against the one he suspects of planning injury to him. The person who expresses suspicion of others in a consistent pattern should be given a psychiatric examination.

When people are disoriented and confused and the memory is not functioning properly, they should receive careful medical and psychiatric care. Perhaps in the majority of cases the psychogenic origin of such confusion may not be obvious.

A fantasy reaction indicates a flight from reality in which a make-believe life is substituted for reality. Fantasies usually occur only in the mentally disturbed patient who is seriously ill and needs prolonged medical or psychiatric care. Often such patients are beyond the point of assistance and must remain in state institutions for life despite the skilled psychiatric care that patients receive in such places.

Often a person who is basically stable may have emotional problems because of circumstances in his life that he cannot control. Sometimes very intensive exploration of a patient's life is necessary to discover the basic causes that have made him difficult to live with, uncooperative or antisocial.

Tension, anxiety, resentment, aggression and many other types of behavior may arise from psychologic reaction to circumstances in the family or group in which the child or adult has none of the basic emotional needs satisfied. In such cases it is not surprising that the emotional development of the individual is defective.

Mind and Body

Many people still think of mental illness as wholly a condition of the mind. The fact is, however, that mind and body are not independent; the body and emotions are interactive and inseparable. Probably every case of physical illness has some effect on the health of the mind, and vice versa; a disturbed mind may cause physical illness.

A term used to designate this interaction of mind and body is the word *psychosomatic.*

The phrase *psychosomatic disorders* is used to mean the various physical discomforts that result from or are associated with strong emotion.

Fear, for instance, activates the nervous and glandular systems, producing such reactions as sudden sweating, dry mouth, frequent urination, rapid and erratic beating of the heart, and gasping breathing. Fear can vary from a small boy's fright to an adult's dread of taking a doctoral examination, having an appendix removed or going on trial for evasion of income tax. But the effect on the body is much the same: the brain sounds the gong for "General Quarters!" and the body organizes for struggle. The senses sharpen, so that the individual sees more clearly, hears more clearly, thinks more swiftly; the ductless glands increase their secretion, and the liver pours sugar into the blood to provide energy fuel for the muscles that are now tensed for action.

Equally as upsetting as fear, in terms of their effects on body physiology, are such emotions as strong remorse and guilt.

Often a person feels symptoms of strong emotion, but *doesn't know why he is upset.* This may be because he has repressed feelings of guilt, hate, resentment, fear, envy or inferiority. He has pushed those feelings deep into the back of his mind and hidden them under his everyday awareness of things. He may repress those feelings because they are not pleasant emotions to have, especially when they involve loved and respected people.

Every physician has encountered many cases in which both mind and body are involved in mental illness.

Dr. Desmond O'Neil, of London, has reported twelve cases of abnormal uterine bleeding associated with the presence of anxiety. In all the patients, onset of the bleeding was associated with some emotional crisis and subsequent attacks were correlated with periods of anxiety, depression, headache and fatigue. When the patients were treated with psychotherapy, menstrual function returned to normal in seven of the twelve women. It is difficult to say whether the hemorrhage in these cases was due entirely to psychologic factors. It is very likely, at least, that the bleeding itself heightened the anxiety and tension, which in turn aggravated the hemorrhage.

One of the outstanding medical examples of an illness in which there is a strong association of body and mind is the peptic ulcer. Psychiatrists have long maintained that such ulcers were produced by tension, worry and emotional disturbances. On the other hand, it was known that an excessive amount of hydrochloric acid was produced in the stomach in this illness, and that the disorder could be treated with success in many cases by nutritional measures. It was also common knowledge that an antacid could be effective in controlling the disease.

In recent years proof has emerged that nervous impulses originating in the brain because of worry, tension and other emotional reactions stimulate the flow of hydrochloric acid in the stomach. These impulses are carried over the vagus nerve from the brain to the stomach.

It is possible to measure the amount of hydrochloric acid produced in the stomach of a given patient and to correlate this production with periods of tension. Cutting the vagus nerve (a part of which goes to the stomach from its beginning in the brain) by surgery greatly reduces the amount of hydrochloric acid being produced in the stomach. Surgery has therefore become one of the means of controlling intractable peptic ulcers. Such surgery, however, is reserved for only the most difficult cases.

Some stomach ulcers can be treated successfully by purely psychiatric approaches. Usually, however, a combination of treatments including diet, antacid therapy and moderation of emotional problems is advocated.

Many infectious diseases may produce temporary or permanent disorders of the mind. In pellagra the mind is usually affected in the late stages of the disease. Pellagra is a nutritional deficiency disease that can be treated successfully with vitamin B complex. Sometimes the rehabilitation of the mind is dramatic when massive doses of this vitamin complex are given to patients suffering from this disease.

Definitions of Mental Illness

A neurosis is a mental disorder of a functional nature. By this is meant that the condition represents a state of tension or irritability in which the personality remains more or less intact, without physical damage to the brain. Psychoneurosis is a synonym for neurosis.

Disorders of this kind can be treated by psychiatric methods, often with great success. Hysteria and neurasthenia are examples of neurosis that often respond well to psychotherapy.

The term "psychosis" was once used to identify any type of mental disorder. Nowadays the term indicates a deeper and more serious type of mental illness, such as schizophrenia and the severely depressive types of mental disease. Such disorders respond less favorably than the neuroses to psychotherapy.

Schizophrenia

Schizophrenia is probably the most difficult of the major mental diseases to treat successfully. This is a disease in which there is progressive deterioration of the mind. The degenerative changes are profound and represent a retreat from reality. The person who suffers from this illness is apt to be apathetic and indifferent to problems that concern persons of normal mental health. There are many variations and grades of schizophrenia, as with other types of mental illness. The person afflicted with schizophrenia is particularly dangerous to society if he is of the paranoid type. The paranoiac is convinced that he is being persecuted or pursued by others, which may lead him to aggressive action against innocent persons. Violence to others is justified in the mind of the paranoiac because it represents defensive action rather than simple aggression.

RISE, INCORPORATED. In September of 1959 the first volunteer agency was formed to advance research into the cause, treatment, prevention, and cure of schizophrenia. This organization known as RISE, Inc., fosters the exchange of information among research investigators of this mental illness and supports the training of personnel in that field. The term RISE was selected as a name for the organization because it is composed of the first letters of the phrase "Research In Schizophrenia Endowment."

Psychosis

Psychiatrists use many different terms to qualify a psychosis. For example, an anxiety psychosis is an emotional disturbance characterized by anxiety, restlessness and depression. The term "febrile psychosis" is used by some physicians and psychiatrists to describe a confusion of the mind caused by infection and exhaustion of the patient. Involutional psychosis is a condition of mental disturbance associated with the menopause or with old age. A toxic psychosis is a severe mental illness due to the action of some drug or poison. A manic-depressive psychosis is a severe mental illness in which there is alternation of intense excitement and depression.

Treatment of Mental Illness

Regardless of the kind of mental disease from which the patient may suffer, the best method of treatment is to remove the fundamental cause of the illness and to repair, if possible, the damage done. It is not always possible to do this for the simple reason that not all the causes of mental disease are known. Sometimes when the cause is known, as in the case of brain damage, it may not be possible to repair the injury. Also, it is difficult in many cases to discover fundamental causes of mental illness, even when it is known that such factors may bring about emotional disease.

One point must be emphasized strongly. Treatment of mental disorders is not solely a problem for the psychiatrist because many physical ailments may affect the mind, and little or no progress toward recovery can be expected until the physical causes are discovered and eliminated. The modern psychiatrist always insists upon a careful medical clearance before he reaches the conclusion that psychotherapy is the best or sole means of treatment for the patient.

Some of the many ways in which the mentally ill patient may be treated are discussed in the following paragraphs.

Hypnosis

Hypnosis is not widely used in the treatment of mental disease. It does appear to have some limited value, however, and the procedure is used in some mental hospitals and by some psychiatrists with beneficial effects.

The Council of Mental Health of the American Medical Association reported in 1958 that about 7,000 physicians were using hypnosis in their practices although techniques of hypnosis are not commonly taught in medical schools. These physicians had learned how to hypnotize people through various seminars and short training programs.

A report on medical use of hypnosis was approved in 1959 by the American Medical Association House of Delegates. Some of the important points of this report were as follows:

1. Use of hypnosis for therapeutic purposes should be restricted to those who are qualified by experience and training to fully diagnose the illness which is to be treated.
2. No physician should utilize hypnosis for purposes that are beyond the range of his ordinary competence.
3. Hypnosis should be used on a highly selective basis.
4. Teaching related to hypnosis should be under responsible medical direction. Integrated teaching programs should include not only the techniques of induction, but also the indications and limitations of hypnosis in specific instances.
5. Instruction limited to induction techniques alone should be discouraged.

Some authorities in the use of hypnosis believe that at least 75 per cent of the population can be hypnotized to some degree, but that only about 20 per cent can be deeply hypnotized.

Cooperation on the part of the patient, either conscious or unconscious, is needed in order for hypnosis to be successful. In other words, no one need fear that he will be put into a hypnotic state by any "evil eye" or comparable superstitious notion. The basis for hypnosis is the suggestibility of the individual. A person who is fully aware that suggestions are being made to him, but is resistant to these suggestions, cannot be hypnotized. So long as the patient cooperates with the hypnotist, however, the process can proceed to a state of hypnosis. This is achieved by suggestion and command. Obviously, if a person will not do as suggested or commanded he will not come under the influence of the hypnotist.

The degree of hypnosis, however, is not related necessarily to the curative effects. Emotional participation in the hypnotic experience by the patient appears to be much more important in achieving good results.

Today hypnosis is used mainly as a means of establishing a good relationship with the patient or for obtaining cooperation for a better exploration of background information on emotional problems. Hypnosis is also used to get around psychologic handicaps or barriers that may prevent the patient from expressing his problem fully to the psychiatrist.

Some psychiatrists have reported that the use of hypnosis often cuts short the symptoms of hysteria in children and allows a better chance of progress.

Although the dangers of hypnosis appear to be exaggerated, it is true that certain types of patients should not be hypnotized. The mentally ill person with strong paranoid ideas ought not to be hypnotized, for this type of illness is characterized by feelings of persecution and the patient may already have the delusion of being under the influence of another person. This may lead him to take aggressive action against the hypnotist. Such treatment may also reinforce his belief that his mind is being tampered with and that he needs to defend himself, which may lead to aggression against innocent persons because of the mistaken idea that such a person is responsible for the subjugation of the mind of the paranoid.

Brain Surgery for Mental Illness

In 1936 Egas Moniz of Portugal began to experiment with brain surgery as a new treatment for mental illness. Moniz later received the Nobel Prize for the development of that type of brain surgery known as lobotomy.

Lobotomy, also known as prefrontal lobotomy, is a type of brain surgery in which certain nerve pathways are cut after holes have been drilled through the skull. It has been found that emotional tensions are released after this type of surgery in many patients. The patient is apt to be happier after his operation even though he has not been cured of his illness.

In the United States various surgeons and psychiatrists have reported on the use of lobotomy in the treatment of the mentally ill. One such study, conducted by Dr. Watts and Dr. Freeman, of the George Washington University School of Medicine, gives an idea of the kind of results that may be expected from this treatment. These surgeons have reported that approximately 2 per cent of those who undergo this type of surgery die from the operation. Approximately 12 per cent have had convulsive attacks at a later date. In a follow-up study lasting about ten years it was found that about 40 per cent of those who underwent brain surgery for mental disease showed good results. A smaller number showed moderate improvement. These surgeons concluded that unless the patient's condition is serious, the risks of brain surgery are not justified. Its value is restricted to certain types of disorders in which there are strong indications of severe tensions and antisocial behavior, and even then the operation is advisable only in extreme cases. Surgery is not without risk and is to be avoided when possible.

Electric Shock

Electric shock treatment for mental disorders was apparently first used in Rome in 1938, and has been used in the United States since about 1940.

Electric shock treatments are often given about twice a week for several weeks, although there is variation in the frequency such therapy is attempted. From about twenty-five to thirty treatments may be given. The amount of current sent through the brain is carefully controlled.

Because electrical stimulation of the brain tends to send nervous impulses to the muscles, there may be a violent contraction of the latter during this treatment. In past years this led to a number of fractures due to intense muscular contraction, but in recent years curare has been used to prevent this complication, as has low amperage current. This has resulted in a great reduction of broken bones, although when the drug is not used in conjunction with electric shock treatment fractures may be expected to occur in about 5 per cent of the cases if standard levels of current are used.

Another complication from electric shock treatment is a temporary loss of memory. Memory loss is not permanent and is usually spotty; it is related only to certain factors such as names, places and dates.

The patients treated by electric shock do not have any recollection of the therapy and are not afraid of the treatments if they are properly prepared in advance by sedation and are protected adequately against injury and discomfort during treatment.

The treatment is most effective against the depressive types of mental illness. With patients suffering from such illness, improvement may be rapid and sustained. In some instances patients have been brought out of a severe depression and have remained in a relatively normal state of mind for many years. Some authorities have indicated that it is possible that a person who suffers from this mental illness may have no more than one or two severe attacks during a lifetime. In such cases the great value of electric shock treatment during the few attacks the patients do have is obvious.

The exact manner in which electrical shock brings about improvement is not known. Changes in blood sugar have been observed in other types of shock treatments such as with Metrazol and insulin. Whether this is the fundamental factor in electric shock treatment is not certain.

Electric shock treatment has tended to replace other forms of shock therapy, although insulin shock is still used by some psychiatrists. This form of treatment is relatively safe and does bring considerable improvement in many patients, although its value depends upon the type of mental illness involved. In short, electric shock treatment is one of the modern and effective ways of treating the mentally ill patient.

Drugs and Mental Illness

Many drugs have been used in the treatment of mentally ill patients. Their principal value, however, seems to be in the temporary alleviation of symptoms rather than in any permanent control of the illness.

Recently much attention has been given in the public press to the use of so-called tranquilizing drugs and their use in the treatment of mental illness. The earliest of these drugs were reserpine, chlorpromazine and azacyclonol, although there are now many varieties of tranquilizing drugs on the market.

Reserpine is a drug derived from the snakeroot plant. In India the drug was used long before the physicians of the United States became aware of its values. Reserpine is used in the treatment of some of the more serious types of mental disease, such as schizophrenia (dementia praecox), in which it appears to be of considerable help in about 60 per cent of the cases. The great value of the drug appears to be in its calming of the overactive and restless patient and in the reduction of antisocial behavior. The drug does not appear to offer permanent cure, although it does make psychotherapy more effective.

Chlorpromazine, like reserpine, has been used as a tranquilizing drug. It has the same general value as the latter. Azacyclonol has been reported as having little or no effect upon a normal person, so that its use has been confined to treatment of major mental illnesses.

Recently the medical literature has begun to include reports that the foregoing drugs sometimes cause serious reactions involving the liver, nervous system and other organs and systems of the body. In some cases patients have become so depressed after treatment that suicide became an actual or potential problem. It should be obvious that such drugs should be taken only under the careful supervision of a physician if expected benefits are to outweigh possible complications.

Meprobamate (Miltown) is an example of a tranquilizing drug that has been widely used for the relief of nervous tension in persons not suffering from serious mental disease. Such a drug should be used with caution and only under the guidance of a physician.

Military experience in the treatment of combat fatigue has shown the great value of sedative and analgesic drugs in the treatment of emotionally disturbed patients. Paraldehyde, hyoscine, hydrobromide, chloral hydrate, sodium bromide and other drugs given under strict medical supervision are often effective in relieving the acute symptoms of mentally ill patients.

Patients with mental illness due to syphilis of the nervous system have been treated with some success by fever, large doses of penicillin, and other drugs. The success of the treatment appears to depend on the speed with which the patient receives medical help. The effects on the nervous system may be permanent if treatment is delayed too long. In former years arsenic and bismuth were used in the treatment of syphilis of the nervous system, but are not commonly used nowadays since the antibiotics have become available.

Several drugs are available for the successful treatment of epilepsy. The most important of these is Dilantin. Proper use of this drug in the grand mal type of epilepsy may produce a restoration to virtually normal health. In epileptic patients who do not have actual brain damage the drug may make it possible for the patient to live a normal life.

Many other drugs have been used, either experimentally or on a proved basis of value, in the treatment of the mentally ill. There is no single drug, however, that can be counted upon to cure mental illness. Relief from symptoms and signs of emotional disturbances is the major effect of this type of medical treatment.

Nutrition and Mental Illness

It is a well established fact that nutritional deficiencies may result in mental disturbance. When this is the case, it is obvious that the best possible treatment is correction of the nutritional deficiency.

Many cases in which the brain has been affected because of allergy to certain foods have been reported in recent years.

Severe migraine headaches have been repeatedly traced in particular instances to an allergy to a particular food.

When ninety-five specialists in allergy were consulted for information regarding the effects of this disorder upon the nervous system, they reported 122 cases in which the most common symptoms were irritability, restlessness and tendency to quarrel. Some children had been taken out of school because they were considered incorrigible. Later, when the nature of their allergy was discovered and proper steps were taken to correct the condition,

these children became friendly and happy and took an active, cooperative part in playing with others.

The great value of vitamin B complex in contributing to the stability of the nervous system has been demonstrated repeatedly. One should remember that not all cases of mental illness stem from the same cause. In particular cases, however, mental illness has sometimes been cured with dramatic rapidity when B complex has been used in the treatment of the disease.

It has been shown consistently that a deficient diet may adversely affect the emotional health. An important part of treatment in most diseases of the mind is therefore a well balanced diet.

Psychotherapy

Psychotherapy is widely misunderstood. The psychotherapist in a sense neither makes decisions for the patient nor solves problems for him. Essentially, psychotherapy is the process of working together with the emotionally disturbed person for better solutions to existing problems. According to Dr. Kenneth E. Appel of Philadelphia psychotherapy is "helping the patient develop solutions, capacities, confidence, and respect through discussions, guidance, talking things out, and the release of pent up feelings. It is a cooperative, searching, prospecting adventure from which confidence, resourcefulness and help develop."

The value of psychotherapy depends primarily on the experience and skill of the psychiatrist, the severity of symptoms of the patient, the patient's intelligence, the quality of his early home situation, and the capacity of the patient for achieving insight into his own problems.

Psychotherapy is essentially the treatment of disease by the power of suggestion, or by guidance and assistance in exploration of relationships and experiences significant to the illness. The modern psychiatrist, however, does not necessarily restrict his treatment solely to psychotherapeutic measures. He may use drugs, electric shock treatment, medical treatment for concomitant illnesses, diet, and many other factors in the treatment of his patient.

The value of purely psychotherapeutic approaches to the treatment of mental illness has been demonstrated in some patients but not in others. Obviously, the value of this approach must rest upon the nature of the mental illness. When the disorder is predominantly of the mind rather than of both mind and body (linked with physical illness), there should be a better chance of cure by psychotherapy. Often, however, it is difficult to evaluate the effectiveness of this form of treatment because the criteria for judging improvement are often intangible.

A recent study by three investigators of the effects of psychiatric treatment on sixty-two patients diagnosed as suffering from an anxiety neurosis (a form of mental illness in which there is a predominance of morbid and unjustified dread or fear) revealed that 23 per cent of the group had improved markedly, 35 per cent were definitely better, and 42 per cent were essentially unchanged after a period of two to twenty years.

Of major importance in psychiatric treatment is the relationship between the psychiatrist and the patient. The latter must have confidence and faith in the psychiatrist, or little can be expected in the way of improvement. This is so fundamental that unless confidence can be attained in such treatment and in the particular psychiatrist involved, there is little value in seeking such treatment.

Studies of anxiety have shown that one of the most successful methods of handling this emotional disturbance is by communication and sharing with someone else. If the person with whom the anxiety is shared responds with a calm attempt to solve the situation, there is progressive reduction of anxiety in the other person. Ability in expression on the part of the calm person appears to be an important part of this type of treatment. The psychiatrist, with his professional training and realization of the importance of reducing anxiety by personal contact with another, can be of great assistance in the treatment of this disorder.

People with phobias (persistent abnormal fears) are often greatly helped by psychiatric treatment. Most phobias or fears could have been prevented in childhood, but when children are basically apprehensive and do not have the opportunity to develop confidence, independence, or understanding of their difficulties, such phobias may persist throughout a lifetime. As the patient gains insight into his condition, usually with the assistance of the psychiatrist, progress in this disorder can be expected.

Group psychotherapy calls for sharing and increased socialization by members of a group. Group discussions often bring about a better understanding of one's own emotional problems. Frequently there is relief of symptoms from psychologic sharing with others. Group psychotherapy often leads to more effective acceptance of suggestions from the psychiatrist. The value of this form of psychotherapy has been demonstrated by the patient's own opinion of the value of such an experience to him as well as by the opinions of fellow patients, psychiatrists, and objective personality tests used before and after treatment.

Nondirective therapy, in which the psychiatrist or counsellor makes no attempt to advise the patient directly, but merely assists him to a better understanding of the immediate situation as well as past events, has also been of value with certain patients. In this type of psychiatric treatment the approach is based upon the concept that many maladjustments result not from a lack of knowledge, but from the emotional satisfaction that a person may achieve because of his present disturbance.

Nondirective therapy is not preparation for further psychiatric treatment, but is regarded as treatment itself, since the patient often undergoes change while he is participating in this treatment.

Although there are different schools of psychiatry, and this fact may at times confuse the individual patient, their value lies not in the particular brand of psychiatry that is fostered or followed, but in the quality of the relationship that is established between the psychiatrist and the patient (in the kind of mental illness that does not involve structural or biochemical damage to the brain). When this is good, then constructive results may be expected from almost any of the various types of psychotherapy. It must be remembered, however, that many forms of mental illness are due to factors that remain untouched by psychiatric approaches.

It is of great importance that the college student realize that most of his emotional problems will not be due to fundamental and unalterable organic changes in the brain, but are of precisely the same kind and quality as those of other normal scholars.

This realization is an important step toward solving those problems. Sometimes knowledge that a problem is commonplace is sufficient to dissipate the intensity of that difficulty. However, when an emotional problem is severe and persistent, regardless of whether it is commonplace with others, it is advisable to seek competent help.

The value of counselling and psychiatry lies in the prevention of mental illness and in dissolution of the emotional problems of people who are relatively stable and fundamentally sound. The psychiatrist, in other words, should not be looked upon as a last resource for a person who is out of his mind and gravely ill. He should be looked upon as a friend, counsellor, and specialist in the field of emotional problems. He should be consulted in problems pertaining to the mind as freely and openly as the help of the physician is sought in ills of the body.

Suicide

Although suicide is not a major problem during childhood it begins to assume more significance during adolescence and early maturity. Attempted suicide in college is common enough to cause students, faculties, and college health services to be concerned about the problem, although it is not a major cause of disability or death at that time of life. In almost every college, however, during the four-year undergraduate life of the student he will hear of a suicide or attempted suicide by one or more members of the student body.

Most suicides by young people are the result of severe emotional problems or mental illness. Dr. Leonard M. Moss and Dr. Donald M. Hamilton, of New York City, studied 50 persons who had made serious attempts to commit suicide, but who had survived.

These two physicians found that in order to prevent further attempts at suicide major changes had to be made in the social environment of the persons involved. *The life situation of these people had to be changed so that they gained hope for a better future.* Some of the factors that needed to be changed were concerned with work, study or occupation, domination by restricting parents, unsuitable engagements, poor sex orientation and narrow social contact and recreation. It would appear that for the college student who attempts or contemplates suicide, attention should be given to producing changes in these areas.

The person involved in a suicide attempt should be brought to the realization that suicide is an expression of an emotionally disturbed personality. Help and changes are needed.

Dr. Norman L. Loux has identified some of the signs or indications of an impending suicide as follows:

1. Depression, with expressions of self-accusation, hopelessness, retardation, or agitation.
2. Any *talk* of suicide, either of committing suicide

or unsolicited denial of it. Such denial of intent is frequently as important as the expression of the wish.

3. Concern that others might commit suicide is frequently an evidence that a person himself is preoccupied with the thought of suicide but projects his concern onto others.

4. Previous attempts at suicide. It is a simple rule that the likelihood of suicide is greater in a person who has made a previous attempt.

5. Close relationship with someone who did commit suicide. Frequently, people who have experienced the suicide of a person important in their lives during the formative years are more likely to commit suicide themselves.

6. Excessive and unrealistic worry over physical health, frequently in combination with excessive concern over sleeplessness, fear of losing the mind, or of losing self-control.

Psychiatric Emergencies

There are certain psychiatric or emotional conditions that require emergency action. These mental or emotional conditions may be a serious threat to the person who is suffering from the disturbance or they may be a danger to others.

These disorders of the mind that need immediate attention by qualified medical and psychiatric personnel may be of brief duration or they may reflect a more permanent and long-lasting mental illness. The urgency of the situation is not altered by these facts.

Some of the leading conditions in which emergency care is needed are as follows:

1. DEPRESSIONS constitute the leading form of emotional reaction in which there is danger to the individual himself. The patient may be suffering from such severe self-deprecation, guilt or general feelings of inferiority that he may be a hazard to himself. In severe depressions the patient may have retired from normal channels of living into a state of physical and mental inactivity. The greatest hazard of depression is *suicide*.

Mental and psychiatric care is needed for the patient in a substantial depression.

Fortunately, electroshock treatment tends to be very helpful in this form of emotional distress.

2. The PARANOID REACTION is a psychiatric emergency because the patient suffering from this disorder may attack, injure or even kill others. The paranoid is apt to brood in a state of heightened sensitivity to a point where he misjudges even the most casual remark made by others. Because the paranoid individual believes that he is being persecuted he may strike back at those he believes to be his enemies. The person who suffers from unfounded suspicions and is belligerent to the point of attacking others is a hazard to even an innocent person. To neglect the need for medical and psychiatric care for such a patient is to permit the hazard of serious assault on others by the paranoid patient.

3. ACUTE INTOXICATION from drugs or other substances may result in hallucinations, violent behavior, symptoms similar to those of inflammation of the brain, semi-consciousness, coma or death. The person who is suffering from an over-consumption of alcohol, barbiturates, bromides or any one of a number of drugs may thus be in danger of his life. Prompt medical treatment is needed and psychiatric care may also be advisable.

4. DELIRIUM AND HALLUCINATIONS represent a severe disorientation that needs prompt medical attention. Sedative and tranquilizing drugs may be needed in such an emergency followed by psychiatric care until orientation is re-established. A careful medical or psychiatric search for the origin of such behavior is basic to proper treatment, although emergency care may temporarily tranquilize the patient.

5. HYSTERIA AND PANIC represent emergency conditions with different foundations although the average person may find it difficult to distinguish between

these two reactions. The panic state arises from an overwhelming reaction because of intense fear. The patient suffering from panic may need sedation and reassurance.

The hysterical person, on the other hand, represents an immature and impulsive effort to get attention. Hysteria is apt to occur only when others are in the immediate vicinity. The person who has suffered an hysterical fainting spell is best brought back to consciousness by a clearing of the room of all people.

6. The CATATONIC REACTION is another psychiatric emergency in which there is relative immobility of a physical nature. The patient does not talk or respond in any way to attention or care. When the catatonic reaction is maintained for a sufficiently long period of time nutrition may become a problem. Such a reaction must be considered a psychiatric emergency because the individual himself may be further harmed by his failure to participate in normal activities.

Questions

1. What are the arguments against mercy killings of people who suffer from incurable mental illnesses?

2. Why are some families ashamed to admit the presence of mental illness and reluctant to employ psychotherapy for treatment, although they may openly complain of physical ailments?

3. From the viewpoint of society, what should be done with the mentally ill person who is a danger to others?

4. What is the distinction between "social remission" of mental illness in contrast to a medical cure of the disease?

5. Why is shock treatment inadequate in the treatment of mental disease? What are its advantages?

6. Does menstruation have anything to do with mental health?

7. Is a person who attempts suicide because of disappointment in love a stable person? Would such a person be a good risk as a lifetime mate?

8. How can society protect itself against mental illness in a leader? Should society establish standards of stability for election to popular office?

9. What should a college student do who thinks that a friend or associate is contemplating suicide?

For Further Reading

1. Dewan, J. G.: *The Organic Psychoses*. Toronto, Canada, University of Toronto Press, 1959.

2. Katz, Barney, and Thorpe, Louis P.: *Understanding People in Distress*. New York, Ronald Press, 1955.

3. Lemkau, Paul V.: *Basic Issues in Psychiatry*. Springfield, Ill., Charles C Thomas, 1959.

4. May, Jacques M.: *A Physician Looks at Psychiatry*. New York, John Day Company, 1958.

5. Smith, Jackson A.: *Psychiatry: Descriptive and Dynamic*. Chicago, Williams and Wilkins Company, 1960.

For Advanced Reading

1. Arieti, Silvano: *American Handbook of Psychiatry*. 2 vols. New York, Basic Books, 1959.

2. Pasamanick, Benjamin, editor: *Epidemiology of Mental Disorder*. Washington, D.C., American Association for the Advancement of Science, 1959.

4

STRESS AND TENSION

PEOPLE who live in a state of stress and tension run significant risks of destructive body changes as well as emotional disturbances that may produce profound changes in behavior.

Stress implies a physical or emotional exertion or intense effort beyond the normal or usual. Tension is a related phenomenon that reflects nervous anxiety and the body's reaction to stress.

Stress is a source of anxiety, tension, apprehension, worry and fear when a person is unable to adapt or adjust successfully to the threatening emotional situation. Emotional reactions due to stress may aggravate pre-existing health problems or they may produce new ones such as peptic ulcers, ulcerative colitis, migraine headaches, asthmatic attacks, heart disease or other disorders.

Adaptation to Stress

The body has definite ways of reacting to stressful situations.

Hans Selye, a leading modern exponent of the significance of stress and body adjustments to this phenomenon, postulates that the body is able to increase its capacities to withstand pressures or strains to a considerable extent. According to Selye, the body meets stress by the discharge of certain chemicals from the adrenal glands. These chemicals, known as corticotropins, appear to affect virtually every part of the body. Tissue metabolism is altered, blood sugar levels may change, blood capillaries may become more permeable, alterations may take place in the digestive tract, resistance to inflammation may be increased and still other changes may occur.

If these physiologic reactions of the body are successful in meeting the stress or strain that occurs, then adaptation to the distressing external or internal forces serves to protect the body against damage. When the body changes are unable to increase the capacity of the tissues of the body to withstand stress, individual tissues may be damaged to such a point that human health is impaired.

It is impossible to live without stress at some level of intensity. This is particularly true of the ambitious person such as the business executive, the aggressive go-getter, or anyone else in whom ambition is coupled with drive and energy. When the body cannot successfully adapt to the fatigue and body changes that may result from stressful situations, injury to health may occur.

The Significance of Tension and Anxiety

Tension and anxiety are symptoms that a person is under stress. Anxiety is a signal of emotional disturbance and difficulty even though it may be of unconscious origin. Tension and anxiety in themselves do not indicate the nature of the problem other than that it is emotional in origin.

Anxiety develops only in the presence of conflict which centers around dissatisfaction, frustration, hostility, aggression and other forces of like nature.

The total personality of the individual suffering from tension and anxiety must be examined as well as the environmental circumstances under which he functions. Some individuals have personalities that are more apt to be involved in conflicts than is true of other people. Sometimes this is because of immaturity; at other times it may be a consequence of driving ambition coupled with frustrations that may arise because of a lack of professional education or other advantages that might enable a person to achieve success in chosen fields.

Mild Anxiety Is Beneficial

One must not assume that society should provide situations in which there is no stress but only complete security and tranquility. In the first place, it is impossible to achieve such an emotional environment. Even within himself, man can create stressful situations by his interpretations of the emotional environment around him. If he imagines a state of *tranquility* to be a hazard to him, then a stressful situation may be created.

It can be safely assumed that it is impossible to produce a society that creates no anxiety or tension in anyone. In fact, a mild degree of anxiety is probably beneficial to both the individual and to the society in which he lives. This is because when a person is in a mild state of tension he is apt to be in a condition of heightened consciousness in which there is more incentive and desire to accomplish. The person is more apt to have ambition and drive and to accomplish constructive things by hard work, good thinking and strong motivation than a person who is placid, secure, satisfied and, possibly, even indolent in his security and adjustment to his environment. It is only when stress and tension reach high levels and become excessive burdens that they become dangerous to human health. When the individual cannot make satisfactory adjustments to his problems, further maladjustments may occur and the efficiency and productivity of the individual may be impaired.

STRESS AND SOCIETY

"... if we study the natural history of mankind we cannot help noting that tension, alertness, alarmedness, fear, worry, anxiety and apprehension have been, are, and always will be important elements in the shaping of progress. As a nation we Americans have been strong ... because we have been able to rise to the occasion ... in the presence of stress, tensions, and apprehension ... (But now) we see a malignant tendency ... forcing us to believe that no one should ever be afraid, no one should ever feel anxiety ... rather we are to be completely tranquil."

Dr. Herman A. Dickel and
Dr. Henry H. Dixon, 1957

Stressful Situations

Stress for one person is not necessarily stress for another. The emotional problems of an individual will depend to a large extent on what he thinks they are. If a person makes the interpretation that a particular situation is a threat or danger to him, a stress reaction may be precipitated. To put the matter more simply, there can be no stress disease unless the stressful situation is recognized by the individual and is not successfully resolved by him. In other words, a man who cannot handle stress is the one who suffers from stress disease.

People in some professions are more apt to suffer from stress and tension than those in other occupations. Business executives, physicians, students and those in positions where decisions must be made are often subjected to greater stress than people in other fields.

Any group of people in whom there is a high incidence of peptic ulcers, high blood pressure, migraine headaches, fatigue, insomnia and heart disease should be suspected of being confronted with stressful situations.

Studies with experimental animals have shown that when monkeys live under a constant fear of punishment (such as with an electrical shock), many of them will not live long unless they make prompt decisions that will protect them against such punishment. Autopsies performed on animals that have died in an environment of continuous emotional stress and tension have revealed extensive damage to the digestive system. Hemorrhages, ulcers, erosions of the stomach and other damage to the digestive system have been revealed. Medical observations suggest the same conclusions for humans.

Some Symptoms of Stress and Tension

Stress, tension and anxiety can produce many different physical symptoms. Some of the commonest symptoms involve the inability to sleep at night. Frequently people suffering from stress and tensions occupy their minds with the problems of the day to such an extent that they are unable to get to sleep. If they do fall asleep they are apt to awaken sometime during the night in a startled condition with the heart beating fast and with a feeling of terror or panic. Often this awakening is followed by a period of rapid breathing.

Sometimes the symptoms of anxiety appear to be restricted almost entirely to the digestive system. The person under stress may experience a loss of appetite, may have a feeling of nausea and abdominal distress. He may develop the habit of swallowing air and may subsequently belch a great deal. Sometimes the person experiences diarrhea and in extreme cases may develop a condition known as chronic ulcerative colitis.

One of the commonest symptoms of stress and tension involving the digestive system is the production of a peptic ulcer. It has long been known that peptic ulcers are associated with worry, apprehension, fear and other disturbing emotional experiences. The turmoil that takes place in the brain may be transmitted through fibers of the vagus nerve to the stomach where the nerve impulses cause an increase in the secretion of hydrochloric acid. This acid, in sufficient strength and amount, erodes the linings of the stomach and nearby intestinal tissues.

Persons suffering from anxiety may experience severe headaches or may be unable to read or think effectively. Strength of memory and the power of concentration may be substantially impaired.

Often the symptoms of anxiety center around the functioning of the circulatory system. As mentioned earlier, the anxious person may suffer palpitation of the heart, but he may also experience a tightness in the chest which is sometimes mistaken for a heart attack. Dizziness and faintness may be associated with a disturbance of the circulatory system, and it may be difficult to bring about an association of these circulatory disturbances with mental activity.

Almost any functioning of the body can be impaired if the person under stress associates his difficulties with a particular part of the body.

Stress and Heart Disease

Many physicians and heart specialists believe that stress, especially in the form of psychoneurotic reactions to social environmental situations, is related to heart failure. It has long been known that an acute emotional disturbance may result in a heart attack. Emotional stress raises the blood pressure, which increases the work load of the heart.

STRESS AND THE HEART

"Intense frustration, disappointment, anger or hostility, as well as guilty anticipation or attainment of forbidden pleasure are the stresses which most often precipitate heart attacks ..."

Dr. William Dock, 1959

Some physicians and psychiatrists believe that a great many persons with coronary heart disease can be classified within a compulsive personality group. Often these people are leaders and executives because of their ambition, drive, energy and compulsions to get a job done and to do it well.

Dr. Henry I. Russek, consultant in cardiovascular research for the United States Public Health Service, has reported that stress and tension appear to be related to a disturbance of fat metabolism which in turn results in changes in the blood and in the walls of blood vessels. These changes appear to be linked with the greater likelihood of coronary heart disease. In studying a group of patients with heart disease, Dr. Russek found that there were about five times as many men with this condition who were under stress and tension than was found in a similar group of persons without heart disease. Such findings have been substantiated by other investigators.

Two physicians at the Mount Zion Hospital in San Francisco found that coronary artery disease was seven times more common among men with greater economic and social ambitions. They found that in a group of men between the ages of 30 and 60, able, alert, intelligent and gifted men who had ambition and drive and a strong competitive spirit had definite physiologic differences from other groups of men who did not have the same sense of work urgency.

Blood cholesterol levels were higher in the intensely ambitious men and heart disease was seven times greater. These investigators also found that men under stress because of occupational and social ambitions smoked more and drank more than other men.

Stress and Tranquilizing Drugs

The tranquilizing drugs have come to be widely used for the reduction of anxiety, emotional stress and nervous tension.

Those who are under stress and tension would do well to concentrate their efforts on the reduction of the causes of stress rather than to resort to the use of tranquilizing or other drugs.

Two Portland physicians studied the effects of tranquilizing drugs in approximately 8,000 patients in whom anxiety and tension were the major complaints. These people were physically normal, of average intelligence and were working steadily but were under emotional stress.

In this group of patients the doctors found that serious problems were *created* by the use of the tranquilizing drugs in 1,700 instances and that in 827 more cases emotional reactions were aggravated. Irrelevant symptoms appeared in 96, general toxic effects in 78, habituation to the drugs in 72, severe liver disturbances in 31 and other severe symptoms in 97 of the patients. Two of the persons committed suicide. The idea that stress and tension should be reduced by drugs rather than the application of intelligence to the causes of anxiety is dangerous.

The Relief of Stress and Tension

Dr. Dwight L. Wilbur of San Francisco found, in treating a group of executives in that community, that they were suffering from an emotional or situational stress involving overwork, tension and anxiety that resulted in extreme fatigue and nervousness. This physician found that psychotherapy did much to help the patient understand his situation and the stress that

it involved. It was often necessary to achieve philosophic changes in the thinking of these executives before they were able to control the ambition, drive and desires which helped to create the stress under which they were working.

Simple but important changes in the daily habits of these executives were found to be helpful. Daily rest (often consisting of simply relaxing in a chair, lying down or sleeping) and regular physical exercise of a pleasant nature were helpful in overcoming the fatigue and tension associated with the stressful situation.

It was also found necessary to improve the diet of these executives and to reduce their smoking and drinking. Medical corrections involving anemia, low metabolism, vision, infection and other conditions improved the patient's capacity for standing up under stress.

A STRESS DISEASE

"Heavy smoking may reasonably be regarded as a stress disease . . . It is the clear duty of the medical profession to try to prevent young people from acquiring the habit of heavy smoking . . ."
Dr. John Lister, 1957

In Chicago three physicians studied 50 business executives under the age of 50 who sought medical care for various reasons. Fatigue and exhaustion were two of the outstanding complaints of these executives.

The life situation appeared to play a very important part in the exhaustion of these business leaders. Many of them were chain smokers and this depleted the blood sugar levels, which in turn aggravated the stressful situation. These chain smokers, as a rule, were irritable and showed evidence of high tension. Many of the executives had turned to alcohol as a means of relaxing from stress, but this in itself had begun to create problems.

The relief of stress and tension depends upon a careful appraisal of the factors causing distress, but it also involves corrections of poor health habits as well as the removal or amelioration of emotional problems. Often, poor habits of rest, eating, drinking, smoking and a deteriorating sense of values are as important in the continuance of tension and stress as the frustrations and conflicts that were originally involved.

Questions

1. How do you explain the fact that emotional tension and stress often affect the digestive system adversely?
2. What is a stress disease?
3. What are the origins of nervous fatigue?
4. Which carries the greater hazard: extreme tension and stress or tranquilizing drugs that may be used for this condition?
5. Why is it that some people cannot assume responsibility or make decisions without emotional distress?

For Further Reading

1. Basowitz, Harold: *Anxiety and Stress.* New York, Blakiston-McGraw-Hill Book Company, 1955.
2. Funkenstein, Daniel H.: *Mastery of Stress.* Cambridge, Harvard University Press, 1957.
3. Laborit, Henri: *Stress and Cellular Function.* Philadelphia, J. B. Lippincott Company, 1959.
4. Selye, Hans: *The Stress of Life.* New York, Blakiston-McGraw-Hill Book Company, 1956.
5. Stevenson, George S., and Milt, Harry: *Master Your Tensions and Enjoy Living Again.* Englewood Cliffs, New Jersey, Prentice Hall, 1959.
6. Wolff, Harold George: *Stress and Disease.* Springfield, Ill., Charles C Thomas, 1953.

For Advanced Reading

Wolstenholme, G. E. W., and O'Connor, Cecilia M.: *Neurological Basis of Behavior.* Boston, Little, Brown and Company, 1958.

5

PHYSICAL FITNESS

PHYSICAL fitness has many definitions. This is because the ability to perform effectively in a physical way depends upon a great many factors. If the will to make a strong physical effort is weak or absent, the results will not reflect a high level of physical fitness. If strength is slight, this will be reflected in the level of fitness achieved. If the nutrition is deficient, then sustained vigorous physical effort will be limited in duration and intensity. If the body mechanics are faulty, the physical effort will lack potential. The simple physics of mass and energy will be reflected in physical performance. No one expects a 260-pound shot-putter to be a champion in the one-mile run. Size and body mechanics make such a performance impossible or highly unlikely. A person may be physically fit for one task, but almost completely unfit for another.

It is for such reasons that it is difficult to define physical fitness, but, generally physical fitness is the ability to perform a specific physical task at a high level of effort.

CONCEPT OF FITNESS

"A true concept of fitness includes the mental, the moral, the social and the emotional, as well as the physical."

Editoral, Journal of the American Medical Association, Feb. 23, 1957

In 1958 a special joint committee of the American Medical Association and the American Association for Health, Physical Education and Recreation issued a statement on the role of exercise in fitness which helps to clarify the meaning of this term.

It was pointed out in this report that fitness has many components and that emotional and intellectual factors are involved, as well as physical exercises.

This committee stated that: "Fitness for living rests first of all upon a solid foundation of basic good health . . . fitness for living implies freedom from disease; enough strength, agility, endurance and skill to meet the demands of daily living; reserves sufficient to withstand ordinary stresses without strain; and mental and emotional adjustment appropriate to the nature of the individual. Physical fitness is but one element in total fitness."

Members of the National Association of Intercollegiate Athletics issued a statement in which it was stated that physical fitness is not an end in itself, but represents a part of total fitness. The members of this organization believe that total fitness is achieved when the student:

". . . is free from handicapping health defects.
. . . has ample strength, endurance and agility to exert the maximum efforts demanded by workaday living.
. . . is competent to perform his daily tasks skillfully, efficiently and with the minimum expenditure of energy.
. . . is socially and emotionally well adjusted, able to live harmoniously with others, and cope successfully with the worries and tensions associated with modern urban living.
. . . is able to relax and conserve energy at appropriate times, sleep soundly, and arise feeling refreshed.
. . . has developed a sense of belonging and of performing useful work.
. . . has an interest in, and enthusiasm for, life and living."

Physical Fitness Requires Physical Exercise

No person can be physically fit unless he engages in the physical movements that are necessary for a particular task. To run swiftly, a person must train at running. To swim rapidly, an athlete must train at swimming. To run long distances effectively, a person must train at running long distances. No one can achieve his utmost potential in physical performance without engaging in whatever vigorous physical exercises may be needed to achieve excellence in the activity.

Physical fitness cannot be attained by determination alone, nor solely by the application of intelligence to the task; nor can physical fitness be achieved solely by good habits of nutrition, by freedom from disease, by moral precepts, good sportsmanship or by any other process. Vigorous physical activity must be a part of this pattern.

Physical Fitness Is Partly a Matter of Ethics

To be physically fit is not enough. The justification of fitness lies not only in the satisfaction or joy of performance that it brings us, but also in the quality and meaning of the physical effort as it concerns those around us.

In a wholesome society there is no place for the physically fit but unscrupulous person who uses his strength and agility to assault the innocent. There is no justification in physical fitness that is used to defeat and humiliate those of willing spirit but of far inferior physical ability. There is no moral strength in the debasement of the less gifted.

Physical fitness must have ethical associations if it is to be respected. Good sportsmanship on the part of the better conditioned athlete is an example of such an association. To lose with good grace, humility and self-respect is another such association.

When there is a deliberate attempt to injure an opposing player in order to remove him from a game, physical fitness is without moral justification. In sports there is no social, ethical or moral justification for the intentional injury of a competitor. Such conduct on the playing field can never be condoned if respect for physical fitness is to be maintained.

Physical Fitness Is
Partly a Matter of Spirit

When a person excels in physical performance, it is partly a matter of determination and spirit. The basic good health, good body structure, coordination and other attributes may be present, but if a person lacks spirit and determination, he will never use his potential to the fullest; he will never attain maximum physical fitness.

The sports world is replete with illustrations of underdog teams that have scored stunning upsets because of the determination, courage and will to win of the players. Many a less gifted athlete has beaten a superior rival simply because he refuses to be beaten. The determination to win exalts and extends a person's physical capacity.

Attainment of a high level of physical fitness and success in athletics is related to the attitudes and satisfactions that the participant may have about himself and the physical activities in which he engages. In other words, when an athlete likes a sport and has a favorable attitude about his participation in it, he is more apt to succeed. This was shown in a study at Cornell University where a comparison was made between 59 athletes who had won letters in varsity sports and 59 athletes who did not win letters. The letter winners had strong feelings of personal satisfaction regarding team spirit, esteem of their fellow students and participation in general in varsity sports.

Physical Fitness Is
Partly a Matter of Nutrition

Many famous athletes have reported unusual diets as a source of their athletic abilities. Various athletes have emphasized such things as sunflower seeds, nuts, seaweed, beer, royal jelly, raisins, black strap molasses and various other foods in their training programs, but medical and nutritional experience has shown that these foods do not have certain value in the promotion of physical fitness.

Jean Mayer, Head of the Department of Nutrition at Harvard University, points out that even the training table for athletic teams is unnecessary from a nutritional standpoint. "If a school's food is bad for athletes, it's bad for everybody," he states. Thus, if a training table is needed by athletes for nutritional purposes, it is needed by all the students of a college.

Nutritional experts and medical groups emphasize that there is no food that is especially valuable in the promotion of physical fitness. A well-rounded, normal diet will supply all the food essentials that are needed by the athlete. Some physicians have reported that the calorie intake should be higher than the average diet provides and that greater amounts of vitamins and proteins are important in the promotion of physical fitness.

Although there is no magic diet for the

achievement of physical fitness, there is abundant evidence that a well rounded diet is necessary for high levels of physical competence.

Man's capacity for physical effort has been measured by scientists many times under the stress of starvation or insufficient food. Josef Brozek, for example, studied men during a period of four days in which they went without food. During this time the amount of physical effort that these men could perform was measured by having them run on a treadmill, and by other tests. Although intelligence tests showed little or no impairment of the mind, there was a pronounced fall in endurance and the ability to exert physically. Fatigue, muscle weakness and soreness of muscles were prominent symptoms. The men also deteriorated rapidly in tests of speed and coordination.

For maximum physical fitness there must be adequate amounts of proteins, carbohydrates, fats, minerals, vitamins and water. If the diet is deficient in vitamins, there may be great deterioration in the ability to perform physical tasks. The vitamin B complex group has been especially studied in relation to physical effort. Although it is well established that a deficiency of these vitamins reduces physical fitness, there is no substantial evidence that a surplus of the vitamin B complex will result in superior endurance or capacity for physical effort. Some investigators have concluded, however, that in vigorous physical activity there is as much as a fourfold increase in the need for B complex vitamins because they are used in biochemical reactions during physical effort. Other researchers have recommended an increase in the intake of B complex vitamins if the person engages in vigorous physical activity over a period of time.

Sometimes it is necessary for athletes in training to increase the amount of salt in a diet. This is especially true when there is considerable loss of salt in the perspiration. An adequate amount of salt is necessary for proper functioning of the heart and circulatory system and for the prevention of muscle cramps.

In general, it can be concluded that good nutrition is an essential and necessary part of physical fitness. In most cases, however, the food needs of the athlete can be attained through a good well rounded diet.

Breakfast is an important meal for the attainment of capacity for physical effort. W. W. Tuttle and others of the College of Medicine at the State University of Iowa have done much research on the physical effects of the omission of breakfast or the eating of an inferior breakfast. It was found consistently that the omission of breakfast resulted in a significant decrease in the ability to perform physical work. The studies also revealed an impairment of reaction time, as well as a consistent increase in fatigue following strenuous exercise. Further studies showed an increase in tremor and a decrease in strength and endurance. Half of the men in the study were found to need more oxygen to perform a measured physical effort.

Physical Fitness Is Partly a Matter of Freedom from Injuries

Competition in sports calls for intense and even violent physical activity. In body-contact sports, the opportunities for injury are usually increased. Sprains, muscle strains, head injuries, bruises, damaged tendons, broken bones and many other injuries may result from vigorous physical activity.

Since physical injuries cause a prompt and sometimes complete reduction in physical fitness, the prevention of injury is a major necessity if physical fitness is to be achieved and maintained at a high level. The injured athlete may be unable to train properly over a long enough period of time to qualify him for the maximum physical effort of which he is capable. The well conditioned and highly trained athlete, at the peak of physical fitness, may be incapacitated completely by an athletic injury.

The prevention of injuries in sports is probably just as important as the conditioning program in the achievement of high levels of physical fitness.

The kinds of injuries that occur in some of the major sports are described in a later chapter (preventive measures are indicated when known).

Physical Fitness Is Partly a Matter of Freedom from Infections

Physical fitness is partly a matter of remaining free from infectious diseases. All infections can temporarily and often dramatically lower the capacity for physical effort. Certain infectious diseases may permanently impair the level of physical fitness. Poliomyelitis has been known to result in partial or complete paralysis and to greatly reduce the capacity for physical effort.

Infectious hepatitis, a virus disease of the liver usually spread through contaminated water, is another infection that causes severe deterioration of the capacity for physical effort. Medical experience has shown that during convalescence from this disease exercise must be curtailed for many months to prevent relapse; any physical activity undertaken is of low quality with substantial lack of endurance.

Influenza is another infection that often causes regression in strength and endurance that may persist for weeks.

There are, in fact, no infectious diseases that do not impair the level of physical fitness to some extent, although effects may be of slight duration and intensity in mild disorders.

To achieve a high level of physical fitness a person should protect himself against communicable diseases to the best of his ability.

The Value of Exercise

The value of exercise and physical fitness has long been established by the medical profession and other groups.

In medicine a program of physical activity following illness and surgery has been found to be most valuable in the prevention of complications such as blood clots and pneumonia. It has also been found to restore the morale of the patient and to bring about a more rapid recovery. From the economic standpoint, the restoration of physical fitness may reduce the period of hospitalization by 20 to 50 per cent at considerable saving to the patient.

Physicians and surgeons prescribe physical exercises for the patient after virtually every medical or surgical treatment. In many surgical conditions, diligent exercise is the only way of preventing disability of joints and muscles.

> **VALUE OF EXERCISE**
>
> "... exercise of almost any kind, suitable in degree and duration for the particular individual concerned, can and does play a useful role in the maintenance of both physical and mental health ..."
>
> *Dr. Paul D. White, 1957*

Physical exercise has been found to stimulate the growth of collateral blood vessels in the heart of patients with coronary disease. Exercise has been found to be highly effective in the treatment of patients with gangrene of the legs or feet. It has been found to prevent the formation of blood clots in the legs and to be of value in many aspects of health and disease.

In general, it can be said that physical activity develops and helps to maintain the effective functioning of the heart and circulatory system, aids in relaxation and release of nervous tension, improves digestion (probably through the reduction of nervous tension), helps to control obesity, improves the capacity of the respiratory system and is valuable even for the older person.

Dr. Hein and Dr. Ryan, of the American Medical Association, have recently summarized the contributions of physical activity to physical health under four major categories:

(1) The prevention of obesity and degenerative diseases that are associated with overweight; (2) the prevention of circulatory degenerative changes characteristic of coronary heart disease; (3) preservation of the physical characteristics of youth; and (4) maintenance of the ability to meet emergencies more effectively and thus to help in the avoidance of disability and perhaps death.

A study of college wrestlers at the University of Maryland revealed that after participation in wrestling matches there was an alleviation of neurotic tendencies and aggressive feelings. Participation in the sport, as measured by a standardized test of personality, revealed that the activity served the release of tensions whether the individual athlete won his match or not.

periods of sitting at the wheel during automobile trips. Others have reported cases of blood clots in the same part of the body from long sitting while watching television.

It has long been known to physicians that when a patient lies inactive in bed during an illness that he is more apt to develop pneumonia, blood clots, bed sores and other consequences.

At the University of Minnesota Dr. Henry L. Taylor has studied the effects of lack of exercise on heart disease. There is evidence that low levels of physical activity over a long period of time contribute to the development of heart disorders.

For youth perhaps the major hazards of inactivity lie in the area of developmental failures. Inadequate physical endurance, inferior physical structure and unimproved coordination are some of the physical deficiencies that may follow long inactivity. Often these deficiencies lead to psychologic problems of inferiority and low self-esteem, so the consequences are not restricted to physical effects.

The Hazards of Inactivity

Medical research has revealed many associations between the lack of exercise and poor health.

Sitting with the legs crossed for long periods of time has resulted in frequent damage to the peroneal nerve and partial or complete paralysis in one or both legs. Some physicians have reported the formation of blood clots in the legs from long

---

BLOOD CLOTS

"Prolonged sitting in one position . . . may result in venous thrombosis in the legs. . . . tall men are peculiarly susceptible. . . . Three patients developed major thrombosis in the legs . . . following prolonged sitting in awkward positions while viewing television programs. . . . Viewers should get up and move about at least once an hour, in addition to moving the legs frequently . . ."

Dr. Meyer Naide, 1957

Tests of Physical Fitness

Because there are many definitions of physical fitness, it is most difficult to establish a satisfactory test of this condition.

Several years ago a great deal of publicity was given to the so-called Kraus-Weber tests of physical fitness. When these tests were applied to large groups of American and European children, it was found that the Europeans made better scores than the Americans. It was found that approximately 9 per cent of the European children between the ages of six and sixteen failed the test, whereas approximately 58 per cent of American youth failed the test.

The Kraus-Weber test of physical fitness consisted of measuring the fitness of six muscle groups including those of the upper and lower back and the abdominal and hamstring muscles of the legs. Many physical educators criticized the results of this test because it left out other aspects of physical fitness such as reflex action, endurance, speed and emotional stability.

In Eugene, Oregon, the test was used on 1,195 elementary school children and 38 per cent failed. However, it was found that almost 80 per cent of the failures occurred on the item of the test which pertained to flexibility. Twice as many boys as girls failed this part of the test, which made the girls appear to be more "muscularly" fit than the boys. Studies in Japan with large numbers of children led to the conclusion that the failure of American children in this test was due largely to the length of the legs in proportion to the torso and that rather than being a satisfactory test of physical fitness, the Kraus-Weber standards were actually a measure of body build.

Two states have produced more widely accepted tests of physical fitness.

The California Physical Performance Test consists of performances on the standing broadjump, a jump and reach exercise, a modified or standard pullup (depending on the age of the child), a pushup for boys and a pushup from the knee for girls, the situp, the 50-yard dash for certain groups and the 75-yard dash for others, a shuttle race for girls and a throw for distance with softball, basketball or soccerball. Performances on these activities are standardized and can be scored easily.

The New York State Physical Fitness Test is an individual test of seven different items that measure posture, accuracy, strength, agility, speed, balance and endurance. Scores of the performances on the New York State Physical Fitness Test have been standardized so that each individual can be rated with a physical fitness score relative to large groups of other children.

Probably no single test of physical fitness can ever be evolved to measure the capacity to engage in all physical activities. Perhaps the best test of physical fitness is the actual performance in a specific physical effort. The best measure of fitness for putting the 16-pound shot is the distance that the individual can actually put the shot; the best measure of fitness for throwing a baseball is the distance that a person can throw the baseball. It may be that no complete or more satisfactory test of physical fitness can be developed.

Drugs and Physical Fitness

In recent years there has been occasional publicity given to the use of drugs by athletes.

There are no known drugs that improve the levels of physical fitness. There are certain drugs that can significantly improve athletic performance for a brief period of time, but these have been strongly condemned for two primary reasons: (1) their use is inconsistent with good sportsmanship, and (2) they may, according to the medical profession, seriously damage the user.

The American Medical Association established a special committee to investigate this problem. This group conducted two years of investigation in which studies were made under controlled research conditions of the use of "pep pills" containing amphetamine sulfate. Experiments were carried out on swimmers, runners and weight throwers and it was found that most of the athletes did improve their performance, but the committee concluded that the regular use of drugs for athletic competition may expose the user to well established harmful effects.

A nation-wide survey of colleges and high schools by this medical committee showed that less than one per cent of the coaches had *ever* advised athletes to use pep pills. The use of such drugs was found to be rare, although sugar pills and vitamin pills have often been mistaken for drugs by sports fans.

Some trainers have asserted that many professional athletes use stimulants or tranquilizers during the competitive season. Many of these claims have not been substantiated, but there is some evidence that, under certain circumstances, athletes have used drugs. This has not always worked to their advantage in sports, however. During the 1960 Olympic games, it was alleged that a cyclist who died in competition had been stimulated with a drug; this was later denied and the full truth may never be known.

The athlete is well advised to leave drugs alone. The American Medical Association strongly condemns their use in any form of sports participation. Little if any good may come from their use and much harm and even death may be the result.

Hypnosis and Physical Fitness

Newspapers in recent years have included stories of athletes who improved their performances after hypnosis. Hypnotists have contended that although hypnosis cannot improve the basic capacity for physical performance, it can make possible more complete use of this capacity. This is thought to be true especially if the attitude of the athlete is a handicap to his performance.

Dr. Conrad K. Gale, diplomate of the American Board of Hypnosis, believes that tensions at the conscious level in some athletes can be relieved and that this may result in improvements in performance. This hypnotist also points out that there is the possibility of over-exertion under hypnosis that may be dangerous to an athlete or team.

The Committee on Hypnosis of the American Medical Association condemns the use of this psychologic method for the improvement of athletic performance. The chairman of the committee expressed the belief in 1960 that this practice is equivalent to injecting a race horse with a stimulant to make it run faster.

This important medical committee has called attention to the fact that the per-

formances of some athletes have deteriorated under hypnosis and that the dangers involved outweigh any advantages. The committee maintains that hypnosis may aggravate physical impairments of which the athlete is unaware and that he may become exhausted to the point of harm; that he may ignore safety measures and that, at best, hypnosis can do no more than help the athlete play up to his basic ability.

Medical Recommendations for Physical Fitness

The Joint Committee of the American Medical Association and the American Association for Health, Physical Education and Recreation has made the following recommendations regarding exercise:

1. All persons should be shown by medical examination to be organically sound before . . . strenuous exercise.

2. A program of exercise started at an early age may be continued throughout life with certain adjustments. . . .

3. An individual in good physical condition and training may appropriately participate in an activity that might be harmful to another person of the same age not in a comparable state of fitness.

4. Hard, fast, sustained, or highly competitive games and sports should not be played by persons beyond the age of 30 unless they have maintained or can attain by systematic training an appropriate state of fitness.

5. Persons who are out of training should not attempt to keep pace in any vigorous sport with persons who are properly conditioned.

6. Persons should not compete in body-contact sports or endurance activities with others of disproportionate size or skill.

7. Persons long out of training, or "soft" (who have not practiced strenuous exercise regularly) will need an extended period of conditioning to facilitate gradual return to full activity.

8. The ability to recuperate after physical activity is a good guide to the desirable severity of exercise at any age. Recuperation should be reasonably prompt.

9. Exercise, regardless of its nature or extent, cannot provide immunization against infectious illness nor cure communicable disease.

10. Sports involving body contact or traumatic

hazards necessitate the provision of protective equipment.

11. Boxing is a controversial activity because of the problem of brain injury from blows to the head.

12. Careful preparation and maintenance of playing fields and other arenas of sports is essential to reduction of injuries. . . .

Fatigue

Fatigue is one of the most common complaints of college students. According to some student health service directors, more students have reported in for medical examinations with a leading complaint of fatigue than for any other single reason. In business and homemaking activities also, fatigue is one of the commonest complaints that the physician hears from his patients.

There are different patterns or characteristics of fatigue in different patients, and these have great significance in the diagnosis of underlying causes.

Treatment of fatigue is most effective when a specific cause or causes of the condition can be found, although it is possible to bring considerable relief through a general improvement in the patient's daily activities. When the patient rests more, reduces the intensity or amount of physical effort, takes life more philosophically, eats better, resolves emotional conflicts and makes other adjustments in the way he lives, it is often possible to bring about a considerable reduction in the extent of fatigue which such a person experiences, regardless of the presence of a more fundamental cause.

Three Basic Types of Fatigue

There are three general types of fatigue. It is important for both the physician and the patient to recognize differences in the various kinds of fatigue if medical treatment and advice are to be sound.

These three types are as follows:

1. PHYSICAL FATIGUE. Fatigue in the healthy person is a normal physiologic phenomenon. Fatigue, in a sense, is nature's way of securing rest in order that the body may balance its physiologic resources and waste products. The person suffering from normal physical fatigue shows a pattern somewhat as follows:

He awakens in the morning feeling refreshed. He is able to do a good day's work. In this process, however, he becomes tired. His fatigue is quickly alleviated by rest, by meals, to some extent by coffee and by other measures (in other words, he shows a quick rebound). By evening he is sufficiently tired so that when he goes to bed his fatigue assists him in falling asleep and securing a good night's rest. By morning he has recuperated so that he is again able to carry on another good day's work.

2. PSYCHOLOGIC FATIGUE. When fatigue is of psychologic origin, it has a different pattern from physical fatigue. The person is apt to awaken in the morning feeling tired. This exhausted feeling is not due merely to an accumulation of the results of sustained physical effort. As the day lengthens, the person with psychologic fatigue begins to feel better. By evening he or she may feel greatly rested and prepared to engage with pleasure in social or other activities. Also characteristic of psychologic fatigue during any time of the day is the sudden development of a feeling of exhaustion at the prospect of some task which is either consciously or subconsciously disliked by the patient. The recovery from this brief interval of fatigue is rapid once the task has been cleared out of the way.

Since psychologic fatigue has its origins in the emotional and mental life of the individual, it must be approached from a different standpoint from that of normal or physical fatigue if improvement in the patient's welfare is sought.

3. FATIGUE FROM DISEASE. There is a third pattern of fatigue in which the pa-

tient awakens in the morning with a feeling of tiredness which continues throughout the day, although it may be accentuated by evening. When there are persistent complaints of fatigue on the part of the patient, without recovery or periods of freedom from exhaustion, the physician suspects the presence of some illness.

One of the classic symptoms of tuberculosis, for example, is a feeling of fatigue on the part of the patient for months before the disease may be finally diagnosed. In general, it can be said that almost any sickness will result in a sustained fatigue until the illness is diagnosed and treated or until the patient recovers spontaneously.

It is sometimes possible, however, that a person who has no basic illness is pushing himself by hard physical effort to the limits of his physical capacity. In such a case there may be accumulated fatigue from day to day and week to week so that he is in a constant state of tiredness even though no disease is present. Only a careful medical examination coupled with an analysis of the person's daily activities can be expected to distinguish between these two origins of chronic fatigue.

Nervous or Psychologic Fatigue

Acute fatigue of nervous or psychologic origin often results from a combination of factors, such as insufficient rest, limited physical endurance, poor nutrition, mild health disorders such as slight anemia, visual disturbance and so on, in addition to some tension or anxiety based upon circumstances or the inherent level of stability in the person involved.

Dr. J. E. Finesinger, Psychiatrist of the University of Maryland Medical School, compared a group of 100 neurotic persons with 100 fatigued patients. He found that both groups felt tired, tense, sleepless, depressed and restless a good part of the time. Both groups experienced headaches, shortness of breath and sexual difficulties. Finesinger found that almost always the fatigue could be boiled down to anxieties

over jobs or family, rejection by a loved one, or guilt feelings. The fatigue of these patients improved in one third to one half of the cases when they were treated by psychiatric means.

Dr. Dwight L. Wilbur of San Francisco found that the relief of fatigue in business men was best achieved by teaching about the effects of uncontrolled ambition, by emphasizing the need for developing a better philosophy toward life, and by convincing such people that they need rest during the day and extra sleep at night or a few days of complete change of environment. He found that rest for the exhausted person could often be obtained by relaxing in a chair, lying on the bed or sleeping during the day.

Dr. Wilbur also found that regular exercise of a pleasant type, a better food intake and correction of mild physical disorders helped a great deal in overcoming fatigue of nervous origin. Young people with emotional and environmental problems which could be solved often improved remarkably and recovered completely from their fatigue. This physician stresses that an improvement of even 10 to 20 per cent in reduction of fatigue may be enough to make life worth living again for some patients.

A group of Chicago doctors studied fifty business executives, all under fifty years of age, and found that fatigue was one of the outstanding complaints. A major source of this fatigue was depletion of the blood sugar level by excessive smoking, which often correlates with a high level of nervous tension. Many of the executives were chain smokers. One investigator found that 62 per cent of the executives smoked more than a pack of cigarettes a day. Dietary deficiencies were also found in this group of executives.

One of the outstanding characteristics of psychologic fatigue is that it is apt to be worse in the morning. It is also apt to be associated with certain activities for which the patient has either conscious or unconscious dread. Such patients often have a strong desire to lie down and rest, but find that they cannot relax or sleep when they do make the attempt.

Three doctors at the Massachusetts General Hospital studied a group of seventy patients from the psychiatric wards and outpatient service whose major complaint was fatigue. These investigators gathered fifty specific indications that fatigue was related to events in the lives of the patients. One patient who would argue with his father suddenly became greatly fatigued when he reflected that it was wrong to argue with one's father. Another man having conflict with his wife would get extremely tired on opening the door and seeing his wife. A business man became very tired in the morning whenever he saw the office building in which he conducted his business, because he was in conflict with his fellow workers. Psychiatric help or good sensible counselling and advice is often of considerable help in this type of fatigue.

Dr. Frank N. Allan of Boston studied 300 persons who came to him with complaints of fatigue and weak spells. He found that a physical disorder was at the root of the fatigue in 20 per cent of the cases, but that a nervous condition was the source of the tiredness in 80 per cent of the cases. He found that most of the relatively mild nervous conditions which were the fundamental cause of fatigue in his patients did not properly fall within the field of psychiatry. In other words, they were not of such severity as to demand psychiatric treatment, although the removal of a cause of worry was a specific remedy for the fatigue.

Fatigue from Disease

Almost any disease, if it is serious enough, will produce a feeling of fatigue. Often this fatigue may persist for years before its origin is discovered.

Although tuberculosis and other chronic diseases will more often be the source of fatigue which is pathologic, there are certain disorders in which fatigue is the outstanding symptom or sign.

Myasthenia gravis is one of these disorders. People with this disease are apt to suffer excessive fatigue from even the ordinary functions of living such as climbing stairs, chewing food, talking, keeping the eyes open and holding up the head. Often the weakness may affect all of the body or may be observed first in specific muscles such as those of the arm, leg or face.

The disorder appears to be due to a failure between nerve and muscle, so that the nerve impulse to the muscle fails to pass a chemical junction. The chemical substance normally found at this juncture is acetylcholine. The most effective treatment for this disease appears to be rest and the use of neostigmine, which is a substance that restores the normal content of acetylcholine at the juncture of the nerve and muscle. The nerve impulse can then get through to the muscle and stimulate it to normal contraction.

Patients with an underactive thyroid gland often complain of fatigue as a major symptom. Dr. Henry H. Turner of Oklahoma City, for example, found that 86 per cent of his patients who suffered from hypothyroidism complained of fatigue.

Other disturbances of the endocrine glands often have fatigue as a main feature. Patients with arthritis, neuritis and other disorders sometimes complain of fatigue in which specific muscle groups are involved.

The important point in considering the relationship of fatigue to disease is that a person suffering from a chronic and long-lasting condition of this sort should consult his physician for a thorough medical examination. There are so many diseases that might be involved in the production of this type of fatigue that only a physician should be trusted to diagnose the disease involved.

Combat Fatigue

In recent wars it has been observed that under certain battle conditions there may be a high rate of battle fatigue. The men experiencing this fatigue have been listed as psychiatric casualties, for psychologic factors have been found to be partly responsible for the condition. Usually, however, a combination of factors has resulted in the ultimate breakdown of the person who suffers from this disorder. In all such cases there has been an extreme, deep fatigue associated with a lack of sleep or disturbed sleep for long hours of time and with inadequate nutrition. During action in the field, especially when troops are pinned down by enemy gunfire, deficiencies in food supplies may develop to the point where rations are considerably reduced. Many persons with combat fatigue have reported that they have gone two to three weeks on a minimum of food.

In addition to lack of rest and poor nutrition, combat fatigue symptoms have been found to be related to psychologic factors such as fear of death, unusual enemy tactics, noise and blast concussion. Military psychiatrists have stated that even the most stable person may be expected to have a breakdown if he is subjected to sufficient enemy gunfire in an exposed position for a long enough time under conditions of poor rest and poor food. If friends and companions are killed in military action, the chance that a given soldier will become a psychiatric casualty under battle conditions is increased still more.

In some battle areas the true battle fatigue casualty was treated with great success in so-called exhaustion centers close to the front lines. At these stations the soldiers suffering from this type of exhaustion were given rest and sedation, and on recovery from their extreme fatigue were rapidly returned to military duty. From 75 to 80 per cent of such casualties were returned successfully to battle.

Insufficient training, lack of confidence in military leaders, lack of confidence in the troops with whom he is closely associated, and combat service under great physical fatigue have been the four outstanding factors related to the production of combat fatigue in any one soldier.

The true combat fatigue case is not a frank psychiatric disorder. Recoveries are excellent. If the patient is not well after two months of proper treatment, he probably suffers from some psychiatric condition, rather than combat fatigue alone.

Noise and Fatigue

Noise in the home, at the office, in the factory or on the battleground is often a great source of fatigue. The Noise Abatement Commission of New York City found that the body metabolism of typists was 19 per cent greater in noisy surroundings than in a quiet environment. One task was performed 7.4 per cent faster when noise was reduced by one-half.

Studies in industrial efficiency have shown repeatedly that noise can be a source of fatigue.

The problem of fatigue from noise plus the damage to hearing from gunfire on naval vessels and in other military situations caused the National Defense Research Committee to conduct research aimed at the production of an ear protector. The sum total of this research was embodied in an ear protector called the V-51R Ear Warden. This device not only gave considerable protection against fatigue from noise, but also saved many persons from ruptured eardrums and other injuries to the ear from concussion waves from big guns.

Excessive noise not only causes fatigue, but also may actually damage hearing. Although no precise standards have been established for the prevention of injury from noise in industry, experts in this field agree that hearing may be permanently damaged by sustained exposure to noise of 75 to 100 decibels.

The National Noise Abatement Council carries on a national program of giving awards for outstanding achievements in this field. Chicago, for example, is one of the cities that has won a Grand National Award for outstanding achievement in the fight against unnecessary noise.

Alternation of Work and Rest

Often fatigue is simply a matter of sustained physical, emotional or mental effort. One of the most valuable lessons learned from studies in industrial fatigue and competitive athletics is that efficiency and work output can be measurably improved if work and rest periods are alternated.

Sometimes an amazing increase in efficiency and production can result from less work. In one of the early industrial fatigue studies conducted in the United States it was found that efficiency rose 212 per cent in the loading of heavy material when the workers labored for eight minutes and then rested for twelve minutes throughout the eight-hour day.

The tough industrial policy that a man must work a full eight hours throughout the day is not based upon biological law. A sounder principle would be that a man should work and rest at whatever particular ratio will preserve his efficiency most effectively.

The British public health authorities learned the value of rest in relation to work output in World War II. After Dunkirk, English workers were staying at their jobs twelve hours a day for seven days a week in order to produce needed defense materials. Public health authorities and physicians found that the workers were soon near the breaking point. When working hours were reduced, production went up steadily. From eighty-four hours a week down to sixty hours, then fifty-six hours and even lower, it was found that more and more war materials were produced. In other words, production improved rather than declined when the employees worked for a shorter time. In one

process the highest production peak was achieved when the workers stayed at their jobs only 43½ hours per week.

The ideal ratio between work and rest is apt to be different for practically every kind of job. On-the-job studies are needed in order to discover the best combination of work and rest in terms of total output. Only when such studies are made will the working hours of human beings be established on a sensible basis. In the meantime each person can conduct his own research to discover the combination of effort and relaxation which permits him to function at maximum efficiency.

Posture and Body Mechanics

The way you sit, stand and work may have much to do with the fatigue you experience. Good body mechanics should be based upon alternate use and relaxation of certain parts of the body.

When people work, they should make themselves comfortable. Often comfort is a matter of changing body position rather than continuing effort in one particular manner. Sometimes very little consideration is given to the comfort of the worker. During World War II, for example, the Women's Bureau of the United States Department of Labor made a study of women workers in war industries and found that a chief complaint among these employees was one of fatigue and back strain. Obviously both these complaints would reduce working efficiency. It was found that many of the workers had to stand continuously through the entire working day. Sometimes when stools were provided for the workers to use, they were of the backless type and did not give the support necessary for relaxation.

Long standing carries certain other hazards to health besides that of fatigue production. Studies have shown that varicose veins are more common in workers who stand throughout the working day.

It has often been observed that the workbench or table at which a person may be employed is not of the proper height. A difference of even a few inches may make marked differences in the amount of fatigue that the worker feels before the day is over.

Working efficiency can definitely be improved by better posture. Good body mechanics in sitting, standing, walking or working in any position will pay dividends in efficiency and well-being, as well as in work production.

Fatigue and Relaxation

Many persons find it most difficult to achieve physical relaxation. It has been shown, however, that relief from tension and fatigue can be considerable if a person learns to relax the muscles of the body.

Those who have specialized in the field of teaching people how to relax find that it often takes from three to six months of instruction to develop this ability in tense persons. Relaxation can be achieved best by stretching a particular part of the body and then suddenly relaxing this portion of the body. Slow, rhythmic stretching movements are desirable. Many people have to be taught the feeling of tension in order to develop the ability to relax. When the sense of a fully relaxed musculature has once been realized, the person thereafter finds it much easier to recognize tension.

Good results have also been obtained by concentration on one part of the body until that part has been relaxed. For example, once relaxation has been achieved in the right wrist, attention can then be shifted to another part of the body such as the right shoulder. In a gradual progression over the entire body it is then possible to secure general relaxation. Some patients have been taught to start by concentrating on the top of the head, the scalp, and then to progress down the body.

It has been found important to relax small muscles as well as large ones. For example, tension is often sustained by contraction of the muscles around the mouth and eyes. One must learn to relax all parts of the body if a maximum prevention of fatigue is to be achieved by this means.

What To Do about Fatigue

The first step in the relief of chronic and long-lasting fatigue is to consult a physician for a thorough medical examination. The possibility of disease must be ruled out. If physical illness is a basic cause of fatigue, treatment must be directed at the former.

If no physical ailment is discovered, attention should be directed to the possibility that the person suffering from excessive tiredness is living at a pace beyond his capabilities or that his habits of rest, nutrition, smoking or other behavior may be at fault. Only by a careful appraisal of the hygienic habits of the person can a sensible conclusion be reached as to whether these factors are related to the fatigue.

The possibility that psychologic factors may be involved in the production of fatigue must also be explored. Discussion of this with the physician at the time of the medical examination may bring to light certain significant possibilities. Sometimes psychiatric assistance may be advisable.

In addition to the foregoing, no matter what the source of the fatigue, some relief can be sought by the development of a philosophy that permits moderation in work or other activities. The encouragement of frequent brief rest periods during the day in an alternation of work and rest, and emphasis upon the improvement of the eating habits of the fatigued person, often bring good results.

In the last analysis, however, each case of excessive fatigue should be thoroughly appraised by the physician in terms of the individual patient.

Questions

1. When is a person physically fit?
2. Why is it that a person who is physically fit for one activity may not be fit for another?
3. How does physical fitness have a relationship to general health?
4. What are some of the hazards of physical inactivity?
5. Why it is unethical and unwise to use a drug to improve athletic performance?
6. Why does the American Medical Association discourage the use of hypnosis in athletics?
7. What relationship does fatigue have to physical fitness?
8. What are the three basic types of fatigue?

For Further Reading

1. Darrow, May Goodall: *The Posture Problem Up to Date*. New York, Vantage Press, 1959.
2. Gutwirth, Samuel W.: *How to Sleep Well—The Cultivation of Natural Rest*. New York, Vantage Press, 1959.
3. Hilliard, Marion: *Women and Fatigue*. New York, Doubleday and Company, Inc., 1960.
4. Karpovich, Peter V.: *Physiology of Muscular Activity*. Philadelphia, W. B. Saunders Company, 1959.
5. Lowman, Charles LeRoy, and Young, Carl Haven: *Postural Fitness: Significance and Variations*. Philadelphia, Lea & Febiger, 1960.
6. Morehouse, L. E., and Miller, A. T., Jr.: *Physiology of Exercise*. St. Louis, C. V. Mosby Company, 1959.
7. Morehouse, L. E., and Rasch, Philip J.: *Scientific Basis of Athletic Training*. Philadelphia, W. B. Saunders Company, 1958.

For Advanced Reading

Licht, Sidney H., Editor: *Therapeutic Exercise*. Physical Medicine Library, Vol. 3. New Haven, E. Licht, 1958.

6

NUTRITION AND HEALTH

THE STUDY of nutrition is no longer only a problem of learning the nutritional content of foods. Food has become a field of research for the psychiatrist; the disposition of food surpluses has become a concern of the political scientist; the multiple effects of nutrients on the human body is an unlimited field of investigation for the biochemist; the wise purchase of foods has become a necessity for the consumer; food continues to be a primary means of livelihood for the farmer and agriculturist; and for the many industries concerned with the marketing of food, the field of nutrition is a vital business unmatched by other interests.

Food for Peace

In the summer of 1960 the United States government advocated a program to distribute the food surplus of the United States to "help feed the hungry of the world."

The plan calls for distributing the food through the United Nations. Countries such as Canada, Australia, New Zealand, the Argentine, France and the Scandinavian nations were invited to pool their surplus supplies for distribution by the United Nations to those countries in need of food.

The concept that sharing of food surpluses will promote the cause of world peace emphasizes anew the importance of nutrition in world politics.

WORLD FOOD PROBLEMS

"I believe that the real food problem in the near future is not whether there will be a world shortage but whether shortages in particular countries will have serious repercussions on international relations."

Warren S. Thompson, Ph.D., 1960

Nutritional Standards

It has been found that the nutritional status of any population depends upon several different factors. First, the agricultural resources and production of the country must be sufficient to meet the needs of the population. Second, there must be an adequate means of transporting food from the place where it is grown to the places where it is needed. Third, there must be sufficient economic resources, in terms of purchasing power, so that people may buy foods of good quality. Fourth, education is needed on the importance of nutrition to human health and in the selection and preparation of foods. Obviously, the food habits and traditions of any group of people will also be a prominent factor in the determination of the nutritional status of that group.

Not all foods are equally nutritious. Some foods, such as certain varieties of mushrooms, are actually dangerous to consume. In this age of eating out there is the possibility of transmission of disease through improperly sterilized eating utensils. The improper cooking of food may destroy certain of its valuable nutrients or may permit the transmission of diseases such as trichinosis.

FOOD LIKES

"Our food likes and dislikes are often keyed to our emotions and are conditioned by our culture, religion, parents, friends and other factors; they may change. . . ."

Dr. William Kaufman, 1959

Some people skip meals, whereas others nibble continually between meals.

The modern processes of canning, dehydrating and freezing foods have simplified the problem of getting an adequate diet the year round. On the other hand, questions may arise as to the effects of processing and refining upon the nutritional value of foods. Confusion may exist as to the safety of chemicals used in agriculture and the food industries in terms of their effects on human health. There may be controversy between those who favor raw milk for its purported nutritional values and those who favor pasteurization because of its importance in preventing the spread of disease through milk.

Food faddists grow rich in certain sections of the United States. Extravagant claims are made for certain health foods, and so-called health food stores flourish in many communities.

In some families the dinner time is an emotionally disturbing period which becomes an occasion for conflict between parents and children.

Knowledge of foods occupies a position of great importance in the modern world; understanding its relation to human health has become almost a necessity if we are to achieve nutritional values without encountering the physical and emotional hazards that can be found in the field of nutrition.

The Six Basic Food Essentials

There are six essentials for a well rounded diet. No person whose diet is deficient in any of these six essential groups can be considered a well nourished person. A serious deficiency in any of these groups is bound to be reflected in a reduction in working efficiency or in the appearance of nutritional disease.

The six basic essentials are: (1) proteins, (2) fats, (3) carbohydrates, (4) vitamins, (5) minerals, and (6) water.

Proteins are highly complex compounds containing nitrogen, which is essential in the building and repair of cells and tissues. Fats are a combination of glycerol and fatty acids that serve primarily as reserve energy. Carbohydrates are compounds containing carbon, hydrogen and oxygen, which are used as primary sources of energy. The most important carbohydrates are the starches, sugars, celluloses and gums. Vitamins are substances occurring in foods in small amounts which are necessary for normal functioning of the body. Minerals are elemental substances also needed for normal functioning and structure of the body.

Proteins

Proteins are necessary for the creation of life, for growth, for maintenance of body tissues, for improved immunity and resistance to disease, for wound healing, for convalescence after surgery or illness, for the formation of blood and bone, for the production of milk in nursing mothers, for the prevention of a variety of deficiency diseases, and for a number of other health reasons.

Some authorities maintain that a typical American breakfast, which is apt to be high in carbohydrates, is likely to be followed by hunger, fatigue and sometimes weakness within about three hours. Experimental research has shown that the addition of protein to the breakfast improves

human efficiency and postpones fatigue. Such studies show that the blood sugar is better maintained when protein is consumed in the breakfast.

Some of the main results from a diet deficient in protein are as follows:

Resistance to numerous infections may be seriously lowered, because antibodies, which are produced for the specific purpose of fighting disease, are largely composed of proteins. For example, gamma globulin, which has been used to immunize both children and adults against a number of diseases, is an antibody composed mostly of protein.

Amino acids are the building stones for the construction of protein in the body. It has been found that human gamma globulin contains at least five different amino acids, namely, lysine, methionine, tryptophan, threonine and leucine. The body is handicapped in the manufacture of gamma globulin if the diet is deficient in the basic amino acids and proteins. It has been shown that the ability of the body to produce antibodies can be quickly restored by a diet of high-quality protein.

Amino acids are manufactured into proteins primarily in the liver. There is some evidence that the body may synthesize proteins from amino acids in other tissues as well, but this has not been clearly established. Milk, egg and meat proteins are generally considered superior to other sources of the essential amino acids.

Undernourished persons are more susceptible to tuberculosis, rheumatic fever and various respiratory and intestinal infections. In hookworm, for example, improvement of the diet may be as important as medical treatment of the disease.

Both medical and experimental research has demonstrated the importance of a high protein diet for resistance to many diseases.

Anemia may also be due to protein deficiency. Hemoglobin, which is needed for the transportation of oxygen from the lungs to various tissues of the body, is about 95 per cent protein. Anemia may come from many other causes, but a deficiency of protein may be just as important as a deficiency of iron, or even more so, in the creation of nutritional anemia.

During pregnancy and nursing there is a greater need for protein. Medical studies have shown that pregnant women who consume a diet rich in protein have fewer complications at childbirth, have healthier children, suffer less anemia, and are better able to nurse their babies after childbirth than mothers whose food intake is low in proteins.

It used to be thought that in kidney disease it was necessary to reduce the intake of proteins, but this has been shown to be false in most cases. In fact, treatment of kidney disease is sometimes a matter of correcting the deficiency of protein in the blood rather than the condition of the kidneys themselves, according to some physicians.

Some association between protein deficiency and peptic ulcers has also been demonstrated. In the treatment of ulcers the need for proteins is increased, and a diet rich in this food element facilitates recovery from this disease when used in conjunction with other measures.

About one gram of protein is needed each day for each 2.2 pounds of body weight. In growing children, pregnant women, and mothers who nurse their babies, as well as in patients recovering from illness, the need for protein is greater.

One of the first symptoms of severe protein deficiency is a swelling of parts of the body. The swelling appears to be strikingly dependent upon body position. It is most apt to be present in the hands and face in the morning and in the legs at night. The swelling is painless and is present on both sides of the body. Pallor, anemia and weakness tend to appear as later symptoms of protein deficiency. Of course, all these signs may be due to many other disorders. It must therefore not be assumed that protein deficiency is at the root of such signs, although the dietary history may be very important in leading the physician to suspect that a protein deficiency may be the cause of such disorders.

Good sources of protein are meat, poultry, fish, nuts, milk, eggs, peanuts, dried yeast, and cereals. Fresh peas and beans contain about 7 to 15 per cent protein. Meats and fish usually range from 10 to 30 per cent in their protein content. Soybean flour is also a good source.

Although many people believe that a diet high in protein will cause high blood pressure, this has not been apparent from medical studies. Experimental and laboratory research on animals, as well as medical observation of humans, indicates that dietary protein is not apt to be the cause of high blood pressure. There has been no general medical acceptance of low protein diets in the treatment of high blood pressure.

Fats

Fats are a more concentrated source of energy than carbohydrates or proteins. One of the values of fats in the diet is that they are apt to contain one or more of the fat-soluble vitamins such as A, D, K and E.

Some authorities believe that fats in the diet are related to the health of the skin, since one of the most characteristic findings from diets deficient in fats, so far as experimental animals are concerned, is a change in the appearance and character of the skin.

Treatment of skin disorders by diets rich in certain fats, however, has not given uniform results. In one study of 120 patients it was found that the condition of the skin improved in about half, whereas in the other half, improvement was either absent or not significant.

Fatty acids from the diet can be changed in the human body to more complex fats, may be deposited as a fat reserve, excreted into the intestines, used in the production of milk fat, or burned in the body to carbon dioxide and water with the liberation of energy.

Plant and animal fats are equally well digested and absorbed. Whole milk, butter, oleomargarine and meat are among the better sources of fat.

The American Medical Association has accepted oleomargarine as being equivalent to butter when vitamins A and D have been added to the former. Studies carried on under the auspices of the American Medical Association showed that fats from either butter or oleomargarine were of comparable quality. Some investigators, however, have maintained that milk and butter contain fat of a superior quality. Nevertheless, there appears to be little basis on which to recommend one in preference to another.

Within recent years it has been discovered that, when the blood levels of cholesterol and associated fatty materials are high, there is a greater incidence of atherosclerosis (hardening of the arteries) and heart disease, with an accompanying decrease in length of life.

Whether dietary fats, especially in regard to foods rich in cholesterol, are a main factor in these disorders *has not yet been fully ascertained.* We do know that some other factor than blood cholesterol alone is involved in the deposition of fat-like materials in the walls of the blood vessels. This other factor has not yet been discovered.

Some nutritionists and food research persons wonder whether the kind of high blood pressure and heart disease described in the preceding paragraph can be prevented or controlled by avoiding foods rich in fats and cholesterol. *This has not been determined for certain,* although some investigators recommended that the diet should be modified toward lower levels of saturated fats. Saturated fats are those that are solid at room temperatures, such as butter and oleomargarine. More research is needed on this problem as well

as on the general relation of fats to human health.

Carbohydrates

Carbohydrates are the indispensable fuel for the body when reduced to simple blood sugar. The tissues are constantly using this substance. Unless the continual need of the body tissues for carbohydrates is met by the eating of proper foodstuffs, fats and proteins in the body will be converted to carbohydrates.

Carbohydrates exert a protective influence on human health in a variety of ways. A liver rich in stored carbohydrate has greater resistance to injurious agents in the body. In other words, the liver is better protected against alcohol, arsenic or any one of a variety of poisons if there is an abundant supply of stored carbohydrate. Apparently the carbohydrate substances combine with many injurious poisons and transform them into harmless substances.

Protein, too, may be very important in protecting the liver against injury and in some cases is superior to carbohydrates.

The functioning of nervous and brain tissues is dependent upon an adequate supply of blood sugar. No other substance can be used.

In infectious hepatitis, a virus disease of the liver, high carbohydrate feeding is a part of the medical treatment. Recovery from this disease appears more rapid and more complete when the diet is rich in carbohydrates.

Although in diabetes the blood sugar rises, this is secondary to a deficiency of insulin. The liver fails in its regulation of blood sugar in diabetes because in the presence of an insufficient amount of insulin the individual cells of the body are unable to utilize the sugar, so that it accumulates in the blood. Liver disease may also interfere with the carbohydrate metabolism of the body, since it is primarily in this organ that carbohydrates are stored in the form of glycogen and made available as blood sugar when body needs are established.

Vitamins

Scientific proof of the relationship of vitamins to human health is so extensive that it is apparent that every part of the body may be influenced by vitamin deficiencies.

Vitamins are related to vision, the health of the liver, health in pregnancy, resistance to infections, color blindness, anemia, mental reactions, endurance, muscular activity, bone growth, health of the teeth, clotting of the blood, fatigue, health of the skin, cellular respiration, the functioning of many glands, and many other body activities and structures.

According to Dr. Thomas E. Machella: ". . . data are available to indicate that vitamins play important roles in many vital processes, including the . . . metabolism of fat, protein and carbohydrate; antibody formation; resistance to infection; detoxication processes; tissue healing; certain aspects of vision; resistance of small blood vessels to rupture; appetite; integration of certain mental and nervous functions; adequacy of hematopoiesis (formation of blood); clotting of blood and maintenance of . . . intercellular substances as well as calcium-phosphorus relationships in bone."

Overdosages of some vitamins may be harmful. Massive doses of vitamin D can produce weakness, exhaustion, nausea, loss of appetite, excessive urination, diarrhea, mental disturbances, and growth and developmental defects of the jaws and teeth.

An overdosage of vitamin A can produce symptoms somewhat similar to those of an underactive thyroid gland. Vitamin A is an antagonist to thyroxin, the hormone produced by the thyroid gland.

In general, however, large quantities of vitamins can be consumed without damage to the human organism. There is much more scientific evidence of vitamin deficiency than of vitamin overdosage, but it

should be kept in mind that either can occur under certain circumstances.

Vitamins differ tremendously in their physical appearance, chemical properties and effects upon the body. Even within the same vitamin complex, the specific vitamins may be vastly different. Thiamine, for example, is a white crystalline substance with a nutlike, salty taste and a yeastlike odor, whereas riboflavin is an orange-yellow, crystalline compound with a yellow-green fluorescence in aqueous solution. This latter vitamin is easily destroyed when exposed to light. Niacin is a white, needle-like substance with a bitter taste. Vitamins A, D, E and K are all oil- or fat-soluble vitamins, whereas many others are soluble in water.

The body can manufacture some of its own vitamins. For example, intestinal bacteria can produce a considerable amount of riboflavin. In one nutritional study with twelve human subjects, from five to six times as much riboflavin was recovered from the intestinal discharges as was present in the food consumed. Somewhere in the body riboflavin was being produced at better than a ratio of 5 to 1 as compared to the quantities of this vitamin present in the food eaten. It was subsequently proved that the vitamin was being synthesized in the intestinal tract by bacteria.

In general, a person should plan to secure the needed vitamins from a well rounded diet. This is important because he will then be more likely to obtain an adequate amount of proteins, carbohydrates, minerals, fats and water as well. He will also be more likely to secure those vitamins that exist in foods and are necessary for good health but have not yet been identified by medical science. On the other hand, if he follows a faulty diet and attempts to replace the missing vitamins with drugstore preparations, he may find in time that his diet has not been adequately corrected, even though some value from the vitamin supplements may be apparent.

There are times when it is advisable to add vitamins to even a well rounded diet. If there has been a previous deficiency, recovery on a well rounded diet will be more rapid if there is a vitamin supplement. After certain illnesses, too, the physician may prescribe vitamins. Some people feel better when they add a small supplement of vitamins to a well rounded diet. The average physician has no objection to this practice, provided the primary sources of food elements come from the diet.

People who engage in severe physical effort may also be advised by their physicians to consume larger amounts of vitamins, especially the vitamin B complex, since experimental research has shown that the need for this group of vitamins is greatly increased by sustained vigorous physical activity.

Vitamins are tremendously significant in human health, but even so, their importance has often been overemphasized in the popular mind. It should never be forgotten that all the other basic food essentials may be just as important as any of the vitamins.

Vitamin deficiencies may develop in a variety of ways. The food that is eaten may be deficient in vitamins, or the body may be unable to absorb vitamins from foods for one reason or another. There may also be excessive excretion of vitamins, such as in the stool or the perspiration. Sometimes there is a greater need for vitamins in the body, so that a deficiency may result merely because the body uses all of the normal supply and needs more.

Vitamins are present in most kinds of foods. Although it is commonly said that fruits and vegetables constitute the main source of vitamins, meat, eggs, milk and almost any kind of food will contain certain vitamins. The whole grain cereals are a major source of the vitamin B complex. Meat may be an excellent source of vitamin B as well as of other vitamins. Fats may contain vitamins A, D, E and K. Only

by a well rounded diet will the vitamin intake be adequate in most cases.

Vitamins are important, but they constitute only one part of a well rounded diet.

Minerals

Minerals are tremendously important to human health. Calcium, phosphorus, iron, sodium, potassium, chlorides, iodine and a number of so-called trace elements such as copper, zinc, fluorine, manganese and cobalt are all essential to human or animal health. Traces of many other minerals have also been found in the body, although the exact function of most of these has not been determined.

Calcium and phosphorus are both related to the health of the bones as well as of other parts of the body. A deficiency of blood calcium, for example, in relation to a disorder of the parathyroid glands can cause the onset of convulsions, especially in infants or small children.

The relation of iron deficiency to anemia, a condition in which the blood is deficient in either quality or quantity of red blood cells, has long been known. Sodium, potassium and chlorides are particularly important in the maintenance of water balance, acid-base balance, the prevention of muscle cramps, and a number of other conditions. An inadequate amount of potassium in the blood plasma causes extreme muscular weakness in the disease known as familial periodic paralysis. These minerals are also important in the prevention of shock because they help to maintain an adequate amount of fluid or plasma within the circulatory system.

It has been known for more than a hundred years that a deficiency of iodine will cause goiter, a disease of the thyroid gland. In some parts of the United States and of certain other countries there is such serious depletion of iodine in the soil that water and plants in these regions do not contain enough of this mineral. In such cases it is necessary to supplement the water and food intake with some form of iodine.

In Colombia, for example, it was once reported that about 50 per cent of the school children in the interior of that nation suffered from goiter. As a result of the observation that the intellectual and physical development of the children was inferior to that of normal children, a national program of iodization of salt was started.

The use of iodized salt in iodine-deficient areas has brought remarkable improvement in the health of the inhabitants of such areas. In Michigan, for example, it led to a decline ranging from 75 to 90 per cent in the number of goiters in different counties in the state.

When iodine deficiency is severe and persists for a long time, the activity of the thyroid gland may become so impaired as to cause more serious disorders such as the disease called myxedema. When the deficiency begins early in life, cretinism may be prevalent among the infants and children affected by an inadequate amount of iodine. In this disease the individual remains a dwarf and suffers from considerable mental deficiency. Growth and development of such a person is seriously impaired through the entire body.

Even in adult life a deficiency of iodine may bring serious consequences. The lack of vitality, overweight, lowered mental activity, and inability to keep warm are some of the signs and symptoms of a reduction in thyroid activity.

Copper is often helpful in the treatment of certain types of anemia. Cobalt is a part of the vitamin B_{12} molecule and therefore has an important relationship to pernicious anemia. In animals a deficiency of cobalt creates disease, but in humans the only clear-cut evidence on the function of this mineral is its association with vitamin B_{12}, which is needed in the treatment of pernicious anemia. Fluorine is present in the bones, and has an important protective effect against dental decay. In animals a deficiency of manganese results in deficiencies in the reproductive process, but

no such association has yet been observed in humans.

Minerals are highly important to human health. In some individual cases it may be more important to restore deficient minerals in the diet than to provide vitamins, proteins or other components of the nutrition which may be fairly adequate.

Water

In an adult slightly more than 70 per cent of the body is composed of water. In a sense, we are still water animals, for the individual tissues and cells of the body are dependent upon water for their very life. Water is a part of the individual cells and the spaces between cells and tissues, as well as of the blood and lymphatic systems.

Water is lost daily in the excretion of both urine and feces, in breathing, and in evaporation from the skin. In hemorrhage, burns and various other disorders there may be extensive loss of water.

If 10 per cent of the body water is lost without replacement, serious signs and symptoms of illness will be produced. It is estimated that a loss of 20 per cent will result in death.

The maximum time that a person can go without any water is about seven to ten days. Infants will live only about half this long.

Water is especially important for carrying sodium, chlorine and potassium in solution. It is the concentration of these salts in the body fluids that controls water balance and the acid-base balance of the body. The blood volume depends upon the amount of water contained in the circulatory system, but the volume may be affected by the shifting of fluids from other parts of the body.

In burns there is a severe loss of water from the oozing of fluid through the injured surface. There is also extensive loss of fluid in diabetes, since urination is greatly increased in this disease.

In any illness in which there is diarrhea there may be serious loss of water from the body. Unless this water is replaced adequately and repeatedly, it may make the difference between life and death. The discovery that water replacement was very important marked a substantial step forward in the treatment of cholera.

In shock, hemorrhage, high fever and many other conditions there may be a substantial disturbance of the water balance or water content of the body. For life and health such losses must be replaced.

The amount of water that a person should drink each day depends on a number of factors. In hot climates where there is excessive sweating, there must be substantial replacement of water and salt. In other environments water needs will be related to the amount of food consumed, for even solid foods contain much water. Still other factors may be involved in the determination of water needs. In general, it is wise to drink several glasses of water daily.

The Antimetabolites

Researchers have found that there are certain substances that resemble, from a chemical standpoint, natural essential compounds in the body such as vitamins, hormones and amino acids. Because antimetabolites so closely resemble needed substances they can cause important nutritional deficiencies, since the body may use the antimetabolites instead of the vitamins or hormones that are needed.

Sulfanilamide, for example, is an antimetabolite for para-aminobenzoic acid, one of the vitamin B complex needed by certain bacteria and all animals and humans. When sulfanilamide is present it may be used instead of the vitamin by the bacteria. This is the reason why sulfa is effective in certain illnesses. The bacteria causing the illness need the vitamin para-aminobenzoic acid but do not get it because of the presence of the sulfa drug which has a close chemical resemblance to the vitamin. Since the bacteria need the vitamin for their growth the effect of the sulfa drug is to disturb the growth pattern of the microscopic organisms and the bacterial infection can be brought under control.

Sulfanilamide does not create a deficiency of para-aminobenzoic acid in higher animals or humans in contrast to its action on some bacteria. The reasons are not fully understood.

The complete role of antimetabolites has not yet been determined, but research has already revealed their significance in human health and nutrition.

Retention of Food Values

The value of foods can be impaired by the manner in which they are preserved or cooked.

Most foods, however, retain their values very well when they are canned, dehydrated or frozen.

In dehydrated foods there is apt to be some loss of minerals, proteins and water-soluble vitamins during the blanching process. In the United States many vegetables are steam-blanched before being dehydrated. Losses of vitamin C and thiamine may be considerable in dehydrated vegetables. Since it is unlikely, however, that dehydrated vegetables will constitute a main part of the diet under ordinary circumstances, this is not apt to cause a serious nutritional impairment.

The dehydration of foods has been mostly a war measure. Under certain circumstances in which men may have to subsist on dehydrated foods for a long time, there might be serious vitamin deficiencies. There have been no cases of food poisoning from dehydrated foods.

The homogenization of fruits, vegetables and cereals is advantageous from the nutritional standpoint because it increases the digestibility of these foods. There appears to be no impairment of the nutritional content of foods when they have been homogenized. The cooking of vegetables in small amounts of water preserves the nutritive content more effectively than when they are cooked in large amounts of water. As might be expected, in large amounts of water there is apt to be a greater loss of water-soluble vitamins and minerals.

In general, fresh vegetables will have a higher vitamin content than stored or frozen ones, although quick-frozen vegetables which have been processed in the field immediately after picking may have a higher vitamin content than foods that are sold fresh, but not delivered to the table until a day or two after they have been taken from the field.

There is high retention of whatever food value is present in foods at the time they are canned or frozen. The heating of foods before canning is a protective feature against such disorders as botulism, but this is apt to cause destruction of certain amounts of vitamin C and nutrients such as thiamine and riboflavin.

Home cooking methods appear to have little effect upon amino acids and proteins. Excessive heat, however, can be expected to lower the nutrient value of any food. Pasteurizing, evaporating, canning or cooking milk has little effect upon the quality of its proteins. The quality of food proteins is seldom impaired by ordinary cooking.

Little difference has been found in the nutritive contents of foods cooked by the radio-frequency heating or electronic cooking methods. Although some slight differences between individual food elements have been found, the general effect is about the same whether the food is cooked by standard methods or by electronic techniques.

The commercial packaging and canning of foods in the United States has been a definite contribution toward better nutrition. The same can be said for quick-frozen foods and most of the other means of presenting foods to the American people. The practical effect has been to bring summer vegetables to the table during the winter and permit the preservation of foods by these methods that might otherwise be wasted because of surplus conditions or low profits.

The Importance of a Good Breakfast

The need for a mid-morning meal or snack decreases if a good breakfast is consumed. Numerous studies have shown this to be the case.

In one investigation with men working on a treadmill, the advantage in the ability to do physical labor went to those who had eaten a breakfast containing both proteins and carbohydrates. In other words, a breakfast containing eggs, milk or bacon in addition to fruits and cereals appeared to maintain the energy levels for a greater length of time than breakfasts without a high protein content. Adequate amounts of cereal proteins assist in the maintenance of energy levels also. It was shown that in about 50 per cent of those who skipped breakfast entirely, there was measurable tremor and weakness, although in the remaining 50 per cent no effects could be observed.

Men in some of the study groups indicated that without breakfast they actually felt weak to the point of illness, whereas other men could observe no difference in their feelings.

It appears that certain persons definitely should not skip breakfast. Even in those who do eat breakfast the staying power is improved if proteins form a part of the breakfast.

Eating Between Meals

Some years ago it was shown that the eating of five meals a day was more beneficial in terms of energy and vitality than eating the traditional three times a day.

In industry, between-meal feedings have become commonplace. When properly controlled so that a great deal of time is not lost, the provision of a mid-morning snack or mid-afternoon feeding has resulted in measurable improvements in work output. In one shoe factory, for example, the provision of a glass of milk and a cracker at 10 o'clock in the morning and 3 o'clock in the afternoon resulted in a 12 per cent increase in the number of shoes produced.

Blood sugar studies have also shown that for many people it is wise to eat between meals. There is a tendency in many people for the blood sugar to fall two to three hours after breakfast. Elevation of this blood sugar by the consumption of food often brings a rapid improvement in vitality.

In some cases mental hygiene may be improved by between-meal feedings. In one nursery school experiment it was observed over a six-month period that a group of children who received mid-morning fruit juices had fewer quarrels, did less crying, were more energetic and more cooperative than a control group of children who did not receive such mid-morning nourishment. When these two groups of children were reversed after a six-month period of observation, the symptoms of irritability, emotional disturbances and other indications of low blood sugar levels were also reversed.

Whatever food is provided between meals should be wholesome and should make a definite contribution to a well rounded diet. The between-meal feedings should not be simple additions to the food intake in terms of quantity. In other words, if a person decides to eat five meals a day instead of three, he should not continue to eat the same quantity of food as he did at each of the three meals. Otherwise, obesity is apt to become a problem.

Foods and Mental Health

When a person goes without food, he is apt to become quite irritable in a matter of hours. Many a mother has discovered that she can reduce quarrels among her children by giving them an early dinner. Adults, too, become irritable as the blood sugar level falls, whereas their personality improves after eating. Some people are more affected than others when food intake is delayed.

Dr. James A. Harrill of Winston-Salem, North Carolina, studied seventy-two patients who had headaches and dizziness, nausea and nervousness, and whose symptoms were relieved shortly after the diet was improved, especially by the addition of proteins. From his studies Dr. Harrill concluded that the symptoms of these patients were related to low blood sugar levels and that supplementary feedings and the addition of protein to the diets of the patients were effective in bringing relief.

Sometimes outright mental illness has been treated by nutritional means. For example, Dr. Tom Spies has reported a case in which an old man was brought into the hospital with a diagnosis of mental illness. Study revealed that the patient's mental disorder was due to dietary deficiency and that he was actually suffering from the end stages of pellagra. Massive injections of vitamin B complex brought about a dramatic clearing of the patient's mind, and continued treatment brought restoration to stability.

Other physicians have reported cases in which patients suffering from fatigue and depression because of inadequate food intake improved dramatically in their mental health with massive doses of vitamins and other food elements. The ultimate correction of such conditions, of course, rests upon the provision of an adequate diet over an extended period of time.

When emotional illnesses are due to dietary deficiencies, they are apt to indicate a general low level of nutrition rather than a specific deficiency of any one food element. There can be little doubt, however, that the level of mental health depends to a considerable extent on the quality of the nutrition.

For example, Dr. Annette C. Washburne has reported a study in which fourteen out of fifteen patients suffering from mental depression showed considerable improvement when they were treated with vitamin B complex. Improvement in the patients was noted within twenty-four to forty-eight hours.

Typical remarks from the patients, according to Dr. Washburne, were as follows:

"I have a sense of well-being. I can think more rapidly and clearly. My sleeping is improved. Life seems more like living."

"I feel fine; I am no longer bothered by the voices."

"I began to feel as though life was worth it. It started quickly. I feel energetic and like going."

Comments of other patients were similar. They indicated, in general, a lightening of depression, improved speed in thinking, increase in and desire for social activity and return of work interests.

Doctor Washburne found no relapses while they received treatment with the vitamin B complex.

Anxiety at the Table

In many families the eating of a meal is often accompanied by emotional distress for one or more members of the family. Some authorities have estimated that about 85 per cent of American children have psychologic problems associated with eating. It should be remembered that the emotional needs of human beings are exactly the same at the table as anywhere else.

Scolding a child for not eating a particular food is psychologically a rejection of the child; the scolding affects his sense of security, denies him acceptance by the group and in a small way impairs his self respect. Forcing a child to eat produces somewhat the same emotional effects. Telling a child what to eat deprives him in a small way of independence and removing

dessert from the table because the child fails to eat other foods is to expose him as a failure before the group.

When anger and emotions centering around the child's eating habits reach a more intense level actual physiologic changes may occur. There may be a reduction of digestive juices; there may be a lessening or cessation of the flow of saliva; there may be disturbances of intestinal function and an outpouring of epinephrine into the blood stream causing disorganization of judgment and other effects.

Studies have shown that when parents make no emotional issue over the child's eating, in time his eating habits will be better than when the parents attempt to control his eating. Knowledge of the nutritive qualities of food and parental desire to have well nourished children may lead to the creation of tension at the table and a poorly nourished child.

In the long run the best nourished child will emerge happy from the table. Parents can better control the nutritional soundness of the diet by putting only wholesome foods on the table and then leaving the child alone in his food selections.

EATING HABITS OF CHILDREN

"...food is to be removed immediately if the child is playing with it, which is unlikely to happen if the helpings are kept at teaspoon size and any extra helpings given on the demand of a child, not the adult."

Dr. Allen P. MacKenzie, 1958

Food Infections

Many epidemics of disease that are spread through foods can be traced to poor sanitation and poor hygiene on the part of food handlers and in methods of handling food.

Many times food epidemics will be due

to poor refrigeration of such food as cream-filled pastries, meats and salads. Especially when food handlers are suffering from some illness such as sore throats, colds, diarrhea or open sores on the body surface, they may cause outbreaks of disease through contamination of foods. If the foods are not refrigerated, there is much greater opportunity for the growth of bacteria once the food has been contaminated.

Some idea of the hazard from food infections can be gained from an analysis of epidemics spread through foods during any single year. In a typical year, outbreaks of disease can be traced to milk, ice cream, poultry, meat, eggs, processed hams, beef, custard-filled pastries (such as eclairs, cream puffs or cream pies), salads, fish, sandwich fillings or spreads, creamed vegetables, shell fish, and a variety of other foods.

FOOD POISONING
". . . food poisoning is frequently associated with acute illness of short duration. When the physician arrives in response to a telephone call, convalescence may be well underway."
                                                Dr. G. M. Dack, 1960

Diseases spread through these foods include staphylococcal food poisoning, typhoid fever, salmonellosis, mastitis, trichinosis, dysentery, diarrhea of the newborn, and other disorders.

Public health authorities have found that the most effective way of reducing disease spread through food is by health education of food handlers. When people understand the importance of sanitation and personal cleanliness in respect to foods and when they are shown how to be careful in the handling of such foods, there is a general tendency toward cooperation with public health authorities. Experience has shown that the educational approach is more effective than the passing of legal requirements in an attempt to force sanitation in the serving of foods.

Pasteurization of Milk

Because milk is such an important part of the average diet in the United States and because this product is an almost ideal substance for the growth of many kinds of bacteria, it is especially important that milk be protected against contamination by microscopic organisms that cause disease.

In addition to the improvement of sanitation in dairies, the pasteurization of milk has helped greatly in reducing epidemics spread through milk and milk products.

During a period of twenty-three years the public health authorities were given an account of 955 epidemics traced to milk and milk products. More than 40,000 people had disease, and 804 died from infections spread through milk in these epidemics. The diseases most frequently involved during this period were typhoid fever, scarlet fever, septic sore throat, dysentery, diphtheria, brucellosis (undulant fever) and paratyphoid fever. The risk of developing a communicable disease from raw milk was approximately fifty times as great as from pasteurized milk.

During recent years most of the larger cities in the United States have adopted laws specifying that only pasteurized milk shall be sold in those cities.

As of today, public health authorities are agreed that diseases spread through milk are not nearly so common as those spread through other foods.

It has often been claimed by adherents of raw milk that the pasteurization process destroys the food qualities of milk. The American Medical Association, however, and other responsible groups have investigated this problem and found that there is virtually no reduction of food values except in the case of thiamine and vitamin C. From 3 to 20 per cent of the thiamine and about 20 per cent of the vitamin C are destroyed by pasteurization. Milk, however, is not a rich source of either of these vitamins; therefore, the moderate loss from pasteurization has no great significance. Foods other than milk must be consumed in order to get adequate amounts of thiamine and vitamin C anyway. The Council on Foods and Nutrition of the American Medical Association has concluded: "It appears obvious that American physicians and health authorities are justified in recommending that all milk be pasteurized."

The pasteurization process itself consists in heating the milk to 143° Fahrenheit for about thirty minutes or to 160° for fifteen seconds. The latter method is known as the flash pasteurization technique.

In conclusion, it can be said that pasteurization of milk gives extensive protection against many of the communicable diseases that can be spread through raw milk and that the food value of the pasteurized milk is practically the same as that of raw milk.

Restaurant Sanitation

At one time it was customary to judge the level of restaurant sanitation by attempting to estimate the actual number of bacteria found on eating utensils. Nowadays the practice is to determine the number of *colonies* of bacteria that can be grown from scrapings or swabs from the dishes being tested. In one study wherein eight soda fountains were investigated, the lowest count on any spoon was found to be 2800 bacteria. An average of 7,000,000 germs apiece was found on beer glasses. High bacterial contamination is still found in many restaurants, soda fountains and bars.

Numerous food epidemics have been traced to public restaurants in past years. Many have also been traced to food served on picnics and at church festivals, military encampments, schools, and other places where food has been served to the public.

Within recent years the widespread use of mechanical dishwashers has made possible a better sterilization of dishes in public restaurants. For example, in New York City a bacteriological survey of slightly more than 1000 restaurants revealed that only 10 per cent of the restaurants in which the dishes were washed by hand met the public health standard of no more than 100 colonies of bacteria per utensil. On the other hand, when dishwashing machines were used, 36 per cent of the restaurants met the sanitary standards.

It can be expected that with more widespread use of automatic dishwashing machines, restaurant sanitation will be improved so far as the cleanliness of eating utensils is concerned.

The problem of the hygienic habits of the food handler remains, however, as a constant challenge to public health authorities. This is primarily a problem of continuing public health education. Excellent results have been achieved in cities like Los Angeles where a sustained effort has been made to educate food handlers in proper restaurant sanitation.

Food Allergies

Some people are allergic to certain foods and should learn to avoid them.

Skin tests for sensitivity to foods are generally not reliable. When there are symptoms that suggest to the physician that the patient may be suffering from a food allergy, the most effective way of identifying the particular food appears to be by means of the elimination diet. In this diet the patient stops eating all but a minimum of one or two foods. Slowly, additional foods are added and the condition of the patient is followed by observation. As symptoms of headache, skin rash, asthma or other reactions develop they can then be related in many cases to the specific food causing the disorder. A further check can be made by eliminating the offending food from the diet and observing whether the symptoms disappear.

In one instance a graduate nurse had

severe headaches for which she was hospitalized twenty-five times in a period of eighteen months. The headaches were associated with dizziness, nausea and vomiting, and great sensitivity of the eyes to light. The head pain was so severe that the patient almost lost consciousness. After extensive study it was found that she was allergic to milk and beef. When these two foods were eliminated from the diet, all headaches disappeared. During an experimental period when she was fed either milk or beef in such a way that she could not recognize either of the two foods, she always had headaches. Strict removal of these foods from the diet always caused improvement. Complete relief of symptoms was obtained when these foods were left out of the diet permanently.

Dr. T. W. Clarke of Utica, New York, has reported the case of a fifteen-year-old boy who suffered from acute inflammation of the brain due to food allergies. When it was found that the boy was allergic to oats and wheat and these were eliminated from his diet, there was a dramatic change in his personality. Previously he had had violent attacks of excitement in which he raged around the house smashing china and furniture. These attacks lasted about thirty minutes and would be followed usually by sleep. After discovery and removal of the foods to which he was shown to be allergic, the boy became friendly, cooperative, happy and well adjusted.

According to Dr. Carl Mauser of Oakland, California, a history of allergic disease during childhood is found in about 50 per cent of the adults who have bronchial asthma. Mauser found that allergic sensitivity to foods in children was of great importance in the subsequent development of this disease.

Some authorities in the field of allergy believe that from 3 to 5 per cent of the general population suffers from various forms of food allergies. The common symptoms of food allergy are blisters on the lips and mouth, swelling of the mouth and throat, canker sores, abdominal dis-

comfort, vomiting, nausea, diarrhea, constipation, intestinal cramps, headache, pain, colic, and itching of the anus. Other symptoms may also be present.

Dr. Albert H. Rowe of Oakland, California, has had patients who had high fevers because of food allergies. One patient was hospitalized for four and one-half months because he was thought to be suffering from some kind of infection. A diagnosis of psychogenic fever was made, but by means of the elimination diet the patient was found to be allergic to milk and some other foods. The removal of the foods brought prompt recovery of the patient.

Dr. Wilfred D. Langley of Pennsylvania has reported the case of a six-year-old boy who was so allergic to carrots that when he received a skin test with a commercial extract of carrot, he went into profound shock. For several minutes it appeared that he might have a fatal reaction to the skin test; however, he recovered within an hour.

Food and Overweight

The problem of the overconsumption of food is discussed in a separate chapter. It should be pointed out here that excessive body weight seriously shortens length of life and increases the prevalence of many diseases such as high blood pressure, arthritis and diabetes.

On the basis of experimental research, Dr. Josef Brozek of the University of Minnesota has recommended that a person should reduce his food intake by 7.5 per cent for every ten years after the age of twenty-five years.

Quackery in Foods

It has been estimated by a district director of the Food and Drug Administration that nutritional quackery costs the American public over five million dollars a year.

The Food and Drug Administration has developed legal cases against many so-called nutritional products which have been claimed as a cure for poliomyelitis, diabetes, heart disease, liver disorders, arthritis, cancer and many other serious illnesses.

According to Gordon R. Wood of the Food and Drug Administration there are currently four primary nutritional myths. These are that: (1) all diseases are caused by faulty diet; (2) soil depletion causes malnutrition; (3) the processing and refining of foods destroy their nutritional values; and (4) every ache, pain, discomfort, and other symptoms of fatigue or illness are caused by vitamin or mineral deficiency.

OUR STAPLE FOODS

". . . the food faddists are spreading the false doctrine that our staple foods are debased and deficient . . . A vigorous campaign of truth about nutrition and diet is needed."

C. W. Crawford,
U. S. Food and Drug Administration, 1951

The Food and Drug Administration does not object to the sale of vitamins and minerals if they are sold honestly and without false claims. Their view is that good health and adequate nutrition can be expected from an ordinary diet that contains fruits, vegetables, meats, fish, eggs, dairy and cereal products.

Food faddists have promoted so-called "miracle" foods such as royal jelly of the queen bee, honey, vitamin E, apple cider and other foods. Medical and nutritional investigations have shown that royal jelly has no practical value for human beings; that honey is a good source of carbohydrates and has a pleasant taste but that it is not a superior food for health; that vitamin E has not been proven to cure heart disease in humans and that apple cider is

not an effective food for the reduction of body weight as has been claimed.

The danger of undue emphasis upon any one particular food is that the diet may actually come to be restricted in nutritional content rather than broadened. The food faddists have been particularly active in emphasizing the health values of certain foods. Many of the so-called health food stores have emphasized the values of certain high-priced foods or the importance of including certain foods in the diet.

FOOD SUPPLEMENTS

". . . if a healthy individual's diet contains the key food groups in sufficient amounts, nutritional supplement is unnecessary."

American Medical Association News,
July 27, 1959

For example, it has often been claimed that blackstrap molasses is a highly superior food that should be included in the human diet. The determination of the vitamin content of blackstrap molasses, however, has shown that of eight of the B complex vitamins only inositol is present in sufficient quantity to make an appreciable contribution to the human diet when compared with other recognized protective foods. After an analysis of 100 samples of blackstrap molasses, a representative of the American Medical Association stated, "Despite the fact that molasses does contain a variety of minerals and vitamins, there is no justification for giving it major recognition as a protective or health food."

Considerable attention has also been given to yami-yogurt. This substance is a fermented milk in which the fat of the milk remains unchanged, but the milk sugar is converted largely into lactic acid or alcohol. The most widely known fermented milk is buttermilk.

Yami-yogurt is an acidophilus milk which is created by fermentation of milk with a culture of the *Lactobacillus aci-*

dophilis organisms. Yami-yogurt is actually a good milk product, but is sold at a price roughly four times that of whole milk. Nothing is added to or taken out of whole milk in the fermentation process; hence yami-yogurt is simply a high-priced milk. It is a good food, but plain milk provides exactly the same nutritional elements.

FOOD FADDISTS

"Food faddists are generally mal-nourished people who eventually suffer from a surprising number of illnesses, age relatively rapidly, and die relatively young."

Frederick Swartz, M.D., 1956

In general, it can be said that there are no health foods. In other words, all staple foods are healthful unless there is some reason to think otherwise, such as an individual allergic reaction to the food. The best guarantee of an adequate diet is a broad intake of staple foods. There is no need for concentrating on any single food. This is especially so when the price of that food has been elevated beyond its significance, as is often the case with so-called health foods.

The Daily Food Guide

There is such a great variety of food available for purchase and consumption that it is almost impossible for any average person to know the specific values of each in terms of various minerals, vitamins, carbohydrates, fats and amino acids.

The calculation of calories from food intake is a difficult process which involves the use of tables of food values and calculations that many people are not prepared to carry out.

Because simple means of judging the adequacy of a person's diet is needed, the daily food guide, or "Essential Four," has been approved by the National Research Council, the National Dairy Council, the American Medical Association, and other groups interested in nutrition. This guide is a simple check list by which an individual can judge whether he is eating a well rounded diet. If an adult uses this guide as a measuring tool for the selection of foods day in and day out, he is almost certain to secure a reasonably well balanced diet. For a person to use this guide it is not necessary that he know the details of vitamins, minerals, amino acids, fats or carbohydrates. The guide provides a balanced selection of different food groups which are almost certain to contain the needed food elements.

The daily food guide, or "Essential Four," is reproduced in the accompanying table in a simplified form.

1. *MILK GROUP:* Four or more servings daily.
2. *MEAT GROUP:* Two or more servings daily.
3. *VEGETABLE–FRUIT GROUP:* Four or more servings daily.
4. *BREAD–CEREAL GROUP:* Four or more servings daily.

Food Additives

In 1958 a food additive amendment was included in the Food, Drug and Cosmetic Act which has given the Food and Drug Administration greater control over the use in foods of chemicals that may be injurious to human health.

Food and chemical manufacturers must now conduct extensive feeding tests on animals before any chemicals can be added to foods that are sold on the market. The results of these tests must be given to the Food and Drug Administration and if the officials of that agency are convinced that the product is safe the manufacturer will then be permitted to market his product. The law also applies to irradiation of foods. Anything that causes cancer in animals or humans is specifically forbidden by the new law. The use of pesticides and coal tar colors in foods had previously been prohibited by law. The new law covers such things as nutrient supplements, sweets (such as saccharin), preservatives, emulsifiers, thickeners, acids, alkalis, buffers, neutralizing agents, flavoring agents and bleaching agents.

In 1959 the Food and Drug Administration prohibited the marketing of certain shipments of cranberries containing the chemical aminotriazole, an effective weed killer suspected of having the ability to cause cancer. The Food and Drug Administration had denied the manufacturer permission to market this weed killer for use in cranberry bogs. The laboratory examination of some cranberries showed that several thousand pounds were contaminated with aminotriazole. This led to the application of the food additives law to control the balance of these contaminated cranberries. Since that episode the use of this substance in cranberry bogs has been discontinued. Some of the food producers have voluntarily withdrawn their products from the market because of the food additives law of 1958.

Questions

1. Why is it that most children dislike certain foods?
2. Does the generation of tension from forcing children to eat outweigh the advantages of a good diet from the nutritional viewpoint?
3. Is there a psychologic basis for overweight?
4. Is international famine a likely outcome of what some authorities call world over-population?
5. What is a "health" food?
6. What are the hazards of food additives?

For Further Reading

1. Byrd, Oliver E.: *Nutrition Sourcebook*. Stanford, California, Stanford University Press, 1955.
2. Bogert, L. Jean: *Nutrition and Physical Fitness*. 7th ed. Philadelphia, W. B. Saunders Company, 1960.
3. Cooper, Lenna F., Barber, Edith, Mitchell, Helen S., and Rynbergen, Henderika J.: *Nutrition in Health and Disease*. Philadelphia, J. B. Lippincott Company, 1958.
4. Dack, G. M.: *Food Poisoning*. Chicago, University of Chicago Press, 1956.
5. Food and Drug Administration: *What Consumers Should Know About Food Additives*. Washington, D.C., Superintendent of Documents, 1960.
6. Keys, Ancel, and Keys, Margaret: *Eat Well and Stay Well*. New York, Doubleday and Company, 1959.
7. McHenry, E. W.: *Foods Without Fads. A Common Sense Guide to Nutrition*. Philadelphia, J. B. Lippincott Company, 1960.
8. Wilson, Eva D., Fisher, Katherine H., and Fuqua, Mary E.: *Principles of Nutrition*. New York, John Wiley, 1959.

For Advanced Reading

1. Burton, Benjamin T.: *The Heinz Handbook of Nutrition*. New York, Blakiston-McGraw-Hill Book Company, 1959.
2. Davidson, Stanley, Meiklejohn, A. P., and Passmore, R.: *Human Nutrition and Dietetics*. Baltimore, Williams and Wilkins, 1959.
3. Wohl, Michael G., and Goodhart, Robert S.: *Modern Nutrition in Health and Disease*. Philadelphia, Lea & Febiger, 1960.

7

OVERWEIGHT AND UNDERWEIGHT

ONE IN EVERY four women and one in every five men is at least 10 per cent overweight by the age of 20.

The foregoing information is based upon data obtained from the most important study ever made in this country on the prevalence of obesity. During 1959 the Society of Actuaries published the results of a *Build and Blood Pressure Study* that covered the experience of several million people. The table on page 78, which is based upon this study, gives more complete results in terms of both obesity and underweight for men and women in the United States and Canada.

Obesity is an individual problem in terms of the basic cause and in respect to the degree of overweight.

In medical history there are accounts of some twenty persons who weighed over 700 pounds. Smith Poti, who died in South

Africa in 1942, weighed 756 pounds. His waistline measured 6 feet, 8 inches. For a human equator, that is impressive. Mrs. Ruth Pontico of Tampa, Florida, was even fatter. Just before her death in 1941 she weighed over 800 pounds. But she was not the fattest person on record.

SURPLUS FAT

"The worst enemy of health today is surplus fat. Obesity aggravates cardiovascular degeneration, diabetes, biliary and renal ailments, arthritis and many other disorders, and increases surgical risks and accident proneness. An educational campaign is needed. . . ."

Dr. Martin G. Goldner, 1958.

In 1857 a man in Tennessee named Miles Darden weighed a little over 1000 pounds at his death.

These are extreme examples. Nevertheless, each of us has good reason to think seriously about his weight. A surplus of flesh has much to do with health and length of life.

Causes of Overweight

Many people believe that the chief cause of obesity is overeating. This is an oversimplification. Overeating is not a cause, it is the means to obesity.

Probably the two commonest causes of overeating in childhood are habit overeating and emotional overeating.

The eating patterns of a family often establish a social environment in which the child finds it difficult to avoid overeating. In many families mothers and fathers may actually force food on a child, even though he may already have exceeded his normal physiologic needs in the food he has already consumed. Studies of fat children have shown that nearly three-fourths of all fat children have one or both parents who are also fat. Once the habit of heavy eating has been established by the child it may be very difficult to break.

Emotional overeating results from a de-
sire for the satisfactions and securities that food may bring to a person. Lonely, unhappy, frustrated, bored and rejected children often turn to food. In many adults who are overweight the basic problem is not one of overeating but of finding the psychologic problems that cause the overeating.

There are other causes of obesity. Heredity is an important factor. Studies show that three out of four fat people have a family history of overweight. People with such heredity must take special pains to eat only what they need and not what they crave. It's not easy to follow such a rule, but it is wise.

Some people believe that becoming fat is due to some disturbance in the functioning of body glands. This may be true, but only to a small extent. One study of 275 obese patients revealed that less than 3 per cent of them had a glandular disorder. Admittedly, glandular deviation can cause a person to put on weight, to gain girth like a snowball rolling downhill. And when a person does gain many pounds in a very short time, his doctor will suspect glandular imbalance, one of the potential causes. But otherwise, it is the rare cause of obesity which can be blamed upon the endocrine glands.

Even rarer are cases in which a brain disorder has caused overweight. Researchers have found instances in which a disturbance in that part of the brain known as the hypothalamus has resulted in a person putting on excessive weight. This is very unusual.

Occupation may be a factor. Overweight is an occupational hazard of cooks, nutritionists and food handlers, who often overeat merely because they cannot resist temptation.

Consequences of Being Overweight

Life insurance companies have made extensive studies on the dangers of overweight. Dublin's analysis of the influence

FREQUENCY OF OVERWEIGHT AND UNDERWEIGHT

Age (Years)	Proportion of Insured Lives with Weights Deviating by Specified Degree Above and Below Average and "Best Weight"							
	MEN				*WOMEN*			
	Per Cent Deviating from Average Weight							
	Overweight			Under-weight	Overweight			Under-weight
	10% or More	10-19%	20% or More	10% or More	10% or More	10-19%	20% or More	10% or More
20-29	21	14	7	23	21	11	10	29
30-39	19	13	6	24	25	13	12	35
40-49	21	16	5	22	27	15	12	31
50-59	21	16	5	21	26	15	11	30
60-69	21	15	6	20	27	18	9	31
	Per Cent Deviating from "Best" Weight							
	Above "Best"			Below "Best"	Above "Best"			Below "Best"
	10% or More	10-19%	20% or More	10% or More	10% or More	10-19%	20% or More	10% or More
20-29	31	19	12	13	23	11	12	22
30-39	53	28	25	6	41	16	25	13
40-49	60	28	32	4	59	19	40	6
50-59	63	29	34	4	67	21	46	4
60-69	57	28	29	5	68	23	45	4

Note: The deviations from average weight are taken from the *Build and Blood Pressure Study, 1959*, Society of Actuaries. The data on deviations from "best" weight, derived primarily from that study, have been prepared by the Metropolitan Life Insurance Company, January, 1960.

of body weight on nearly 200,000 established that extra weight reduces the life span from 25 to 75 per cent. By eating unwisely you can cut your life expectancy down considerably.

Life insurance statistics show clearly that overweight shortens life. Obesity increases the death rate, over and above the normal expectancy, by the percentages shown in the table on page 79.

Excessive weight which is well distrib-uted over the body is the least harmful kind of fat in respect to length of life. The most harmful kind of overweight is the potbelly type.

When the abdominal girth is more than 2 inches greater than that of the chest at full expansion, an *extra* mortality (still greater reduction in length of life) of about 50 per cent is found *in addition to the decrease in life expectancy from already being overweight*.

Degree of Overweight	Increase in Death Rate
15–24 per cent overweight	30 per cent
25–34 per cent overweight	45 per cent
35 per cent overweight or more	60 per cent

The fat person, far more than the person of average weight, is subject to heart disease, high blood pressure, varicose veins, flat feet, diabetes, arthritis, hernias, gout, gallstones, gallbladder disease and accidents. Persons who weigh 15 to 20 pounds below the average have a longer life expectancy.

HEART DISEASE. Fat people have more than their share of heart disease. The fat person's heart has to work harder than the lean person's. After all, a person who carries 50 pounds of fat on his body at all times is doing extra work just as surely as the man who carries a 50-pound sack of sand on his back. The man carrying the sand bag can dump it on the ground and sit down to take a short rest if he feels so disposed; the fat person, however, can't slough off his burden of extra weight, so his heart has to keep on pumping blood through all that surplus flesh. The fat man's heart gets less rest.

Increase in body fat also causes an increase in body surface. This requires a great expansion of the circulatory system. Veins, arteries and capillaries must fan out in an ever-increasing system of distribution to supply the added surface area. Inescapably, this growth in the number of small blood vessels imposes a greater work load on the heart. More effort is required to pump the blood.

Sometimes fat may accumulate in the connective tissue beneath the membrane which encloses the heart. This fatty deposit may become so extensive that the heart is encased in fat, which may penetrate between the fibers of the heart muscles. When this occurs, the operation of the heart is mechanically handicapped.

Dr. Smith and Dr. Williams, of Minnesota, studied the hearts of 136 obese patients at autopsy, and concluded that in 7 per cent of the cases the accumulation of fat in the heart was the basic cause of heart failure.

The mortality from coronary heart disease and other degenerative heart conditions among overweight men is more than 1½ times that of men of average weight.

DIABETES. Fat people are at a disadvantage in the prevention of diabetes, a hereditary disease. Not all people with a diabetic ancestry have diabetes. It's possible for such people, mostly by proper diet, to keep the disease from developing, or to delay its onset. If the heredity for diabetes is present, overweight is more likely to bring on the disorder than any other factor. The death rate for diabetes, among those who are 25 per cent or more overweight, is eight times as high as among average-weight persons, and thirteen times as high as among persons who are underweight.

FLAT FEET. Fat people have a greater load on their feet. It is not surprising, therefore, to find that overweight persons have more foot trouble than do leaner people. Fat people are more prone than underweight people to have flat feet.

ARTHRITIS. Similarly, the knees, hips and ankle joints of fat people have heavier burdens to manipulate than do the joints of people of normal weight and consequently suffer from overstrain and breakdown. Fat people have more arthritis than do lean people, partly because of the greater wear and tear on the joint structures.

HERNIA. As fat accumulates in and on the abdomen, the abdominal pressure is increased. If there are weaknesses in the abdominal wall, extra strain may be sufficient to cause a portion of intestine to jut through a weak spot in the abdominal wall. Hernias, therefore, occur more frequently

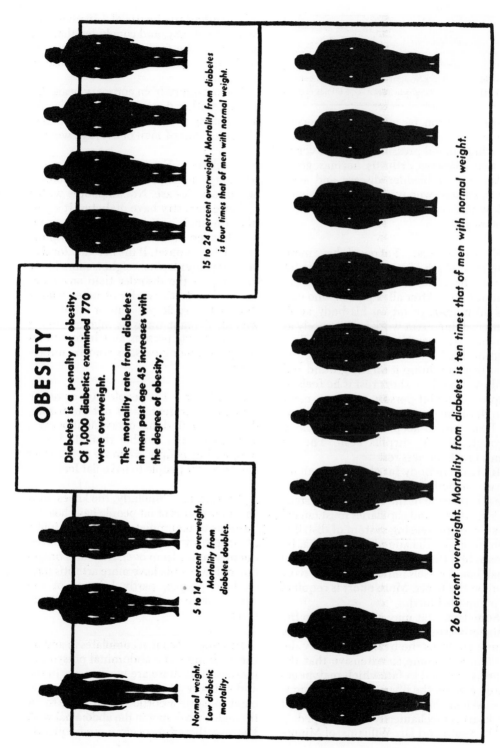

Figure 2. There is a distinct relationship between obesity and death from diabetes. (Courtesy of Eli Lilly and Co.)

among fat people than among average-weight people.

HIGH BLOOD PRESSURE. It is dramatic proof of the danger of overweight that such an affliction as high blood pressure is often relieved merely by the loss of weight.

High blood pressure is more than twice as common among obese men as among average-weight men. The blood pressure tends to go up as fat accumulates. The result is that the fat man's heart often has this extra burden of pumping a stream of blood against a head of pressure at all times. This is like forcing a stream of liquid uphill; it's hard work, it's added hard work for a straining heart. The danger is even more increased when that pressure exists in weakened blood vessels. The deposition of fatty materials in the walls of the blood vessels may weaken these structures. And when they've been weakened, and the pressure against them increases, there is danger that they will rupture and bring on early ill health or death.

PSYCHOLOGIC PROBLEMS. Obesity may *cause* psychologic problems or it may be a consequence of them.

There are two main forms of emotional obesity. Reactive obesity is a condition that usually begins in middle age because of some distressing emotional experience such as the death of a loved one, homesickness, illness or the breaking up of a love affair. The unhappy person turns to food as a comforting reaction to the emotional situation. Often the individual does not recognize that his overeating represents a psychologic reaction to his emotional distress.

Developmental obesity involves the whole personality and often starts in childhood. Overeating is a consequence of insecurity, loneliness, tension and anxiety, defeat and neglect. The person who develops this kind of obesity is apt to give up social contacts and to retire more and more from the company of other people into the psychologic satisfactions of eating.

Psychosomatic problems may also result from overeating and obesity. The young fat person may feel self-conscious, inferior, socially inadequate, ashamed and even unable to participate in many activities of young adults. In such cases excessive body weight may bring about profound changes in the future of a young person.

Obesity Means Shortened Life Span

It is a sad irony that in war time, in countries where the food supply has been limited, there have been surprisingly sharp reductions in deaths from diabetes and from other chronic diseases associated with overweight. The fact is that overweight is often a guarantee of a curtailed life span.

Obesity, especially if it is of considerable degree, strains practically all the vital functions of the body and speeds up the degenerative disorders. The majority of deaths in adult life are caused by chronic diseases of the heart, kidneys and blood vessels—and the mortality rate steps up with the degree of overweight. The fat person will have such diseases earlier than the lean person, and die sooner. The death rate from chronic nephritis, for instance, is 1¾ times as high for overweight men as for average-weight men. Even the death rate from appendicitis is increased by obesity. Childbirth is more risky for stout women than for average-weight women. Almost any operation is made more hazardous by excess flesh; the fat person is, therefore, a poorer surgical risk.

Overweight is so common that it constitutes a national health problem of the first order. Mostly, overweight comes from overeating. And to point up the risks of overeating, it is of interest to repeat the following incident from a Reuter's dispatch of December 4, 1946.

In Bayonne, three men contested for the title of Biggest Eater. They sat down to a meal consisting of an enormous steak, a rabbit, and ten pounds of beans. Shortly after leaving the table, one of the contestants collapsed and died. A second was hospitalized with paralysis. And the third man suffered a heart attack.

How to Reduce Wisely and Well

A primary problem in reducing is to discover the cause of overeating. Unless the cause is alleviated or corrected it is unlikely that reducing efforts will be successful. *An overweight person must try to find out why he is overeating.* He must make changes or adjustments in relation to the cause. Only then is it likely that he will be able to correct his eating habits.

Some people will need the counsel and advice of experts in finding out the cause of their overeating. It may even be wise to consult a good psychiatrist, if the obesity is great enough and the fat person is oblivious to the cause of his overeating. The problem should be discussed with the family physician in terms of causes of overeating.

A second problem in reducing wisely is to lose weight safely and consistently until a desirable weight level is reached.

A case was reported of a woman weighing 479½ pounds who lost 300 of those excessive pounds. She lost it *safely*, because the process was under the guidance of a physician and required a full eighteen months. This time element must be stressed. It is dangerous to lose weight too rapidly. If you set about reducing more than a few pounds, do it under the care of a doctor.

There are a few musts to be observed when starting a program of weight reduction. First of all, discuss it with your physician, and have an immediate physical check-up and arrange for regular check-ups on your progress. Your rate of loss of weight should be slow and steady. Not more than 1 or 2 pounds a week. It is necessary for the heart to receive nourish-

ment; if emaciated, it loses ability to do its necessary work. This is especially true if the heart has some defect before the reducing program is started.

Fasting

Undereating is not fasting. Going without food is a risky business, as is illustrated by a recent case in Birmingham, Alabama. A man weighing 357 pounds attempted to complete a planned 100-day fast. Newspaper reports implied that the man had gone ninety-two days without food, though this is unlikely. At any rate, he lost 112 pounds in ninety-two days—but on the ninety-third day he lapsed into unconsciousness and died. He lost too much in too short a time.

Some physicians do advocate fasting for one whole day as a means of starting a reducing program. This is because the obese person not only gets a good start in reducing his calories, but he also gets psychologic satisfaction in going without food for a day. His success represents a self-discipline that strengthens his resolution at the outset.

Fasting, if attempted, should be under the guidance of a physician. It is not advisable for people suffering from such disorders as tuberculosis, mental illness or heart disease.

Exercise and Reducing

Many people believe that one of the best ways to reduce weight is to *work* it off by exercise. *This is partly wrong.*

Arthur Steinhaus, one of the leading physiologists in the United States, used metabolic tests before, during and after exercise as a basis for calculating the amount of exercise necessary to bring about a loss of 1 pound of fat in a man of 155 pounds. Dr. Steinhaus found that a person of this weight would have to walk 144 miles to lose 1 pound, or would have to run 129 separate hundred-yard dashes, in ten seconds each, if he desired to lose this solitary pound by sprinting. You'd have to work just as long and hard doing other types of physical activity to lose that pound of flesh.

CREEPING OBESITY

"The creeping type of obesity occurs when physical activity is reduced. We have shown that, in experimental animals as in human subjects, when activity is reduced below a certain level, the appetite cannot diminish accordingly."

Jean Mayer, Ph.D., D.Sc., 1958

Despite the foregoing comments about the necessity of a considerable amount of exercise being needed for successful reduction of body weight, it is agreed that physical activity does have a role in weight reduction. A greater amount of energy is expended during vigorous or moderate physical activity than in more sedentary states. If good judgment is used in the intensity of exercise, so that undesirable stress is not placed upon a heart that is already overburdened with fat, and the major emphasis is still upon the decrease of food intake, physical activity may make a worthwhile contribution to weight loss. *The important thing to remember is that you have to eat less to weigh less.*

But, it may be objected, you absolutely *do* lose weight when you go out and sweat yourself dizzy in some vigorous physical effort. It is true that there is a rapid loss of weight from sweating, an appreciable loss, too; but it is a temporary loss of water, not a true loss in weight. Those pounds are quickly regained when you drink so thirstily after all that effort. In a few days your weight is back where it was.

A sensible combination of exercise and diet finding favor with some physicians is that of planning to reduce the food intake by about 250 calories per day and then doing enough exercise to burn up another 250 calories per day. On this schedule of losing about 500 calories a day the average person can lose about one pound of body weight per week.

Dr. Jean Mayer believes that the majority of adolescents do not overeat, but that they get surplus calories from an extraordinary inactivity. For the adolescent or young adult physical exercise can be an important part of any reducing program.

Massage Not Helpful

Massage is mistakenly believed to be an effective method of removing fat from localized areas of the body. Again, the facts are otherwise. Years ago Carl Rosenthal showed experimentally with animals that vigorous massage produces no change in fatty tissue. It may help muscle tone; it may produce some degree of relaxation; it may be pleasurable to have the circulation stimulated by the masseur's deft pummeling; but loss of weight—no. There is no breakdown of fat and no dissolving of fat by this technique.

But sometimes people who pay a masseur for a course of treatments *do* lose weight; do they not? Again, true. But it is not the physical mauling which reduces the weight; it is not the massage which remolds a bulging silhouette nearer to the heart's desire. What happens is that most masseurs, in addition to thumping the adipose tissue of their patients, also put them on a diet. It's the diet that works wonders.

Drugs and Reducing

To reduce weight by taking drugs without medical guidance is a risky procedure. The American Medical Association, through its Council on Pharmacy and Chemistry, has frequently warned the public against the dangers of using drugs to make the body lose excess flesh. Drugs for this purpose should never be used except under the supervision of a physician who carefully watches the patient's reactions to the prescription.

A few years ago, dinitrophenol was hailed as a miracle drug for reducing.

Dinitrophenol steps up the body metabolism, and, in a sense, burns off the excess fat by added chemical activity inside the tissues. There is no doubt that dinitrophenol is effective for reducing weight. However, soon after dinitrophenol had come into use, numerous reports of complications caused by it began to appear in medical literature. Some patients lost their eyesight, and others their lives, before the drug was withdrawn as unsafe for weight reducing purposes.

Hormones, laxatives and stimulants of various kinds are frequently contained in "shotgun" remedies advertised by commercial organizations for use in the treatment of obesity. Some of these have been highly injurious to health and are not safe for indiscriminate use by anyone desiring to lose weight.

The status of the use of drugs in weight reduction was summarized by Dr. Walter Modell, on July 9, 1960, in a report to the Council on Drugs of the American Medical Association. In this report it was said that "... There is really nothing new on the scene ... there are no useful depressants of the appetite. ... Total therapy must consider the psychosocial aspects of eating patterns and the desire to lose weight, as well as the specific psychological or physiological disturbances. ... Insofar as drugs are concerned, at the very best, their potential is secondary to the elimination of the cause. ... Drugs which give assistance along the lines now available provide short-lived symptomatic relief only. These seem to be useful only as adjuvants to a carefully controlled diet and, in many cases, some sort of psychotherapy."

Group Approach to Weight Control

In the last few years much interest has been shown in the group approach to weight control. This method of reducing is based upon a crude, but often effective, form of psychotherapy.

As the plan now operates, sponsorship of the local medical society, public health department or other responsible social agency is obtained for group meetings of persons who are willing to come together for the purpose of reducing their body weight.

At the meetings, which are conducted under the guidance of an effective leader, there is plenty of opportunity for free discussion of the problems of overweight. Applicants are admitted to the group if they have medical approval, have a desire to lose body weight, and can arrange their time so as to be able to attend the meetings.

Scales are available, and those in attendance are expected to keep a record of their weight and to participate in the discussions, the purposes of which are to give opportunities for talking about problems and reaching decisions regarding them.

In Louisville, Kentucky, a weight-control project of this sort brought about an average weight loss of about 5 pounds during the first three weeks of the group meetings. Ninety-six per cent of those in attendance lost weight in significant amounts in the early stages of the project. Attendance records were discouraging, however, and only about one fourth of the group were still attending after twenty-six weeks. In this tenacious group 79 per cent had lost weight to a significant degree. In other words, those who stay with the plan are apt to get good results.

In the Louisville experiment 99 per cent of the people who came to such meetings were women. Separate groups for men and women who are overweight may be a partial or complete answer to this problem. The group plan for reducing may help many, but it will not resolve the problem of overweight for all.

Special Diets

Many people think they have to go on some special diet to reduce body weight. This is not so. In most instances the person who wishes to reduce can do so effectively by *reducing the quantity of all the foods he customarily eats.*

A reducing diet should be well rounded, with correct proportions of carbohydrates, proteins and fats, and rich in vitamins and minerals. Every item of your ordinary diet may be included, even potatoes and bread, just so the total quantity is diminished. In fact, if properly balanced, your reducing diet need not be supplemented with vitamin preparations, although this is usually advisable when dieting is extended over a long period.

Sometimes publicity is given in the popular press to a special diet that has been advocated by a particular hospital or physician. The so-called Rockefeller diet is an example. This low-protein, liquid diet is not the only one used at the hospital of the Rockefeller Institute. Although many other diets are used at this hospital, the Rockefeller diet was the only one that received such publicity. The diet was administered under medical supervision, which does not suggest that hospital authorities were recommending the diet for the general public in their weight-reducing efforts.

In commenting on the liquid, low-protein reducing diet, Dr. Norman Jolliffe, Director of the Bureau of Nutrition, Department of Health, New York City, made this remark: "Fortunately, few people will adhere to . . . these diets for long, so no great harm will be done other than to deplete the . . . protein stores that the body in its wisdom has devised to protect us foolish mortals. But there are compulsive dieters, just as there are compulsive drinkers and smokers and eaters, and in these subjects harm can be anticipated that neither the resources of the publishers nor the ingenuity of the research scientists can always correct. The unqualified recommendation of these diets to the public is a disservice to science and to those it serves, the public."

The Council on Foods and Nutrition of the American Medical Association has pointed out repeatedly that obesity is a medical problem that should be handled by a physician and that he must recommend abnormal diets only after careful investigation. For the average person this means that you should not submit yourself to special diets unless your physician so recommends. A reduction in total food intake is safer and much more pleasant.

OBESITY AND SELF-CONTROL

"In following the development of a large group of obese children into adulthood, an embarrassing contrast between the amount of medical and dietary treatment and the later adjustment became apparent . . . A favorable outcome . . . was achieved by those who had the least amount of medical attention, no endocrine injections, and no enforcement of dietary restrictions. These patients had established control over their weight during adolescence, or in early adult life, on their own initiative, with a constructive goal and without outside compulsion."

Dr. Hilde Bruch, 1958

Most Favorable Weight and Age Relationships

Not all men of the same height should be expected to weigh the same, for there can be wide differences among such men in body structure and heredity. Some six-footers are narrow of shoulder and long of legs, while others have massive shoulders, barrel-like chests, and legs short in relation to the torso. These variations are allowed for in a general sense in the accompanying table, which provides a range of "ideal" weights at each inch of height for three types of frame: small, medium and large.

The table does not differentiate as to age, but applies to all men over twenty-five years. Tables commonly used in the past were based upon average weights, and showed a progressive increase with succeeding years.

Women are more apt than men to be concerned about weight. Not for reasons of health, however, so much as for looks.

To wear clothes well, a shapely figure is necessary.

Ordinary tables of *average* weights for women show considerable increase with age. Short women between the ages of thirty and fifty show a general increase of 13 to 14 pounds, more than 10 per cent. Tall women show an average increase of 15 or more pounds. This augmentation of girth is not beneficial to either health or appearance. *Average* weights are not *ideal* weights.

The Problem of Underweight

Two factors are especially significant in underweight. The first pertains to *heredity and family structure* and the second to the relation between the current degree of underweight and *what has been normal* for the individual.

Some people must reconcile themselves to the fact that they can expect no great success in exceeding the heredity and body structure characteristic of their own families. If you come from a lean, small-boned family, regardless of whether most of your relatives are short or tall, you may find it very difficult to attain average weights based upon the general population. If this fits your situation, be realistic about it. What you cannot change, you must accept, whether you do it willingly or grudgingly.

Underweight that is normal for a person is actually a strong protective factor against diabetes, heart disease, high blood pressure, arthritis, foot disorders and many other diseases, especially those of a type characteristic in old age. The underweight person can expect to live a longer life, provided his slight figure is normal for him.

When heredity or family characteristics are not responsible for underweight, the condition may be due to undernourishment or to some handicap of digestion, or to illness.

Both mental and physical illness may cause a loss of appetite, sometimes over an extended period of time. Obviously such a loss of the desire to eat will bring about a reduction in body weight.

Tuberculosis, severe inflammation of the stomach, disease of the liver, strong emotional disturbances and mental illness, ulcerative colitis (inflammation and ulceration of the intestinal tract) and many other diseases may cause loss of body weight. An overactive thyroid gland may cause underweight because of the high level of chemical activity in the body, which means greater consumption of energy in the individual cells. Persons suffering from such complaints may be eating large quantities of food, but may be unable to gain weight.

Underweight due to illness is, of course, a medical problem. Only when the underlying disease is cured can the person expect to gain weight. A person who drops *well below his normal weight* should consult a physician for a careful medical appraisal of his health and should then follow the advice he gets. Only in such a manner can a swift and reasonable cure be expected.

When underweight is due solely to a lack of sufficient food, in terms of either quantity or quality, undernourishment is the problem that must be faced.

A weight loss of approximately 10 per cent *below your normal weight* due to a deficiency of food intake does not represent serious deterioration. Such a loss indicates slight undernutrition which can be corrected usually by a prompt restoration of an adequate diet.

When a person is from 10 to 20 per cent *under his own normal weight* a moderate degree of undernourishment is involved, provided food deficiency is the only cause. Fatigue is apt to be characteristic of this level of malnutrition, but the person affected can still perform light or moderate work.

When a person is 20 to 30 per cent *below his own normal weight,* he is in a state of severe undernutrition and is liable to

DESIRABLE WEIGHTS FOR MEN AND WOMEN
According to Height and Frame. Ages 25 and Over

Height (in Shoes)	Weight in Pounds (In Indoor Clothing)		
	Small Frame	Medium Frame	Large Frame
	Men		
5' 2"....................	112–120	118–129	126–141
3"....................	115–123	121–133	129–144
4"....................	118–126	124–136	132–148
5"....................	121–129	127–139	135–152
6"....................	124–133	130–143	138–156
7"....................	128–137	134–147	142–161
8"....................	132–141	138–152	147–166
9"....................	136–145	142–156	151–170
10"....................	140–150	146–160	155–174
11"....................	144–154	150–165	159–179
6' 0"....................	148–158	154–170	164–184
1"....................	152–162	158–175	168–189
2"....................	156–167	162–180	173–194
3"....................	160–171	167–185	178–199
4"....................	164–175	172–190	182–204
	Women		
4' 10"....................	92– 98	96–107	104–119
11"....................	94–101	98–110	106–122
5' 0"....................	96–104	101–113	109–125
1"....................	99–107	104–116	112–128
2"....................	102–110	107–119	115–131
3"....................	105–113	110–122	118–134
4"....................	108–116	113–126	121–138
5"....................	111–119	116–130	125–142
6"....................	114–123	120–135	129–146
7"....................	118–127	124–139	133–150
8"....................	122–131	128–143	137–154
9"....................	126–135	132–147	141–158
10"....................	130–140	136–151	145–163
11"....................	134–144	140–155	149–168
6' 0"....................	138–148	144–159	153–173

Note: Prepared by the Metropolitan Life Insurance Company. Derived primarily from data of the *Build and Blood Pressure Study, 1959*, Society of Actuaries.

have a greatly reduced resistance to many illnesses, such as malaria, skin diseases, dysentery and other disorders. He is also likely to be showing signs of vitamin deficiencies, protein starvation, mineral deficiencies, visual disturbances and other conditions. A person in this degree of undernourishment can seldom do more than very light work.

A weight loss of more than 30 per cent *below a person's own normal weight* reflects a condition of extreme undernutrition. This person is ill and unable to do useful work. All the signs and symptoms of illness present in lesser degrees of malnutrition can be found with greater exaggeration at this level of deficiency.

When food deficiency is so great as to cause a loss in body weight of 50 to 60 per cent *below a person's normal weight,* death is apt to result.

Treatment for underweight must rest upon its cause. No treatment is needed or advised when weight is normal in terms of the heredity and body structure of a particular family. If disease is involved, medical diagnosis and treatment for the underlying cause are essential before any gain in body weight can be expected. When lack of sufficient food is the cause of underweight, a better program of feeding is needed. This may be brought about by educational methods, improvement in economic conditions of the family, individual determination or by other measures, depending upon the circumstances.

Questions

1. How can an overweight person develop psychologic strength to reduce food consumption, without the use of drugs?
2. Why should an overweight person not depend on exercise alone as a means to weight reduction?

3. Why is it unnecessary to follow any special diet in reducing?
4. Should the pleasures of eating be denied the overweight person when overeating may be a result of boredom and lack of psychologic satisfactions?
5. What are the psychologic disadvantages of being underweight?

For Further Reading

1. Bruch, Hilde: *The Importance of Overweight.* New York, W. W. Norton, 1956.
2. Gelvin, E. Philip: *Obesity: Its Cause, Classification and Care.* New York, Paul B. Hoeber, Inc., 1957.
3. Jolliffe, Norman: *Reduce and Stay Reduced.* New York, Simon and Schuster, 1957.
4. McHenry, E. W.: *Foods Without Fads. A Commonsense Guide to Nutrition.* Philadelphia, J. B. Lippincott Company, 1960.

For Advanced Reading

1. Society of Actuaries. *Build and Blood Pressure Study.* Chicago, 1959.
2. Wohl, Michael G., and Goodhart, Robert S.: *Modern Nutrition in Health and Disease.* Philadelphia, Lea & Febiger, 1960.

8

COFFEE, TEA AND COLA DRINKS

COFFEE is a mild stimulant, so is tea, cocoa and the myriad cola drinks. Coffee contains caffeine. So do tea and cocoa, but these beverages also contain theophylline and theobromine, respectively.

These drugs, called xanthines (pronounced zan-thines), are stimulants of different parts of the body. They differ only in the *intensity*, not in the *kind*, of their effects in stepping up the action of the nervous system, kidneys, muscles, heart and respiration.

More people drink coffee than tea, cocoa or cokes. More people, therefore, consume caffeine than the other xanthines, but the action of this whole group of drugs is fundamentally the same. A cup of coffee contains about 100 to 150 milligrams of caffeine. A cup of strong tea contains just about as much. Some people have nervous systems which are more irritated by caffeine than others. Children are definitely more sensitive to caffeine than adults and most physicians would suggest that the child should not drink coffee. The average person, to get a "lift," must consume 150 to 250 milligrams of caffeine: 1 to 2 cups of coffee or tea. Some persons, however, get a strong reaction from even one cup of coffee.

Caffeine is not harmful in the sense that it may impair growth or shorten the life span, for it does not have these effects. Theoretically caffeine *could* kill you, if you took enough of it. For fatal effect, you'd have to drink 150 to 200 cups of coffee in a short time. Such drinking has never been reported. Nevertheless, excessive amounts of coffee or tea can have uncomfortable effects upon you, depending on your personality and physiology.

It is not uncommon for some people to drink as many as 20 to 30 cups of coffee a day. When this much coffee is consumed there are possibilities that health may be impaired. A point to consider is whether the person uses sugar and cream in each cup of coffee. A person drinking this much coffee will consume from four to seven quarts of water daily which may create certain problems in itself. Finally, there is the question of the effects of the caffeine contained in this much coffee.

Perhaps the primary effect of the consumption of a great deal of coffee in which sugar is taken is that of dental decay and obesity. Heavy consumption of sugar in any form may be expected to cause obesity and bad teeth. The almost continuous presence of sugar in the mouth would create an oral condition highly favorable to dental decay. From 20 to 60 teaspoons of sugar daily would also constitute a definite problem for weight control.

The fat contained in cream might be of sufficient quantity in 20 to 30 cups of coffee daily to create a hazard, not only in terms of body weight, but also in terms of the health of the cardiovascular system. Research has shown that in certain persons atherosclerosis may be a genuine problem due to the deposition of certain fatty materials in the walls of the heart and blood vessels.

The consumption of large amounts of water, such as are contained in 20 to 30 cups of coffee, would create a health problem in any person suffering from certain disorders, such as high blood pressure, epilepsy, certain forms of heart disease and other conditions. In any health disorder in which a difficulty already exists in the elimination of fluids the consumption of large amounts of coffee would aggravate the water clearance problem.

The consumption of large amounts of caffeine might well produce over-stimulation of the nervous system as well as other systems of the body. A person suffering from ulcers should not drink much coffee, for the reason that caffeine stimulates the production of acid in the stomach to an even greater extent than alcohol. Apparently this stimulating effect is achieved by a direct effect upon certain acid-producing cells in the walls of the stomach.

Some persons are definitely over-stimulated by caffeine to a point where sleep is disturbed, despite contrary opinions held by many people. The likely explanation as to why some people are not stimulated by caffeine to a point where sleep is disturbed lies in individual differences.

Too much caffeine may bring on some sensory disturbance, such as ringing of the ears, and may even cause muscles to be tense and trembling. Too much caffeine may disturb digestion and cause excessive urination, may increase your breathing rate and accelerate your heart rhythm. Also, drinking too much coffee can do real harm in that by satisfying your hunger before you have eaten enough wholesome food, it may work to keep you undernourished. Some people should either abstain entirely from coffee and tea, or restrict themselves to very moderate amounts.

Tense people, suffering from "nervousness," should not increase their irritability by caffeine. Children and adolescents should not drink coffee. People suffering from peptic ulcers may sharpen their pain by drinking coffee, for it increases the hydrochloric acid in their digestive systems. People with thyroid disease may find that the stimulation of caffeine will increase their jittery discomfort. Coffee is considered bad for some forms of heart disease. People who are allergic to some of the ingredients of coffee invite rashes, swellings and illness by drinking it.

One of the advantages of coffee is that it seems to relieve morning or afternoon fatigue. Some people even think that it alleviates their aches and pains. Since caffeine is not a pain-relieving drug its stimulating effects are probably the reason why a person feels better after drinking a cup of coffee. Caffeine does stimulate the central nervous system and this would be likely to stimulate physical movement as well as mental alertness. Such movement might result in better circulation to the muscles and produce relief from muscle stiffness and aching. Perhaps, however, the whole feeling of better health might be psychologic and associated with stimulation of the central nervous system. Such a reaction might mask a state of physiologic fatigue rather than make any real contribution to its elimination. It is far better to seek the cause of fatigue than to disguise it by drinking coffee.

On a hot day, a cola drink is refreshing. Momentarily, it quenches thirst and provides an injection of fresh energy, which is not surprising, considering that some cola drinks contain from 4 to 9 teaspoonsful of sugar. If such quantities of sugar are not appropriate to your diet, it's good sense to avoid such drinks.

Most children delight in cola drinks. However, a sweet drink may spoil appetite to such an extent that youngsters may then refuse to drink milk or eat other wholesome food which is necessary to their health.

Just as important is the effect of concentrated sweets upon dental health. Research has shown that overconsumption of sugars is a primary cause of dental decay. This will be discussed more fully in another chapter.

So far as the drug effects of coffee, tea, cocoa and various soft drinks are concerned, the average healthy adult can drink them in moderation without fear of serious consequences. The effects of caffeine and the other xanthines depend upon the individual level of health. Some people should not drink caffeine-containing beverages, but there is no scientific evidence that coffee will shorten life, impair the growth, induce a nervous breakdown or otherwise be injurious to the average person in reasonably good health. In moderation, coffee drinking can be a pleasant and sociable experience. If coffee appears to disturb you in any way, leave it alone until you consult your medical adviser as to whether you should give it up entirely or moderate your drinking. Most likely he will advise you to use moderation in your coffee consumption unless he finds a real reason for recommending abandonment of the habit.

Questions

1. Would the prohibition of soft drink sales on a school campus make a significant contribution to the solution of the problem of undesirable "snacks" between meals?

2. How can a parent who drinks coffee justify refusal to approve the same drink for children in the family?

3. Does the "coffee break" found widely in industry make a significant contribution to the relief of fatigue?

4. Should the sale of highly sweetened soft drinks be legally prohibited because of their harmful effects on dental health?

5. Does coffee make a contribution to the diet?

9

DENTAL HEALTH AND FLUORIDATION

THE CONTROL of dental decay is passing from the individual effort of the dentist with each single patient to a mass effort at prevention by public health authorities.

Fluoridation of community water supplies is becoming the most important single factor in the prevention of dental decay that has ever been found. Despite this, the individual himself can and should do a great deal toward the care of his own teeth and supporting mouth structures.

To protect himself against dental decay and to give community support to fluoridation of public water supplies, the individual needs to be well informed on dental health matters.

By the beginning of 1960 approximately 1850 communities in the United States, including more than thirty-six million persons, were fluoridating their water supplies. An additional seven million people

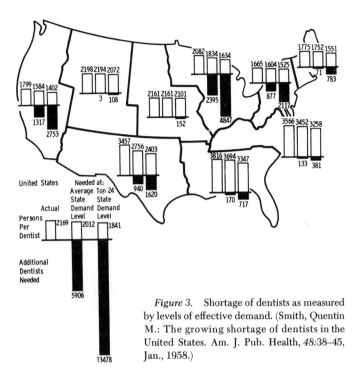

Figure 3. Shortage of dentists as measured by levels of effective demand. (Smith, Quentin M.: The growing shortage of dentists in the United States. Am. J. Pub. Health, 48:38–45, Jan., 1958.)

were living in communities in which there was a natural fluoride content at the approximate recommended level. Thus, a total of more than 43 million people in the United States are drinking fluoridated water. No community has had to discontinue fluoridation because of health reasons; striking evidence of the truth of medical and public health statements that fluoridation of public water supplies is completely safe.

The effectiveness of fluoridation in reducing dental decay will be discussed later in the chapter, as will other aspects of this problem.

Causes of Dental Decay

Scientific research has established that in the great majority of cases tooth decay results from the production of acids in the mouth by bacteria. It is the acid that attacks and destroys the surface of the tooth. When acid-forming bacteria in the mouth have access to sugars, they promptly begin to manufacture acids from those sugars. As soon as the acids are produced they begin at once to destroy the tooth structure.

When a person keeps the foregoing process in mind he can discover many ways to protect the teeth against dental decay. Some of these methods will be discussed in the following sections.

Mouth Bacteria

Various kinds of bacteria may be found normally in the human mouth. Some of these bacteria may produce alkaline substances, but the majority are apt to produce acids.

The microscopic organism which has been proved to be primarily responsible for dental decay is the *Lactobacillus acidophilus.*

A clear-cut relationship has been found between the number of organisms of this type in the mouth and the extent of dental decay found in the same mouth. Studies at the University of California and the University of Michigan have shown that when samples of saliva are collected, incubated under standard conditions, and then studied in respect to the number of colonies of acid-forming bacteria present, if there are under 2000 colonies per cubic centimeter of saliva, very little dental decay will be found. If the *Lactobacillus acidophilus* is found in colonies ranging from 2000 to 10,000 per cubic centimeter of saliva, then moderate dental decay will exist. On the other hand, it has been shown that if more than 10,000 colonies of this acid-forming organism are found per cubic centimeter of saliva, then extensive dental decay will be present.

It ought to be obvious that if the acid-forming bacteria in the mouth can be reduced in numbers, there will be a smaller production of acid and therefore less dental decay even if the diet remains high in sugars.

There are several ways in which the acid-forming bacteria can be reduced.

In one study three investigators examined the effects of thirteen different dentifrices in reducing the number of acid-forming bacteria in the mouth. Of all the tooth pastes and powders used, it was found that powder containing 0.07 per cent penicillin was most effective in cutting down on the lactobacilli found in the saliva. With this substance a decrease of approximately 90 per cent in lactobacillus counts was obtained. Streptomycin and tyrothricin were the next most effective substances. Each of these antibiotics achieved a reduction of slightly more than 50 per cent in lactobacillus counts. The use of antibiotics in tooth pastes is not generally recommended, however, because of the possibility of sensitizing the user to such drugs or for the reason that antibiotic-resistant strains of lactobacilli might be developed. It was also found that ordinary tooth paste, when used consistently, brought about a decrease of about 20 per cent.

Some investigators have attempted to cultivate an alkali-producing colony of bacteria in the mouth. These protect the teeth through the release of ammonia in the saliva. This greatly reduces the number of acid-forming bacteria and also acts to neutralize the acids produced by these organisms.

From the foregoing it does appear possible to change the type of bacterial growth found in the normal mouth. Undoubtedly research will in time suggest even more effective ways of cutting down on the number of colonies of acid-forming bacteria.

Sugars and Dental Decay

Some dentists estimate that if sugars were completely eliminated from the diet, better than 90 per cent of all dental decay would be arrested. Others do not feel quite this optimistic, but most agree that cavities could be reduced by at least 50 per cent or more if sugars were greatly reduced or eliminated from the diet.

It has been proved that sugars are the substances which the acid-forming bacteria use to make acids. For example, two dentists took freshly extracted teeth that had no dental decay and subjected them to various studies to measure the effects of different substances in promoting cavities. They obtained saliva from 100 persons without dental decay and from 100 persons who had from ten to twenty actively decaying teeth. The freshly extracted teeth were thoroughly cleaned and sterilized and then broken into small parts. These tooth fragments were weighed and placed in separate bottles containing the "susceptible" and 'immune" salivas. The tooth particles were removed and weighed twice weekly for three months. The loss of weight of the tooth structure under these experimental conditions was taken as representing a loss comparable to that of active dental decay.

Various substances were added to the

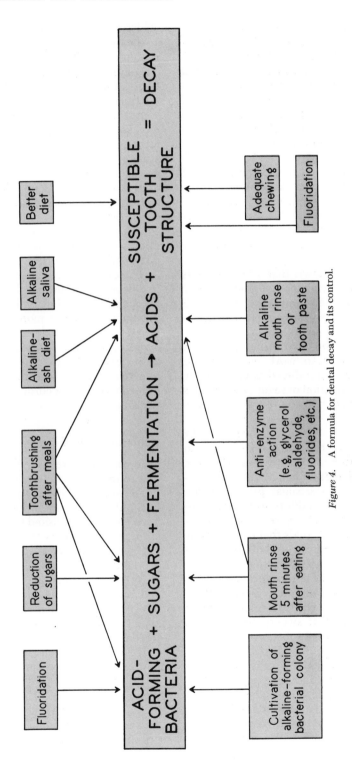

Figure 4. A formula for dental decay and its control.

saliva such as sugar, penicillin and other drugs and products. Of all the substances tested, the greatest loss of tooth structure occurred in the "susceptible" saliva when *5 per cent sugar* was added. In the presence of this sugar, nearly 31 per cent of the tooth structure was lost in twenty-one days. The saliva containing penicillin showed less solvent action that any other substance.

It was also found that certain types of yeast contributed to the chemical processes involved in dental decay and that the *Lactobacillus acidophilus* was the type of organism most prominent in the decay, especially when sugars were added to the saliva.

It was also shown that when sugar is placed in a decaying tooth, the acidity may rise within three minutes to a point high enough to cause damage to the tooth structure. If no sugars are present in the mouth, then the acid-forming bacteria have very little to work with and the amount of acid produced is exceedingly small. The reduction of sugar intake is thus a very effective way to prevent dental decay.

Rinsing out the mouth with water promptly after the eating of sweets can make a significant contribution to the health of the teeth. Such a rinse would remove much of the sugar present in the mouth, and would dilute some of the remaining sugars. The rinse would also remove some of the acids that have already been produced and would dilute some of the remaining acids. Rinsing the mouth promptly after the consumption of sugars is thus very good mouth hygiene. If done consistently and within a minute or two after the eating of sweets, this practice should make a very substantial contribution to the reduction of dental decay.

Dr. L. S. Fosdick of Northwestern University Dental School has suggested that glycerol aldehyde should be added to sugar in order to stop dental decay. Fosdick points out that this chemical substance acts to check the fermentation which causes acid to be formed from sugar in the mouth. Glycerol aldehyde acts as an enzyme inhibitor to retard fermentation. The substance itself is harmless to human beings and is a natural constituent of muscle tissue.

In the dietary treatment of dental decay, sugar should be eliminated entirely, although saccharin may be used as a substitute for sugar. Saccharin has greater sweetening power than sugar, but is not used as a source for the production of acids by acid-forming bacteria, nor does it promote their growth in the mouth. One-fourth grain has the sweetening value of about one teaspoonful of sugar, but does not supply any calories.

The control of sugar in the diet results in a decrease in the lactobacillus count of the mouth. Once the number of acid-forming bacteria in the mouth has been decreased it is again safe to consume carbohydrates and sugar at one meal a day. Such a diet can be followed for six months to two years without any increase in the lactobacillus count, according to some investigators.

Acids and Dental Decay

It was suggested as long ago as 1887 that tooth decay was due to the formation of lactic acid in the mouth as a result of carbohydrate fermentation. It has since been clearly established that the *Lactobacillus acidophilus* is the microscopic organism commonly responsible for acid production and dental decay.

By 1915 it had been shown that in general the saliva of people who were relatively immune to dental decay was more alkaline than the saliva of people who suffered from dental cavities.

It has further been established that the flow of saliva has a connection with dental decay. The more rapid the flow, the less the decay, whereas the slower the flow of saliva, the higher the rate of dental decay. This relationship can be explained on the grounds that the fast-flowing saliva has a rinsing action and a diluting action. If the saliva is on the alkaline side in addition, then a still greater protection against dental decay prevails.

In people who have a high degree of dental decay, acid formation from sugar in saliva is extremely rapid. Enzymes from the saliva or from the tissue itself appear to play an important role in the speed with which acids are produced.

Numerous acids cause dental decay. Citric acid appears to be especially damaging to tooth structure. In one experiment when teeth were deposited in citric acid, the dental structure was dissolved to an extent of about 80 per cent in five days.

Many of the hard candies are made with citric acid. Research conducted at the College of Dentistry of New York University has shown that these hard candies, when put in solution, will actually dissolve tooth enamel. Studies made by the United States Public Health Service have shown that citric, phosphoric, lactic, acetic, benzoic, tartaric, oxalic and carbonic acids will all dissolve teeth. They rank in damaging effect in the order named. Lactic acid, third on the list, is produced in the mouth by acid-forming bacteria.

Some foods that are high in acid content can cause damage to the tooth structure, according to other studies made by the United States Public Health Service.

Two scientists in New York City conducted studies in which they measured the acidity or alkalinity of the tooth surface by the use of electrodes. It was found that rinsing the mouth with water or ordinary dentifrices did not affect the surface pH (acidity or alkalinity) of the tooth. On the other hand, a mouth rinse with a solution containing 3 per cent urea and 5 per cent diammonium phosphate caused a temporary elevation of the pH on the tooth surface (making it more alkaline) for about one hour. When a mouth wash containing 13 per cent urea and 3 per cent diammonium phosphate was used, the surface of the tooth was profoundly alkalinized (maintained at a high pH) for more

than two hours. The importance of this research is that it gives scientific evidence that it is possible to reduce or eliminate the acidity on the surface of the tooth. By alkalinization of the tooth surface it should be obvious that the process of dental decay would be stopped or delayed.

This research is consistent with experimental studies in which children have been divided into different groups for the measurement of the effects of ammoniated dentifrices.

In one large study a reduction of 17 to 20 per cent in dental decay was achieved when an ammoniated dentifrice was used in the brushing of the teeth. This study also showed that brushing with an ordinary tooth paste or tooth powder helped to prevent dental decay, but that protection was greater with the ammoniated compound.

In Glasgow, Scotland, the chief dental officer conducted a two-year study in which he found that the use of an ammoniated dentifrice gave a protection twice as great as that obtained from the use of ordinary dentifrices.

Both on theoretical grounds and on the basis of actual experimentation it does appear that alkalinization by one means or another can help to prevent dental decay.

Diet is also important in this respect. The acid-neutralizing power of the saliva can be changed by a diet that produces an alkaline ash. In a number of cases the control of dental decay by this method alone has been successful.

Elimination or destruction of the enzyme system involved in the formation of acids can also be accomplished by certain substances known as enzyme poisons. Some authorities state that fluorine may act in this manner to protect against dental decay as well as by entering into the actual structure of the tooth and making it more resistant to the action of acids. It must also be emphasized that the elimination of sugars will cut down on the amount of acids produced. This has been discussed in the previous section.

The Value of Fluorides

It was observed some years ago that people in certain parts of the United States had a very low incidence of dental decay. It was also observed that when fluorides were present in the drinking water of an area in high enough concentration, people in that area suffered from mottled enamel. Dental decay in such teeth, however, was definitely below that of the average.

It was not long before scientific studies pointed to the conclusion that fluorides in the water supply had a protective influence against dental decay. It was established that when fluorides are present in amounts of about one part per million parts of water, there will be no blackening or mottling of the teeth, but there will be less dental decay. In general, if no more than 3 parts of fluoride per million parts of water are present in the community water supply, there will be no ordinarily discernible discoloration of the enamel.

In Aurora, Illinois, fluorides in the public water supply resulted in about 95 per cent less dental decay on the surfaces of certain teeth. About six times as many children in Aurora were found to be completely free of dental decay as in most other communities.

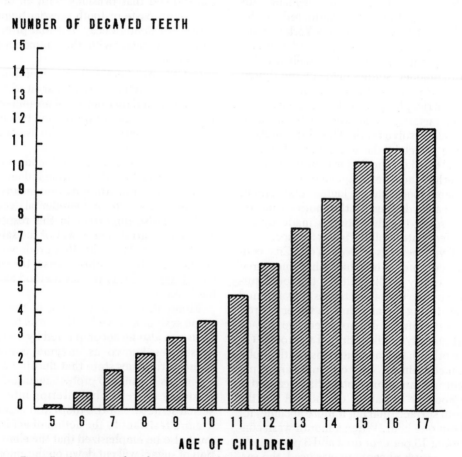

NUMBER OF DECAYED TEETH

AGE OF CHILDREN

Figure 5. Average number of permanent teeth per child affected by decay in nonfluoride California cities. (Richards, Lloyd F., and Loretz, Wayne: Dental caries survey of school children in nonfluoride cities in California. California's Health, *16*:41–43, Sept. 15, 1958.)

In Minnesota early research soon established the fact that children to whose teeth sodium fluoride was applied had much less dental decay than children to whom this protection was not accorded.

In Michigan, as in other states, studies were made of the dental conditions in children brought up in communities in which the water naturally contained fluorine in contrast to other communities where no fluorine was present. It was found in one investigation conducted by the Michigan Department of Health that children in nonfluoride areas had an average of nearly six decayed, missing and filled permanent teeth compared to an average of only two such teeth in the children who lived in the areas where fluorine was naturally present in the drinking water. It was also found that only 13 per cent of the children who lived in nonfluoride areas had no dental cavities whatsoever, but that 39 per cent of the children who lived in fluoride areas had no decayed, missing or filled teeth.

In other Minnesota studies it was shown that the application of a 2 per cent solution of sodium fluoride to children's teeth brought about a definite reduction in dental decay. It was found that the number of treatments with sodium fluoride was directly related to the results obtained. When one application was made, only 5 per cent less dental decay was found, but when two treatments were made, there was a reduction of nearly 15 per cent. When three treatments were given, there was 21 per cent less dental decay in the permanent teeth and 40 per cent less in the deciduous teeth. It was concluded that from four to seven treatments would probably give best results.

In Wisconsin a dental study was made of the school children in Green Bay and Sheboygan. In Green Bay 2.3 parts of fluorine were found to be naturally present in one million parts of water in the public drinking supply. In Sheboygan, on the other hand, only 0.05 part of fluorine was present. In the community with fluorine in the water 30 per cent of nearly 2000 school children had no dental decay whatsoever, whereas in Sheboygan, where there was virtually no fluorine in the water, only 3 per cent of nearly 2000 students had no dental decay.

By 1948 the New York State Department of Health had come out in support of the use of sodium fluoride solutions to reduce decay in the teeth of children. The Department had taken this view after careful and exhaustive study by its Dental Bureau of the research on this subject and after consultation with the authorities of the Public Health Service and others. By this time it had been found that swabbing a child's teeth with a solution of sodium fluoride would reduce dental decay by at least 40 per cent.

In Connecticut, Dr. Basil G. Bibby released a report in which he showed a reduction of 47 per cent in dental decay in a group of adults of an average age of twenty-five years. This group had received four treatments of sodium fluoride. It appears from this that fluorides have values in reducing dental decay in both children and adults.

Milwaukee, Wisconsin, is another of the many communities that have now reported on the value of fluoridation in the reduction of dental decay. It was reported in March, 1960, that the percentage of children *with no dental decay whatsoever in their six-year molars* in this community had doubled, rising from approximately 20 per cent to nearly 40 per cent after fluoridation had been in operation for six years. There was approximately a 60 per cent improvement in dental health in the seven year old children during this period as compared to data from pre-fluoridation years. This improvement in dental health was achieved at a cost of approximately five cents per person over the six-year period.

In the last few years attention of public health authorities has shifted from the swabbing of teeth with a 2 per cent solution of sodium fluoride to the addition of fluorides to the public drinking supply.

Studies have shown a consistent reduction of around 60 per cent or more in dental decay when proper proportions of a fluoride are added to community water supplies.

Fluoridation Safe

There has been some opposition to this procedure on the part of uninformed but possibly conscientious persons on the grounds that fluorine is a poisonous substance and therefore injurious to health. It should be noted that the American Medical Association as well as the United States Public Health Service and the American Public Health Association have all gone on record as saying that when fluorides are added to the water in the proper concentration of one part fluoride to one million parts of water, the effects are beneficial rather than harmful. Not one single case of poisoning from this use of fluorides has been reported, although millions of people are now obtaining their water supply from fluoridated community sources.

A ten-year study of the health of the people in Bartlett and Cameron, Texas, has helped to give scientific proof that fluorides in the drinking water are not harmful. These two towns are quite different in the fluoride content of their water supplies. Bartlett has a natural fluoride content of approximately 8 parts per million. This is eight times the recommended allowance for the prevention of dental decay. Cameron, on the other hand, has a water supply that contains only 0.4 part of fluoride per million parts of water.

A medical and dental team of scientists made a careful health appraisal of 116 persons in Bartlett and of 121 persons in Cameron. Ten years later the same group was studied by medical history, physical and dental examinations, x-rays, blood and urine analyses and other means. Except for some discoloration of the teeth, there were no significant differences in the two groups in respect to heart disease, blood pressure, arthritis, thyroid disease, dis-

orders of the eye, hearing, tumors, cysts, bones and bone fractures, white blood cell counts or general death rates. Absolutely no harmful effects of the fluoride in the drinking water could be found so far as the general health of the persons in these two communities was concerned.

San Francisco was one of the first cities in the United States to adopt fluoridation of the community water supply. Fluoridation of a part of the city was begun in 1952 and total fluoridation was started in 1955. On May 23, 1960, the Department of Public Health reported that throughout all of the fluoridation years not a single doctor or dentist had reported any indications that the health of any person had been damaged by the process in San Francisco.

The California Conference of Local Health Officers in 1959 reaffirmed its endorsement of fluoridation "without any reservations" as a safe and effective way to reduce dental decay.

In another investigation of possible effects on human health, the death rates for five diseases (heart disorders, cancer, brain hemorrhage, kidney disease and cirrhosis of the liver) in 32 cities with fluoridated water supplies were compared with those of 32 cities without fluorides. No significant differences could be found in death rates from these diseases in the two groups of cities.

It should also be pointed out in answer to criticisms of fluoridated water that there are many other areas in the United States where fluorine appears in the water supplies naturally. Millions of people have grown up in these areas without any evidence of toxic effects from the fluorides.

Health and Science Groups Approve Fluoridation

Because of widespread misrepresentation of the attitude of the American Medical Association on fluoridation, that organization was moved, in June, 1955, to make the following statement: "The unscrupulous opponents of fluoridation have spread the impression that the American Medical Association did not endorse this public health measure. The fact is that it did, and that it stands by its endorsement. ... Both the American Medical Association Council on Pharmacy and Chemistry and the American Medical Association Council on Foods and Nutrition expressed themselves definitely to the effect that fluoridation is safe."

By 1955 court rulings in favor of fluoridation had been made in eleven different states and by the United States Supreme Court. There is absolutely no doubt that fluoridation is both legal and safe. Its value in the prevention of dental decay has already been made clear.

Resistance to fluoridation in some communities by poorly informed persons has led the American Public Health Association to stress the value of health education in overcoming this opposition.

On October 21, 1959, the American Public Health Association took the following action:

"RESOLVED, That the American Public Health Association vigorously support and recommend the adjustment of the fluoride content of water supplies as a progressive health measure, and BE IT FURTHER RESOLVED, That the American Public Health Association urge all health authorities to give high priority to public education on water fluoridation . . ."

The Opposition

Efforts to improve the dental health of the national population by fluoridation have met with intensive resistance from certain minority groups. Some communities have been battlegrounds for those who favor and those who oppose fluoridation. Often the vote of the people in a community for or against fluoridation reflects an emotional bias rather than an understanding of the scientific effects of this procedure on human health.

Several years ago John A. Hutchison reported a sociological investigation of a community conflict on fluoridation that illustrates the intensity of emotions that may be involved. In a small New England college town it was voted at the town meeting, on the recommendation of two local dentists, that fluoridation of the public water supply should be started.

Opposition started with letters to the local newspaper in which the charge was made that fluoridation was dangerous and that it was being recommended because of an evil alliance of misguided doctors and companies selling fluoridation equipment and supplies. Another said fluorides were rat poison and predicted the whole town could be silently exterminated by the enemy. Still others made the assertion that fluoridation was a communist plot.

People in the community who were known to oppose pasteurization of milk, compulsory smallpox vaccination and chlorination of water took up the battle against fluoridation. Meetings were held at which scientists, dentists, physicians and public health authorities gave the facts on fluoridation. The opposition claimed the doctors were agents of certain sinister powers and that dentists were promised a share of profits from the sale of fluoridation equipment and supplies.

The opposition heckled and filibustered the meetings where well qualified scientists were asked to speak in favor of fluoridation. One opponent said her ancestors had fought the Indians in the area and it was now time to fight with equal vigor against fluoridation. People who had spoken in favor of fluoridation were called "stinker" and "communist" on the main street of the town.

An antifluoridation association charged that illegal votes had been cast and the whole process was illegal. Petitions were circulated for a special meeting against fluoridation. The main speaker was advertised as a senior dental consultant at a well known nearby hospital. It turned out he was not a member of the hospital staff. A special election was held amid dramatic charges that fluoridation would produce a generation of degenerate and crippled pig-mies. Although six of the seven local doc-tors favored fluoridation and a local col-lege professor pleaded for the triumph of reason over emotion, the public vote de-feated fluoridation.

Fluoridation of Individual Water Supplies

It is estimated that about 40 per cent of our population does not live in towns or communities where the public water sup-ply can be fluoridated.

Although these persons can have fluo-rides applied directly to the teeth by re-questing this service from their dentists, the cost is much greater than it would be if these persons could obtain fluoridated water. The reduction in dental decay amounts to about 40 per cent in contrast to about a 65 per cent result from fluo-ridated water.

Bottled fluoridated water is available in many areas, but in a rural area the cost would be high and problems of delivery would be great.

The adding of fluoride pills to the water supply of individual homes can also be done, but again the cost is relatively high and there is often a failure to add the pills to the water.

Franz J. Maier has reported the produc-tion of a small device that can be installed for the fluoridation of home water supply in an individual home. He estimates that a home system for fluoridating the water supply can be achieved at a cost of about thirty-six dollars a year. This fluoridation unit has been produced by the U. S. Pub-lic Health Service.

Fluoridated Tooth Paste

In 1960 the American Dental Associa-tion broke precedent by recommending the use of a tooth paste containing fluo-ride. After careful examination of the re-search on the results of the use of this product, the national organization of den-tists concluded that the use of a fluo-ridated tooth paste can make a substantial contribution to the reduction of dental de-cay when it is used over a period of time.

Diseases of the Supporting Structures

The prevention of dental decay is not the sole means of preserving the teeth in good condition. Sometimes neglect of the supporting tissues of the teeth, such as the gums and bones of the jaw, may result in the serious loss of teeth, even though the latter may not be defective. Any infection of the mouth should be promptly treated.

Some disorders are more characteristic than others so far as health of the oral tis-sues is concerned. Two examples of this are the disease known as trench mouth, or Vincent's angina, and periodontitis, more commonly known as pyorrhea. To neglect either of these two diseases is to invite serious impairment of the dental health.

Trench Mouth (Vincent's Angina)

In this disease the gums are swollen, spongy and inflamed. If the disease has ad-vanced far enough, the gums may exude a thick, yellow pus which has a foul odor. There may be ulceration of the gums and growth of a thick, grayish membrane.

The disease may spread to the tonsils, throat, bronchial tubes, and lungs. Gan-grene may occur from the disorder in the lungs and bronchial tubes. In this dead tis-sue large numbers of spirochetes and fusi-form bacilli may be found when such tis-sues are examined under the microscope.

These two microorganisms are involved in the production of the disease. Ordinar-ily the body has an extremely high resist-ance to them, and they are found in the mouths of over 80 per cent of all adults even though the persons are in good health. Apparently it is the poor nutritional status of the gums and nearby tissues of the mouth that permits the organisms to become more virulent or more invasive.

Although many cases of Vincent's angina of the mouth have been completely cured with niacin, the modern treatment emphasizes the use of penicillin. Relief of the disease with niacin alone does indicate that poor nutrition is one of the factors involved in development of the disease.

The disease may be treated by penicillin, applied directly to the diseased tissues or by mouth sprays, troches or intramuscular injections. After treatment with penicillin there is usually a rapid clearance of the disease. Within twelve to thirty-six hours the patient is usually without symptoms. In some cases large doses of vitamin C may be necessary, especially when there is severe bleeding of the gums. Niacin is also frequently given along with the penicillin.

Old toothbrushes should be discarded, excessive use of alcohol or tobacco should be avoided, and mouth hygiene in general should be improved.

When the disease spreads to the lungs or bronchial tubes, a severe and critical illness may ensue. Prompt treatment of any case of trench mouth is wise, both for cure of the mouth infection and also to prevent more serious complications.

Bleeding Gums

The most common cause of bleeding gums with recession of tissues is vigorous, improper brushing of the teeth. Vigorous brushing may push the gum back from around the teeth, may expose the root surfaces and cause bleeding.

Bleeding gums may result from irritation in the mouth, serious disease affecting the whole body, nutritional deficiency, blood abnormalities, poor alignment of the teeth and other factors. Tumors, trench mouth, leukemia, diabetes, allergy, scurvy, pellagra and certain types of skin disorders may be reflected in bleeding gums. Both the dentist and the physician should be consulted when a person is troubled with this condition.

Pyorrhea is a major cause of the loss of teeth in persons over the age of 35. Inflammation and bleeding of the gums are the diagnostic signs by which the dentist can recognize this condition. Both for reasons of general health and for protection of the teeth, bleeding gums should never be neglected.

Pyorrhea

Pyorrhea, better known to the dentist as periodontitis, is an inflammation of the gum tissues at the margin of the teeth. The tissues become swollen and inflamed and separate from the tooth structure in such a way that pockets may form between the teeth and the gingival tissues. These pockets then become filled with food and other substances which may cause further inflammation. In time pus may be produced and exude from the pocket. Small abscesses may be created, and these, too, may drain pus into the pocket. There may be resorption of the bone of the jaw holding the teeth in position. The teeth then become loose in their sockets, since they are no longer held firmly by the bone. Sometimes there may be a recession of the gum from the tooth without inflammation or formation of pockets.

Various factors appear to be involved in the production of this disease. Endocrine disturbances, an inadequate diet or general disease may serve as predisposing factors.

When such disease is found by the dentist or physician, there is a problem in drainage of the pockets of pus, clearance of secondary infections, nutritional improvement of the tissues involved, correction of faulty habits of brushing the teeth, removal of mechanically irritating deposits and correction of poorly fitting crowns, bands or fillings, and treatment of any other more fundamental factor that may be involved in production of the disease.

Questions

1. How much dental decay, if any, is justified by the pleasures derived from the eating of sweets?

2. What can the parent do to create a favorable attitude toward the dentist on the part of a small child?

3. Since fluorides are poisonous, is the use of these chemicals in the public water supply justifiable for the reduction of dental decay?

4. Is there a satisfactory answer to religious objections to the addition of fluorides to the community water supply?

5. Should the responsibility for healthy teeth and gums rest primarily with the individual or with the community?

For Further Reading

1. American Dental Association: *Accepted Dental Remedies.* Chicago, 1956.

2. American Dental Association: *Teeth, Health and Appearance.* Chicago, 1957.

3. Bacon, Edgar S.: *Your Child's Teeth.* New York, E. P. Dutton and Company, 1957.

4. McNeil, Donald R.: *The Fight for Fluoridation.* New York, Oxford University Press, 1957.

Recommended Film

Schumaker, J. Robert: *Teeth, Their Structure and Care,* 16 mm., color or black and white, sound, showing time 11 minutes, 1956. Rental or purchase from Coronet Instructional Films, Inc., Coronet Building, Chicago 1, Illinois.

10

CARE OF THE EYES

A PERSON'S whole life revolves around his ability to see. Most learning is related to vision, so that intellectual development is largely dependent upon eyesight. The eyes reflect the general health of the individual to a remarkable degree. Good vision is perhaps man's most precious physical asset.

VISION AND TIME

"If you have trouble reading the numerals on your watch, it is later than you think."

Anonymous

Good vision is partly a matter of heredity, normal development and protection against injuries. It is also a matter of good nutrition, protection against communicable diseases, mental health, sensible use of the eyes and the proper use of medical,

105

ophthalmologic and surgical services when they are needed.

Vision may be impaired because of the presence of diseases such as diabetes or severe anemia. Hemorrhage in the eye, as well as severe bleeding elsewhere, may result in impairment of vision. The eyes may be damaged by heat and radiation, methyl alcohol, cancer and a wide variety of infectious organisms such as the pneumococci, streptococci, staphylococci and viruses. The length of the eyeball may be related to near-sightedness, and the shortness of the eyeball may be a cause of far-sightedness.

Many temporary conditions may affect vision even though the structures involved in seeing are all mechanically sound. Eye tissues are especially susceptible to a lack of oxygen. Headaches may occur because of sustained exposure to glare. Severe headaches and disturbance of vision may be associated with the eating of foods to which a person is allergic. These and still other factors are related to the health of the eyes. The eyes do not exist in isolation, but as a part of the total mind and body. Some visual disturbances are purely psychogenic, but the disturbance of vision is just as real as that caused by physical changes affecting the eye.

How People See

Light is a necessary part of vision. In complete darkness we cannot see. In fact, everything we see is reflected light unless we are looking at a primary light source such as a lamp or a fire. Not only must there be adequate illumination for good vision, but also there should be absence of glare or any other light disturbance which our eyes are not capable of receiving without handicap.

We must have full and normal development of all the structures involved in the process of seeing if we are to perceive properly and interpret adequately the light rays that reach our eyes. If there is inheritance of any defect or handicap involving the pathways of vision or if there is abnormal development of these tissues, it is obvious that vision will be impaired.

There must be proper and effective refraction for good vision. By refraction is meant the bending of light rays. Since light travels in parallel columns, the eye is unable to see properly unless these rays are brought to a focus on the retina of the eye.

Light is bent or refracted when it passes through a curved surface. The curvature of the cornea, or outside surface of the eyeball in front of the pupil, bends the light rays toward each other as they pass inward. When these partially refracted or bent rays reach the lens, which is another curved surface, they are bent still more so that they then have a better chance of being brought together at a focus at the proper point on the retina.

Even if there is plenty of good light and effective bending of the light rays to a proper focus on the retina, vision will still be impaired unless the cells of the retina function in such a way as to create nervous impulses from the light energy that has been delivered to them.

The nervous impulses generated in the sight cells of the retina must be conducted through the pathways of the brain that lead to the optic center. Should there be any interference with these pathways, then the sight impulses may not reach without distortion that part of the brain where an interpretation of them can be made.

Another important requirement for good vision is that the external muscles of the eye be in sufficient balance so that binocular vision is possible. By binocular vision is meant the process of seeing with both eyes. The perception of depth, for example, is largely a function of seeing with both eyes at the same time.

Finally, after the light rays have been changed into nervous impulses and conducted to the occipital area of the brain, good vision still depends upon a proper interpretation of what has been seen. Even experts in the field of vision often overlook the fact that seeing is partly a psychologic process. Even if the eye is mechanically perfect, we will have mistakes in vision if proper interpretation is not made on the nervous impulses received by the brain.

Emotional problems, low mentality and brain injury are some of the factors that may make a proper interpretation of impulses generated in the retina impossible. In such a case there may be severe reading difficulties or visual disturbances in general.

Tests for Vision

There are many different tests for vision. Some are quite simple and widely known to most people, while others are complicated and used only by the specialist who wishes to explore the possibility of more complicated forms of eye disorders.

VISION TESTS FOR CHILDREN

"About four and a half years seems the ideal age for visual testing; earlier, the child's cooperation and the accuracy of response is doubtful . . . at (this) age 20/40 vision is satisfactory; at five or six years, 20/30 is normal, and 20/20 may not be attained before seven or eight."

Dr. Warren A. Wilson, 1959

THE SNELLEN TEST. The Snellen test for visual acuity is perhaps the most widely known of all visual tests. The Snellen chart, or one of its several variations, is used extensively for the testing of vision in school children. It is also used in most doctors' offices, in industry, in military service and wherever mass testing of vision is done.

Letters, figures or drawings on the Snellen chart are correlated in size with distance. The standard reading distance is 20 feet.

The Snellen chart is not dependable for the discovery of many visual disorders, but is effective in detecting near-sighted persons. When used in conjunction with the plus-sphere lens, the far-sighted person can also be detected.

In testing with the Snellen chart vision is recorded in a standard manner. If a person being tested is able to read at 20 feet what the person with normal visual acuity reads at 20 feet, then vision is recorded as 20/20. The top figure always indicates the distance at which the chart was read, namely, 20 feet. The bottom figure indicates the line on the chart which was read correctly by the person being tested. If this line is the one that the person of normal visual acuity reads at 20 feet, the recording is 20 over 20. When a person has 20/40 vision or worse, it is usually wise to have a thorough eye examination by a specialist.

THE PLUS-SPHERE LENS. When the plus-sphere lens is used in conjunction with the Snellen test for the detection of far-sightedness, it is used only at 20 feet for the reading of the 20 foot line. If the person is able to read this line correctly, then he is far-sighted. On the other hand, if the figures are so blurred that he cannot distinguish them properly, then he is not far-sighted.

THE MASSACHUSETTS VISION TEST. The Massachusetts vision test is a battery of tests approved by the American Medical Association for use in schools and with other large groups. This test is composed of the Snellen chart, the plus-sphere lens and Maddox rods. The latter constitute one of the more reliable tests for muscle imbalance. The Maddox rod is basically a glass rod which is set in the center of an opaque disc. This disc is held in front of one eye so that a person looks through the glass portion of the disc with this eye. Vision is directed at a light such as a small flashlight. The Maddox rod converts this light into a streak of light. The position of this streak relative to the image of light seen by the other eye indicates the presence or absence of muscle imbalance. The Massachusetts vision test is therefore a test for near-sightedness, far-sightedness and muscle imbalance.

TELEBINOCULAR TESTS. The telebinocular test requires fairly expensive equipment and has a high rate of error in that it screens out too many people for further examination. Visual acuity, muscle imbalance, fusion, depth perception and color vision are tested with this device. It is probably best used by eye specialists for making special studies of any particular person or of a group of persons needing more than the standard tests.

DROPS IN THE EYES. There are a great number of other tests for vision. In the office of the ophthalmologist the patient may have drops put into his eyes. The purpose of these so-called drops is to paralyze the muscles of accommodation so that a person with impaired vision may not make up for his handicap by extra powers of accommodation.

COLOR BLINDNESS TESTS. Testing for color vision is usually done by use of the Holmgren wools or pseudo-isochromatic or Ishihara plates for color blindness. Basically, these devices test the ability to select and identify colors. In the plates, for example, the person being tested will be able to identify certain numbers written in particular colors if he is not color-blind. On the other hand, if he is color-blind, he may report misleading figures.

BRAIN WAVE TESTS AND VISION. Recently, an interesting study suggested that the electroencephalograph may have an important function in the diagnosis of visual disorders. In a study of 1281 children under sixteen years of age it was found that 30 per cent of the children with stra-

bismus or muscle imbalance had distinctive brain wave recordings, compared with less than 1 per cent of a group of children who had normal vision. It was recommended from this study that children who show certain types of brain wave recordings should have thorough eye examinations for the possible detection of visual abnormalities.

THE OPHTHALMOSCOPIC EXAMINATION. The eye examination made by the eye specialist that includes a look at the retina is known as an ophthalmoscopic examination. This is an eye test in which the ophthalmologist shines a light through the pupil to the inner, back portion of the eyeball where the retina is exposed.

The retina is a unique structure of the body. Under direct observation by the eye specialist, the retina yields many clues to the health of the patient. Changes in the retina may occur in diabetes, high blood pressure, kidney disease, certain forms of heart disease and many other diseases affecting other parts of the body.

Many conditions of the eye itself can be directly observed, such as optic atrophy, inflammation of the optic nerve, detached retina, hemorrhage in the eye, blocking or occlusion of the retinal artery and other conditions.

Testing for visual health is a fairly complex subject. It is a function that should be reserved to those who have adequate professional training in this field. The particular kind of test that will be advocated by the physician or other specialist depends upon the symptoms of the patient and the judgment of the health adviser.

Muscle Imbalance

The cross-eyed person represents the most commonly observed type of muscle imbalance so far as the general public is concerned.

This is not the only type of muscle imbalance, however. When the eyes diverge outward rather than inward, the condition is often called walleye. Both the cross-eyed and the walleyed person are suffering from muscle imbalance, as are many other persons who do not have such extreme divergences and may therefore escape detection unless someone skilled in vision testing makes the examination.

Strabismus is the medical term for muscle imbalance, of which there are two basic types. One is due to a complete or partial paralysis of one or more eye muscles, whereas the other is nonparalytic. It is this latter form of muscle imbalance that is more common. Some causes of the less common paralytic type of muscle imbalance are indicated in the following table.

CAUSES OF OCULAR PARALYSIS IN 1,000 CASES*	
Cause	*Number*
Undetermined	282
Head injury	168
Brain tumors	165
Diseases of the blood vessels in the brain	165
Aneurysm (sac-like dilation of a blood vessel)	109
Miscellaneous	123
Total	1,000
Dr. C. Wilbur Rucker, Mayo Clinic, 1958	

Muscle imbalance should be recognized and treated early in childhood. Babies under the age of four months often appear to be cross-eyed because they cannot fuse images, but the eye muscles may be quite normal. Parents should not be alarmed, therefore, when a baby in the first three or four months of life apparently shows some muscle imbalance.

About 90,000 babies a year are born with inward converging of the eyeballs and it has been estimated that nearly half a million children between the ages of 5 and 9 years are cross-eyed.

Some physicians believe that muscle imbalance in a baby can be detected as early as four months while others think that a definite conclusion should not be reached before 12 to 15 months. In either case it is wise to consult the physician for advice if muscle imbalance is suspected after the age of about 6 months.

Muscle imbalance usually does not improve with age. In other words, there is no spontaneous correction or cure. Treatment must be based upon a proper diagnosis and should be started as early in life as possible once a diagnosis has been definitely established.

The effects of muscle imbalance are apt to be both visual and psychologic. Vision in one eye is usually lowered, although complete blindness does not usually result. Some authorities believe that strabismus becomes permanent at about the age of seven years; hence treatment must be started well before this time.

When a person has muscle imbalance, he tends to see or fixate with just one eye. This is because he finds it difficult to bring the eyes into the joint or common fixation which is necessary in binocular vision. In order not to have vision impaired in the defective eye, treatment usually includes the blocking off of the sound eye for several weeks at a time. This forces the person to use the other eye.

Eye exercises are also important in order to strengthen the defective muscle. These exercises are designed primarily to strengthen the weakened muscle only, so that exact diagnosis of the muscle involved is necessary.

Sometimes muscle imbalance can be compensated for with glasses. The prism lens displaces light toward the base of the lens. It is therefore possible with a prism lens to compensate for the displacement of light rays in the opposite direction by the defective eye. In other words, the lens does not cure the defective muscle, but merely makes it possible for an image to be brought to a proper focus so that the child or adult will continue to use both eyes in seeing. This tends to preserve vision in both eyes.

The use of glasses in conjunction with rotation exercises and periodic blocking off of the sound eye is reported by some authorities as resulting in a cure or strengthening of the weak muscle in about 50 per cent of the cases. If such a program fails to bring definite improvement within six months to two years, however, eye surgery is generally advisable.

One operation alone may not be sufficient, and it is generally better to undercorrect and operate a second time than to make a cross-eyed child walleyed, or vice versa. Eye surgery is painless, safe, and an effective and scientific method for curing muscle imbalance. There should be no hesitation on the part of the parent or the patient in obtaining needed surgical correction for this type of eye disorder.

The correction of muscle imbalance, especially in the cross-eyed or walleyed child, is very important because of the disturbing effect of this condition on the personality of the child. If the condition goes uncorrected, the child is apt to have an inferiority complex based upon his appearance and the ridicule of other small children. Many such children develop into behavior problems because of the psychologic impact of this disorder. Parents should go to great lengths to secure correction of such a condition. Fortunately, muscle imbalance can be greatly improved or completely corrected by proper treatment.

Who Should Wear Glasses?

Glasses should be worn by those who have errors of refraction that are sufficiently great to cause impairment of vision or discomfort in seeing.

An error of refraction means an unsatisfactory bending of light rays by the cornea or lens of the eyes in relation to the location of the retina, in which the cells that perceive light are located.

The near-sighted person has blurred vision at a distance because what he sees there is not brought to a focus on the ret-

ina. For seeing at normal distances the near-sighted person needs glasses that will bend the light rays to a precise focus on the retina.

The far-sighted person can often see well at both near and far distances. He cannot see or read at close range for very long without development of eyestrain, headache or blurring of vision, however. This person needs glasses that will make close work easier. When such glasses cause the light rays to focus directly on the retina instead of behind the retina (this latter, of course, does not actually happen, since the light rays cannot penetrate the coats of the retina), then the far-sighted person can read in comfort and stay with a task requiring close vision for much longer periods without discomfort.

The person with astigmatism has a disturbed focus because light rays are sent in varying directions toward the retina, owing to irregularities in the surface of the cornea or the lens. In his attempts to secure a proper focus on the retina the person with this error of refraction is apt to suffer tension and headache. What he needs is a pair of glasses that bend light rays in such a manner as to compensate for the distortions that occur from the irregular surfaces of his own eye tissues. When such glasses, properly prescribed, are worn by the patient, vision becomes better and easier and symptoms of discomfort disappear.

The foregoing circumstances account for most eyeglass prescriptions. Glasses are worn for other visual conditions, however. As mentioned elsewhere in this chapter, glasses may be prescribed, at least temporarily, in the treatment of muscle imbalance. They may be advisable for other conditions as well, but always their basic function is that of the refraction of light rays except in those instances in which protection against light is needed. In the latter case dark or tinted glasses may be prescribed, although this is often a temporary measure: what is really needed in such instances is a correction of the funda-

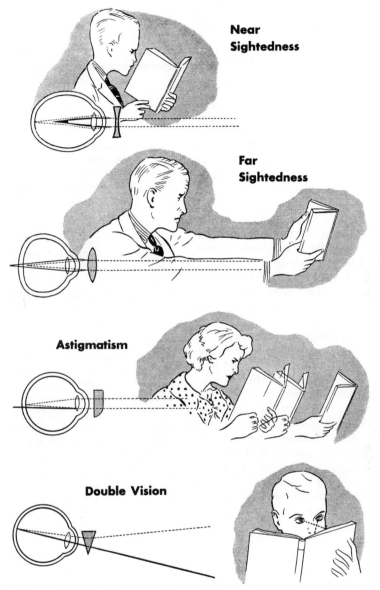

Near Sightedness

Far Sightedness

Astigmatism

Double Vision

Figure 6. Four main defects of the eyes, and lenses which are needed in these conditions. (Adapted from chart of Better Vision Institute.)

mental cause of the excessive sensitivity to light.

The importance of telescopic lenses for certain persons with seriously impaired vision has recently been stressed by some eye specialists. Probably in the future such lenses will be more widely used by ophthalmologists for improving the vision of partially-seeing patients.

Glasses do not correct near-sightedness, far-sightedness or astigmatism. They merely compensate or counterbalance existing errors of refraction. Glasses make seeing an easier and more comfortable experience when they are properly prescribed and correctly used, but they make no fundamental cures.

The proper fitting of lenses is only the first step in the alleviation of eye discomfort and disturbed vision due to errors of refraction. The second step lies in the intelligent use of the glasses that have been prescribed. Spectacles should be kept clean, they should be worn when needed, but not otherwise; they should be protected against scratching or breaking and should be changed periodically as regular eye examinations reveal that such changes are needed. People who wear glasses should also learn to look directly through the center of the lenses, rather than through the top, bottom or sides, since such habits may cause distortion of vision even though the glasses are properly prescribed. Bifocal lenses are constructed, of course, to permit vision through the central portion of the glass and the lower part of the instrument as well, as the need for near or far vision changes.

An important point to keep in mind when children must wear glasses is that they can now be obtained with lenses of hardened glass or plastic that protect against breakage and eye injury. These "safety glasses" may also protect the child against other accidents because he can wear the glasses while engaging in active play without danger of breaking them. With improved vision he would be less vulnerable to accidents in general.

Emergencies of the Eye

All mature persons should be able to recognize when an emergency exists in regard to eyesight. These emergencies of vision may require prompt medical or surgical care if the ability to see is to be preserved. The doctor cannot save the eyesight if the patient comes for help too late.

Eye Inflammations

Chief among the medical emergencies is an inflammatory condition that the eye specialist recognizes as the "red eye." The so-called red or inflamed eye may be identified by the specialist as conjunctivitis, iritis, glaucoma, an allergic condition or one of other conditions.

> **THE RED, ALLERGIC EYEBALL**
>
> "Sometimes a red eyeball will be associated with shiny, tense, and sometimes wrinkled and weepy eyelids. These cases are usually allergic . . . Cosmetics are number one on the list as a cause of red, itchy eyeballs . . . Patients can be allergic to any cosmetic . . . Hair tonics, hair sprays, hand lotions, nail polishes, and after-shaving lotions will cause red eyes in some patients . . ."
>
> *Dr. Ernest H. Dengler, 1959*

The factor that makes the red eye a medical emergency is that the average person cannot be trusted to make a proper diagnosis. Delay in the treatment of glaucoma may result in permanent impairment of vision within a matter of hours. Delay in the treatment of an infection of the conjunctiva or iris may make cure of the disorder exceedingly difficult.

Many persons refer to an inflamed eye as "pink eye" and consider it a relatively insignificant eye disorder. Such a conclusion is not justified. Any infection or inflammation of the eye calls for careful examination and accurate diagnosis in order to secure proper treatment.

Glaucoma, a Leading Cause of Blindness

Glaucoma is a condition in which fluids in the anterior and posterior chambers of the eye accumulate faster than they are drained away. Many people do not even realize that there is a constant flow of fluid through the eyeball, but any interference in the proper balance between inflow and outgo may increase the tension inside the eyeball to such an extent that permanent damage is done to nerves and cells of the retina. When this occurs, partial or complete blindness results.

About 20,000 people in the United States are blind because of glaucoma and about one million persons have the disorder. Since both medical and surgical treatment may temporarily or permanently reduce the tension inside the eye, it is sheer negligence not to seek proper attention for this eye disorder.

The early detection of glaucoma by the physician or eye specialist depends mostly upon two major factors: the regular use of the tonometer in eye examinations by the physician and the description of symptoms by the patient.

The tonometer is an instrument for measuring the tension inside the eyeball. When this instrument is used by the doctor he first puts "drops" on the surface of the eyeball to reduce or eliminate sensitivity to the tonometer. One drop is usually all that is needed. The patient is then asked to fix both eyes on some point and to hold the eyes steady. The flat base or foot of the tonometer is then placed against the surface of the eye and a reading of the pressure is made. A reading of an intraocular pressure of 26 millimeters of mercury or more is generally interpreted by the eye specialist as being within the range of glaucoma.

Symptoms of glaucoma that may be reported by the patient to his physician include complaints that glasses (even new ones) do not help his vision; that he has blurred or hazy vision at times; that he has difficulty in adjusting his vision to a dark room, such as in a theater; that he sees a rainbow halo around lights; that he has frequent headaches; that his field of vision has narrowed and that his eyeballs feel hard and tense when felt through the eyelids. According to Dr. William J. Gibson the foregoing symptoms and signs may make it possible for the physician to make an early diagnosis of glaucoma, especially in persons past the age of 40 when about 2 per cent of the population has this disorder.

Foreign Bodies in the Eye

Foreign bodies in the eye also represent a medical emergency. Pieces of metal, stone, wood or other objects may cause serious damage to eyesight if they are not completely removed. Microscopic particles of metal, for example, may rust, cause ulceration, and eventually lead to the loss of eyesight. It is therefore very important that an eye specialist be consulted for the removal of such potentially serious foreign bodies when they become lodged in the eye.

National significance is given to this type of medical emergency, since about 1000 eye injuries per day occur to workers in industry.

EYE INJURIES TO CHILDREN

"In the case of a penetrating injury . . . it is much better to put the child in a hospital and examine the injury under anesthesia, with adequate preparation for operation. Forceful retraction of the lids . . . may mean the difference between saving and losing the eye and therefore justifies anesthesia."

Dr. Warren A. Wilson, 1959

Chemical Burns of the Eye

Many such injuries consist of chemical burns of the eye. This is another medical emergency that must be treated promptly if vision is to be maintained. Prompt flooding of the eye with water immediately after it has been damaged by any chemical may save the sight of that eye. First aid of this sort should not consist solely in an initial washing of the eye. The flooding with water should be generous and should be repeated over and over again. Some physicians recommend that the head be immersed in a bucket of water between breaths in order to achieve a maximum dilution of any chemical affecting the eye.

Some chemicals can penetrate eye tissues and must be removed by the surgeon if permanent loss of eyesight is not to follow.

Ulcers of the Cornea

Ulcers of the cornea should also receive prompt medical treatment. The cornea has a remarkable power for rapid healing if it is given a chance by good medical treatment. Most ulcers of the cornea are caused by infections. The commonest microscopic organisms involved in this eye disease are the pneumococci, streptococci and staphylococci. These bacteria are apt to be especially damaging after some other injury to the cornea. The ulcer, composed of dead tissue and pus, may spread to other parts of the cornea or may penetrate into the deeper eye tissues. The deeper the penetration, the more serious the complication. If fibrous tissue forms, there may be scarring of the cornea with loss of vision.

Small ulcerations often occur after the removal of foreign bodies, but these heal rapidly within twenty-four hours when properly treated. In general, the possibility of complications from corneal ulcers is sufficiently great so that this type of disorder should be treated by an eye specialist.

Sudden Loss of Vision

Any sudden loss of vision should be looked upon as a medical emergency of the eye, and prompt treatment by an eye specialist should be sought. A loss of central vision, for example, that occurs suddenly has been correlated with spasm of the retinal artery. A deficiency of oxygen and other nutrients to the part of the eye involved may result in rapid loss of vision and permanent blindness if the spasm of the blood vessel is not relieved promptly. The condition is therefore a medical emergency. Prompt antispasmodic treatment coupled with a proper diagnosis and removal of the basic cause of the spasm should result in maintenance of good vision.

Prompt medical treatment of many eye diseases not only makes it easier to clear up the disorder, but also may actually prevent permanent impairment of vision or actual loss of eyesight. Even if a person has to travel many miles to secure proper care for the eye, such a procedure may preserve vision in one or both eyes. A person should not be hesitant to seek the advice and treatment of an eye specialist if he has any reason at all to suspect a medical emergency of the eye.

Eye Surgery

Many persons have the mistaken idea that the eyes are so delicate that surgery on these organs may be exceedingly dangerous. Such is not the case. There are many types of operations that can and should be performed on the eyes with little risk to the patient. Failure to seek surgery for the correction of certain handicapping disorders may have profound detrimental effects upon both a person's vision and his personality.

Surgery is advisable for a number of minor complications such as a turning inward or outward of an eyelid, an individual eyelash that is painful, a small tumor, or for a chalazion, a condition which is essentially a small tumor of the lower eyelid resulting from an inflammation of a small gland.

More extensive surgery is needed for the correction of ptosis, a condition in which there is a drooping of one eyelid, or for support of the lower lid after paralysis of the facial nerve. Sometimes it is wise to obtain a reconstruction of defective eyelids.

Various types of surgery may be advisable for the glands and passages through which tears are produced and pass across the eye into the nasal passageway. It may be necessary to remove by surgery certain adhesions between the eyelids and the globe of the eye or to take off other unsightly attachments to the eyelid. Sometimes the cornea must be penetrated in order to evacuate harmful contents of the anterior chamber of the eye.

Surgery may also be necessary for the relief of glaucoma, a condition in which the tension of fluids inside the eyeball may reach such proportions as to cause permanent blindness.

Surgery for cataract may restore a considerable amount of vision to a person who has been blinded by this development. When there is a detachment of the retina, surgery may be necessary, and early treatment may result in a 70 to 75 per cent chance of cure. Foreign bodies such as metal objects in the eye must be removed by surgery if they have penetrated the eye tissues to any particular extent.

The foregoing conditions and many others can be corrected by surgical means; often they cannot be corrected or cured in any other way. It must be recognized that eye tissues are not as delicate as is often thought. In a sense the structures of the eye are quite tough. Certainly they can be operated on with safety and relatively little discomfort to the patient. Surgery for the eyes should be looked upon as a needed resource for the cure of various disorders affecting structures of these organs.

Eye Specialists

Many persons are somewhat confused on the identification of the various eye specialists available in most communities.

The ophthalmologist is the eye specialist with the greatest amount of professional training. He is a medical doctor who has gone on in his professional training to specialize in the recognition and treatment of eye disorders, and is qualified to diagnose and treat diseases of the eye as well as to prescribe the kind of glasses a person may need. This specialist can also use drugs in the eyes for more accurate diagnosis and is qualified to recognize signs in the eye of diseases elsewhere in the body.

The oculist is precisely the same as an ophthalmologist. The two words are synonyms.

The optometrist is a person who has received professional training in measuring the degree of visual acuity possessed by the patient. Although he does not have a medical degree, he now receives excellent training in refraction and can do a good job of prescribing glasses, a service which is now authorized by license in all fifty states. In most states the optometrist is not permitted to use drugs in making an appraisal of the kind of glasses that a person may need, but the alert optometrist will refer patients who need such service, or who give indication of obvious or questionable eye disease, to the ophthalmologist (oculist). In Illinois, for example, the optometrists and the oculists work together effectively to provide an adequate service to the community in respect to visual health. This cooperation has been especially fruitful in uncovering visual handicaps of school children.

The optician is a maker of optical instruments. He accepts the prescription for glasses which has been written by the ophthalmologist or optometrist and then makes eye glasses for the patient. The optician is therefore a technician in the making of spectacles. He has no training for or legal right to examine the eyes of patients or to make a diagnosis of their health status.

Eye Exercises

Eye exercises can be helpful with certain visual disorders. As indicated in the section on muscle imbalance, the exercise of these external muscles, notably the muscle at fault, may produce beneficial effects. Many patients with poor vision who have been properly fitted with glasses become more comfortable when proper eye exercises are prescribed and followed.

When there is actual damage to some part of the eye that transmits or refracts light, or receives the light impulse (such as in the retina), eye exercises can be of no value. Obviously, eye exercises would be of no value in cancer of the eye or in brain injury involving the sight centers.

Many patients can be taught through eye exercises to reduce the handicap of their defects even though no cure of the defect is achieved.

The psychologic effects of exercising the eye muscles may lead to mistaken conclusions on the part of the patient and others. One study, of 100 patients with cataract, showed that when these patients were given eye exercises for one year, 75 per cent said their vision had improved. However, careful eye tests showed that the vision had actually become worse in nearly every case. Psychotherapy was responsible for the patients' belief that their vision had improved. Merely giving a person medical attention sometimes makes him feel that he is getting better.

Color Blindness

It has been estimated that about six million men in the United States are partially or completely color blind. Only about 100 cases of total color blindness have been reported in the medical literature, however. The commonest kind of color blindness is so-called two-color vision. Most of the people who have this disorder confuse reds, greens and yellows and are unable to distinguish clearly between bluish-greens, blues and violets. The overwhelming majority of so-called color blind persons are actually only partially color blind.

Apparently most color blindness is a sex-linked, hereditary characteristic. The defect travels from fathers to grandsons through the daughters; thus, color blindness is mainly a male defect. The disorder is occasionally produced by damage to the eye, the optic nerves or the visual centers of the brain. There is no known cure or medical treatment for this condition. No training systems for the color blind have ever had medical justification.

It is only occasionally that color blindness may have a relationship to health. Accidents have been known to occur because a color signal was missed or mistakenly interpreted. A classic case is that related to the collision of the steamship *Isaac Belle* with a tug on the night of July 5, 1875. Ten people lost their lives in this collision. The captain of the tug insisted that he had seen a red light and had directed his craft according to that signal, but it was proved that the steamship had been showing a green light. Four years later it was found that the captain of the tug was so color blind that he could scarcely distinguish red from green at a distance of 3 feet. It was judged that his color blindness had been responsible for the collision and the loss of ten lives.

Color blindness in traffic is not as great a hazard as some people assume. The person suffering from this disorder may take his cues from other drivers or may learn the position of colored signal lights so that he is not handicapped by failure to identify the color unless he encounters a street signal with a reversal of colors. Since signal lights are now standardized in most places, it is not likely that color blindness will be much of a handicap so far as traffic accidents are concerned, even when the defect does exist.

Television and Eye Strain

Television viewing in itself does not cause visual discomfort. Effects depend upon the existing quality of visual health and upon the duration and manner in which we watch the television screen. Persons who have muscle imbalance, errors of refraction or other visual handicaps will have discomfort sooner than other people and perhaps to a greater degree, depending upon the length of time they continue to observe.

In general, the television screen should be watched from a distance of about 10 feet and from a position perpendicular to the image. The latter should also be at eye level if possible. Television should not be watched in total darkness, since the contrast between the lighted screen and the dark surrounding area causes eye fatigue more rapidly. Preferably there should be a diffuse light throughout the room so that the contrast between the screen and room is reduced to a minimum. Large screens are better than small ones from the visual standpoint.

It can be said that the effects of television upon vision depend upon the manner in which we view the screen and the length of time we spend in watching it.

Cataracts

Although cataracts have been reported as being due to a number of factors such as vitamin deficiency, diabetes, hereditary disease, x-ray irradiation, electrical accidents, excessive use of corticosteroids, heat and old age, it has not been demonstrated that this condition is due to any single cause.

A cataract is a loss of transparency of the lens of the eye. Obviously, if light can no longer penetrate through the lens, then it cannot reach the retina in the back portion of the eyeball. This, of course, means loss of sight in the eye that is affected.

Although the exact cause of cataract is probably never identified in the majority of cases, it is possible to treat this disease successfully by surgery. Surgery for cataract is a fairly simple procedure for the eye surgeon. The results are often strikingly good, and there is usually a considerable restoration of sight.

No effective drug treatment for cataract is known.

Since the power of focusing the rays of light on the retina will be virtually lost when the diseased lens is removed, glasses must be worn in order to compensate for this impairment of function, although recent research suggests the possibility of substituting an artificial lens in the vacant capsule.

Eye Banks and Corneal Transplants

The eye bank is a modern development. The Eye Bank for Sight Restoration, Incorporated, was organized on April 13, 1945, to collect and preserve healthy corneal tissue from human eyes for transplantation to blind persons who had lost their sight from corneal defects. This organization is now national in scope and is affiliated with many hospitals throughout the United States.

It was estimated at the time of the founding of this organization that between 10,000 and 15,000 blind persons with corneal defects in the United States might have the opportunity to see again if their own defective tissue could be replaced with a healthy cornea obtained from someone else.

Corneas obtained from a dead person must be removed within a few hours after death, and it has become common for certain persons to will their eyes to an eye bank for transferral to some blind person in need of this healthy eye tissue.

Corneal tissue taken from either a living or dead person can be stored for only about three days before it is transplanted; hence, advance planning and organization are necessary to bring together at the proper time the blind person in need of help and the healthy cornea which has been recently removed from another person. In some states permission of the nearest relative is needed for post-mortem removal of an eye even though the deceased may have left written instructions for the contribution of his eye or eyes to the eye bank.

Questions

1. Since visual defects increase with age, is this good evidence that schooling is an important *cause* of such disorders?
2. Does insufficient light ever cause permanent damage to the eyes?
3. Does the wearing of eyeglasses create psychologic problems for children?
4. What is the true explanation when claims are made that visual acuity has been improved by eye exercises?
5. Which is more important for the cross-eyed child: the visual handicap or the psychologic reaction that results from this disorder?

For Further Reading

1. Farrell, Gabriel: *The Story of Blindness.* Cambridge, Harvard University Press, 1956.
2. Norris, Miriam, Spaulding, Patricia J., and Brodie, Fern H.: *Blindness in Children.* Chicago, University of Chicago Press, 1957.
3. Pollack, Philip: *The Truth About Eye Exercises.* Philadelphia, Chilton Company, 1956.
4. School of Public Health: *Light and Vision.* Ann Arbor, Michigan, University of Michigan, 1959.
5. Vail, Derrick: *The Truth About Your Eyes.* New York, Farrar, Straus and Cudahy, 1959.

Recommended Film

Hamilton, Nancy: *Helen Keller in Her Story.* 16 mm., black and white, sound, showing time 48 minutes, 1954. Rental or purchase from Louis de Rochemont Film Library, 13 E. 37th St., New York 16, N.Y.

11

CARE OF THE SKIN

HEALTH problems pertaining to the skin represent one of the leading reasons why students consult the college health service when such is available. At Stanford University, for example, during the first seven months of 1960 a total of 2058 calls were made at the health office for problems of skin health. During the months indicated, skin disorders ranked seventh among all the reasons for consultation with the college physicians.

There are many disorders and diseases that may affect the health of the skin. Viruses and bacteria may cause a variety of skin infections, such as impetigo and boils. Fungus infections of the skin or scalp, such as athlete's foot and ringworm, are commonplace. Inflammation of the skin may result from contact with harmful substances such as chemicals encountered on

119

the job or from poison oak, from overtreatment with improper medicines, from numerous allergens and other causes. The skin may be damaged by accident or may be burned by fire, chemicals or sunlight.

> RESPECT THE SKIN
>
> "We must practice and teach respect for the skin. The skin is a wonderful creation that is a protective, defensive covering, aiding in the temperature control of the body and in excretions. If treated and handled gently its defensive and reparative mechanisms will respond . . . When well cleaned the skin is only clean, never sterile . . . Respecting the skin is basic whether the patient's condition is medical or surgical, and the surgeon particularly should practice and teach it."
>
> *Dr. Egbert H. Fell, 1960*

At birth the beauty of the skin may be marred by unsightly birthmarks or other congenital conditions. Some skin disorders are psychogenic, since the skin reflects the state of the mind. Metabolic and other internal relationships may be reflected in the skin, as in acne, a disorder outranking all other skin problems during adolescence. The skin may act as a barometer for serious generalized disease, or it may have serious disease of its own, such as cancer. It is impossible to discuss in a single chapter the many health problems associated directly or indirectly with the skin. This part of the book should be looked upon as an introduction to the care of the skin, for only a few of the many problems of this organ of the body can be discussed in such a brief presentation.

Overtreatment Dermatitis

One of the commonest skin disorders seen by skin specialists is an eruption or inflammation which comes from overtreatment of a pre-existing skin condition. Many people are advised by friends to use a particular ointment or salve for the treatment of a skin disorder, although no medical diagnosis of the condition has been made. Instead of getting better from such treatment, the patient sometimes suffers an acute inflammation and eruption. Often he will tell his physician that an ointment which he applied to his poison ivy, athlete's foot, infection or other skin disorder has made the condition worse, that it has burned him or caused the eruption to spread.

Skin disorders that have resulted from overtreatment should be given careful attention by skin specialists. Cure may take time and patience even under expert guidance. The important point to keep in mind is that skin conditions should be treated by competent physicians after a proper diagnosis has been made. In no case should skin diseases be treated with ointments, oils or salves which are recommended by friends, drug store clerks or others without special training in the field of dermatology.

The use of substances such as Merthiolate, iodine, sulfa drugs, local anesthetics such as benzocaine, antihistamines and antibiotics often results in overtreatment dermatitis. It is especially important to avoid the use of penicillin ointments in the treatment of skin disorders, for medical experience has shown that sensitization to this antibiotic often occurs. The tendency among physicians is to use only those antibiotics in ointments which are not taken internally. In this way it is possible to avoid sensitizing a patient to an antibiotic that may be useful in treating more serious disease.

It cannot be emphasized too strongly that a person should use only those skin preparations that have been prescribed by a physician and only for the length of time the doctor has recommended. When some of the medicine is left over, it should be destroyed; otherwise there may be temptation to pass it on to others for use on an undiagnosed skin disease.

Dr. L. Edward Gaul of Evansville, Indiana, reported to the Council on Pharmacy and Chemistry of the American Medical Association that at least 150,000 cases of overtreatment dermatitis occur annually, if the number of such cases seen by skin specialists is to be taken as a representative figure. If cases seen by physicians in general are added to this total, it can be seen that this represents one of the commonest of all skin diseases in the United States.

Dr. Gaul concluded from a survey of the medical literature and from polls of skin specialists that organic mercurials, sulfonamides, local anesthetics, antihistamines and antibiotic ointments and salves are the worst offenders in the cause of overtreatment dermatitis.

The first signs of sensitization to such medicines is a gradual onset of inflammation and the appearance of blisters or vesicles (sometimes containing pus). Often this inflammatory reaction occurs around the edges of the previous skin condition to which the patient has added the new and ill-advised treatment. When treatment with the medicine is continued, more severe reactions are likely to occur. Reactions may be hivelike, blotchy and diffuse inflammation may be widespread, and large deeper blisters may form. Commonly the first signs may be seen after the treatment of some trivial eruption, itching, insect bite, poison ivy, sunburn or athlete's foot. Frequently the patient thinks the original skin condition being treated is spreading, instead of realizing that he is suffering a reaction and sensitization to the medicine that is being used.

Dr. Gaul emphasizes that "the lay public must be taught to beware of all semiprofessional advice and ideas. They must learn to use dermatological (skin) preparations as directed by their physicians and not to use anything else. All remedies should be destroyed when a cure is effected, and they should not be given to anyone else."

"Housewives' Eczema"

A skin condition sometimes called "housewives' eczema" by physicians can be traced in most cases to the irritating effects of cleansers or detergents, although other causes are sometimes found. Since housewives are more commonly exposed to such things as detergents and cleaning compounds it is to be expected that they would suffer more than men from allergies associated with these products.

Detergent irritation usually starts on ring fingers, as does an allergic reaction to soaps. Sometimes the ring itself has an irritating effect although more commonly it is only because detergent or soap may be sheltered by the ring in contact with the skin.

To prevent "housewives' eczema" many skin specialists recommend the wearing of cotton gloves inside of rubber gloves for dishwashing or other cleaning. These precautions are not necessary if there is no skin irritation to the products commonly encountered in the kitchen.

Acne

Acne represents a common and sometimes serious health problem for the college student. Acne is important for two reasons. First, if the condition is untreated and if it is severe enough, the disease may leave scars. Second, the disorder may have substantial psychologic effects upon the individual. There may be a tendency on the part of many adolescents to withdraw from social contact because of self-consciousness about this skin disorder.

Acne is one of the most commonly neglected skin disorders because of the belief on the part of many parents that the disorder will, in time, clear itself spontaneously. Unfortunately, this attitude neglects the psychologic impact of the disorder on the young person. Such indifference may also result in permanent scarring of the face which not only distorts the physical appearance of the young person, but has further psychologic effects of an undesirable nature.

Apparently many different factors are involved in the production of acne: heredity, general health, body metabolism, diet and hygiene of the skin. Perhaps a most important relationship is that during puberty the sex hormones stimulate secretions of the sebaceous glands. On the other hand, it is common medical experience that diets rich in fats and carbohydrates often aggravate acne.

At present there is no single, certain method of treatment for acne. The physician cannot guarantee that the disorder will be cleared up in a short time. On the other hand, if medical treatment is neglected, there may be serious scarring of the face as well as the adverse psychologic effects previously mentioned. Many young people are helped a good deal by medical treatment of acne, and this should be definitely attempted.

Physicians recommend the limitation of fats and carbohydrates in the diet when a person is suffering from acne. It is especially advisable to restrict or eliminate chocolate, nuts, ice cream, cheese, gravy and sea foods (because of their iodine content).

Some favorable results in the treatment of acne have been reported by a group of physicians at Syracuse University. These doctors used tetracycline in the treatment of seventy-two patients with acne. All the patients were young university students of both sexes between the ages of seventeen and twenty-two. At the beginning of treatment a count was made of the number of pimples in each specific area of the face, and as treatment proceeded additional counts of individual acne lesions were made for comparison with the beginning data. All supplementary treatment such as special diets, soaps, lotions, ultraviolet light treatments and so on were discontinued and were not used at any time.

At periodic intervals a recount of the total number of pimples for the group showed a reduction in the number of pus-containing blemishes that amounted to 50 per cent within thirty days and sixty-two per cent at sixty days. In only seven of the seventy-two students was there a failure to improve. Thirty-three of the students had a 75 per cent reduction in acne within thirty days or less of treatment with tetracycline, whereas twenty-one students had a 75 per cent reduction in acne after more than thirty days. None of the patients had any observable evidence of sensitivity to tetracycline.

For some young women treatment with the sex hormone estrogen during the last two weeks of the menstrual period has been very successful in preventing the flare-up of acne that often occurs at the time of menstruation. No strong evidence exists, however, that any permanent changes are produced. Improvements seem to be restricted mostly to the period of time that the estrogen is given to the patient.

There are a number of reasons why most physicians prefer not to treat the acne patient with estrogen. The menstrual period may be affected, enlargement of the breasts of a painful nature may occur and some conditions may be aggravated. Young women with uterine fibroids, ovarian cysts, or breast-cancer susceptibility should not be treated with this hormone.

The young woman with acne who receives estrogen treatment should be prepared to abandon this approach to her problem on her physician's advice and should not forsake other methods of treatment.

Dermabrasion is sometimes used for the eradication of scars. In this type of treatment the surface of the skin is smoothed out with sandpaper (under anesthesia). This treatment does not cure acne, but it may alter some of the permanent effects such as scarring of the face.

At the Temple University School of Medicine, Dr. Elmer R. Gross has treated over 5000 acne patients over a period of years. Dr. Gross advocates washing of the face at least three times a day, application of a prescription provided by a physician, keeping the fingers away from the face, plenty of rest and sleep, avoidance of violent exercise, sunburn, foods containing iodine, rich foods, alcoholic drinks, nuts, peanut butter and certain other foods. He also specifies that the face should not be picked if scars are to be avoided and that a cure should not be expected from a few treatments.

Perhaps the principal advice that can be given young people with acne is that the condition should not be neglected. The services of a skin specialist should be sought and his advice followed carefully if improvement is to be expected. Present medical treatment of this condition is better than it has ever been before.

It should be expected that progress in the control or prevention of acne will result from current medical research. Even if you have an acne problem that has failed to respond to medical treatment in the past, hope should not be given up.

Fungus Infections

Fungus infections of the feet are commonly called athlete's foot, which is common among the general population. To the skin specialist or the physician in general, athlete's foot is known as dermatophytosis of the feet. It is not a serious disease. Usually the disorder is of a minor nature, although at times this infection can cause more serious discomfort and disability, especially if secondary infections follow the initial disorder.

A major breakthrough has occurred in the treatment of fungus infections of the skin in recent years. Griseofulvin, an antibiotic produced from several different kinds of penicillium, has been found to be highly effective in treatment of certain fungus conditions of the skin. When one

gram of this product is taken by mouth daily, many fungus infections of the hands, feet or other parts of the body may be cured within about three weeks. Badly infected fingernails and toenails have been greatly improved or cured in a matter of months. Athlete's foot usually responds to griseofulvin treatment within three to six weeks.

The antibiotic appears to be quite safe as no serious side effects have been reported to date, although some patients have found it necessary to discontinue treatment because of digestive upsets.

Rapid relief is usually experienced from itching, normal sweating returns within a short time and normal skin and nail growth follows within weeks or months. One fungus infection of 35 years duration was cured within six weeks by griseofulvin according to one New Jersey physician. Of 107 patients, this physician obtained cures in 80 per cent of the cases.

A number of fungi are found normally on the feet and skin disease from this source occurs only when there is some local condition of lowered resistance. Fungi are so prevalent that it would be next to impossible for a person not to be periodically exposed. That fungus disease of the skin does not develop in most persons is due to the normal resistance of the healthy skin.

There are certain things that a person can do to prevent infection with fungi. There are certain measures that can help to maintain or improve the normal resistance of the skin, such as (1) using a nonalkaline, soapless detergent for washing the feet, (2) wearing cotton or wool socks (which absorb moisture) rather than nylon, rayon or other nonabsorbing materials, (3) using perforated shoes during hot weather for better ventilation of the feet, (4) careful drying of the feet, and (5) using a mildly fungistatic foot powder (such as Desenex or some comparable product containing undecylenic acid) which both dries the feet and tends to destroy fungi.

When fungus disease of the feet or

other parts of the body has already developed, the condition should be treated by a physician or a specialist in skin disease (dermatologist). Self-treatment should be avoided, especially because of the hazard of overtreatment dermatitis.

Sunbathing

Exposure of the skin to sunlight does not bring the unmixed rewards that many young people believe. For some persons aggressive sunbathing may be highly injurious to health; moderation for most persons is desirable.

In discussing the effects of sunlight on the skin, Dr. Beatrice M. Kesten, a dermatologist of New York City, says that for centuries people have assumed that sunbathing is beneficial. However, in a report submitted to the Committee on Cosmetics of the American Medical Association in 1956, she observed that a conservative use of sunlight is probably healthful for most persons, but that the current habit of prolonged exposure to sunlight is open to question.

Sunburn is produced by wavelengths of ultraviolet light rays between about 2900 and 3132 angstroms. (One investigator of the problem of sunburn states that wavelengths below 2900 angstroms are not present in sunshine because of the filtering action of the atmosphere.) It is within this so-called sunburn range that the normal white skin absorbs maximum radiation, about 90 to 95 per cent of the rays being absorbed.

Gradual exposure to the sun is always advisable in acquiring a tan. It permits the skin to build up pigmentation that protects the body from damage. The first period of sunbathing should last no more than fifteen minutes during the middle of the day. As each day passes, the length of sunbathing may be extended by a few minutes. The appearance of the skin cannot be taken as a dependable guide to the length

of time for sunbathing. *Reddening does not occur until more than an hour after actual burning of the skin except in very severe burns.*

Although many people, and especially young persons, look upon a suntan as desirable and attractive, the sun may actually produce harmful effects, including sunburn, allergy, photosensitization and aggravation of a number of diseases, including tuberculosis. Habitual exposure to sunlight can be a cause of cancer of the skin, although the occasional act of sunbathing is not a hazard in this respect. Cancer of the skin is a definite occupational hazard among persons who have long exposure to sunlight because of their work.

The intensity of sunshine is no safe criterion of whether or not a person will be sunburned. Even on a dull day there may be much invisible sunburning radiation. The factors controlling the amount of sunburn that may be received include those of latitude, time of day, time of year, elevation, amount of ozone in the upper atmosphere, turbidity of the air and the reflecting qualities of the surrounding environment.

When a person has been sunburned, redness of the skin usually does not appear for two to three hours, hence a sunbather who watches for redness as a clue of when to seek the shade is using a false criterion. Maximum burn or redness does not appear for 10 to 24 hours, after which it gradually subsides for one to seven days, depending on the severity of the reaction.

Swelling and blistering of the skin may develop after the redness. If the sunburn is especially severe, chills, fever and general illness may occur. Pain, of course, appears with the redness or burning of the skin. Peeling may follow even a mild case of sunburn.

The effects of sunburn last much longer than most people realize. Changes in normal skin responses to heat and cold, for example, may persist for as long as 15 months. Degeneration, premature aging, and development of cancer are some of the more permanent reactions of the skin to excessive sunbathing and sunburn.

Suntan preparations may give important protection to the skin, but not all of them are alike in value. The chemical laboratory of the American Medical Association examined fifty-six different suntan creams, lotions and oils in the Chicago area. Of this number thirty did not list the active ingredients they contained. Two of the suntan oils contained an insect repellent which has little value as a light absorber. According to studies reported in 1954, the suntan preparations that contain p-aminobenzoate and tannic acid are among the best screening agents. It would seem advisable to purchase suntan preparations that have one of these two ingredients listed on the label. Some suntan products cause an allergic inflammation of the skin which may appear shortly after the first use or only after years of application. No suntan lotion can be guaranteed to be either safe or effective for all persons. For best results suntan preparations should be applied at least every two hours, and more often if swimming removes the product or if it is removed in some other manner.

Tanning

True tanning begins about two days after exposure to the same ultraviolet rays that cause sunburn. It depends upon the new formation of melanin in the skin, which reaches a maximum after about two to three weeks and then declines after about one month. Tanning is usually completely gone in about 10 months.

New drugs have come on the market in recent years to promote tanning of the skin. Such drugs, taken by mouth, are reputed to minimize the tendency of the skin to burn because the epidermis is "strengthened." Actually, some of these drugs have been suspected by physicians of causing liver damage, nausea, headache, swelling of parts of the body, and even cancer.

Many of the drugs are too new for proper appraisal, hence the sunbather should use them cautiously, if at all, and only under the guidance of a physician.

The use of compounds that are applied externally to the skin for tanning purposes has also become more general. Whether these skin applications are completely safe remains to be seen. Until their harmlessness has been convincingly established it would be well for the sunbather to exercise caution in their use.

Skin Coloring Agents

One of the most popular compounds used in cosmetic preparations that give the user an artificial tan is dihydroxyacetone. This chemical is used in combination with other products and appears to be fairly safe.

Dihydroxyacetone was first used in medicine in the treatment of diabetic coma, cyanide poisoning and other disorders. Only recently was it found that the product could be used to darken the skin and hair by application to these parts of the body.

The safety of the product is being carefully studied although to date only cases of dermatitis have been reported from its use and even this reaction may have been due to other allergenic substances in the cosmetic preparation.

Other skin coloring products have been marketed for external application to the skin. Alcoholic extracts of black walnut are used in some preparations and combinations with dihydroxyacetone are used in others.

It must be reemphasized that while these products appear to be relatively harmless their safety has not yet been fully established. Caution should therefore be exercised in their use.

Products to be taken *internally* for the achievement of skin color changes *are not recommended for tanning purposes*. Such products as meloxine may have medical uses for persons unduly sensitive to sunlight, but internal medications of this sort should be taken only under the guidance of a physician and are not recommended for indiscriminate tanning.

Skin Cancer

Cancer of the skin is frequently discovered by the physician when the patient seeks medical treatment for other disorders. In general, a physician should be consulted when rapid changes occur in the size or color of a mole or other skin blemishes, when there is some skin condition that bleeds frequently, and when there is a sore that is ulcerated or refuses to heal.

A melanoma is the most malignant of all skin cancers, although a majority of such cancers can be prevented through early diagnosis and proper treatment. The melanoma is a tumor made up of pigmented cells and usually has developed from a mole or birthmark which has begun to grow or change in color.

Unfortunately there is a popular misunderstanding that leads some people to believe that surgical removal of a mole or birthmark may be dangerous. This is a mistaken belief. It is advisable that moles and birthmarks be removed when they are in an area of the body such as the belt line, neck or bearded part of the face where frequent injury is likely to occur from shaving, the pressure of clothes, and so on. Moles and birthmarks on the palms of the hands, soles of the feet, genitals and mucous membranes should also be removed as a precautionary measure. Moles or birthmarks of recent origin which are blue or black should be removed as well as those which undergo change during adolescence.

Usually cancer of the skin is a slow-growing disorder which occurs most often on the face. It is probably the main hazard of excessive sunbathing, but this disease is liable to occur only if there has been continued exposure to the sun over a period of many months or years. With men, cancer of the lower lip has been associated with exposure to the sun, whereas this type of cancer is relatively rare in women, probably because of the protection from sunlight which is obtained from lipstick.

Cancer of the lip is a fairly common disease that can be readily diagnosed by the physician and can almost always be cured if it is treated in time.

The National Cancer Institute has estimated that about 50 per cent of all cancers are accessible to direct examination by a physician through sight or touch. *All skin cancers can be seen by the physician, and most can be seen by the patient himself.* When there is delay in seeking advice from a doctor about a skin condition that is found to be cancer, the patient must usually accept a large share of the responsibility for such delay, for medical experience has shown that many people are slow to consult a physician for skin cancer.

Approximately 95 per cent of all skin cancers can be cured completely if the diagnosis is made soon enough. The National Office of Vital Statistics reported in 1960 that nearly 4,000 persons lose their lives annually from cancer of the skin. More than 20,000 other persons suffering from the same disease are cured because they consult the physician in time. Of the 4000 who die of skin cancer, approximately 2700 *could be saved* if an earlier diagnosis is made. The lesson from such statistics is simple enough. If you have any of the signs of a possible cancer of the skin, consult a physician.

Infections of the Skin

A variety of infectious organisms may cause disease of the skin. This was especially true before the development of the antibiotics. These infections were often difficult to cure. Nowadays, most such disorders can be treated successfully with one or more antibiotics.

When infections of the skin are neglected, they sometimes become chronic and may be difficult to cure even with proper medical care. When a person tries to treat a skin condition that he thinks is a simple infection, he often causes an overtreatment dermatitis or fails to check spread of the disease because the wrong treatment is used. The important thing to remember is that *prompt medical care should be sought for infections of the skin.* Even though the antibiotics can cure many skin infections, they may also cause sensitivities that bring about complications of treatment. The only safe procedure is to consult a physician for such treatment *based upon a proper diagnosis of the condition.*

Psychogenic Skin Disorders

For a number of years psychiatrists have observed that some patients get skin disease because of emotional problems. The same observation has been made by skin specialists.

Evidence of the association between emotional problems and skin disease is forthcoming from such studies as the one made by Dr. Harry M. Robinson, Jr., Dr. Raymond C. V. Robinson, and Dr. John F. Strahan, of Baltimore, Maryland. These physicians treated 159 patients who were suffering from various skin diseases with one of the tranquilizing drugs. Forty-one patients with skin diseases were treated with alternating courses of tranquilizing drugs and a placebo. Objective evaluation of forty-one of these patients led to the conclusion that the tranquilizing drug was a valuable help in the treatment of patients with skin diseases in which emotional tension is a factor.

In another study Dr. Richard J. Ferrara and Dr. Hermann Pinkus, of Detroit, reported that they had achieved improvement in thirty-five out of thirty-six patients when their chronic skin disorders were treated by the daily administration of one of the derivatives of the *Rauwolfia serpentina* root. This tranquilizing drug tended to relieve both emotional distress and the skin disorder.

Three physicians at the University of Pittsburgh have reported favorable results in group psychotherapy among patients with certain types of skin disease. In this study it was found that persons who talked freely, showed the least amount of pessimism and expressed the greatest self-confidence also showed the greatest improvement in their skin diseases after the group sessions.

In England Dr. Hugh Gordon investigated the effect of hypnotism in 144 patients suffering from skin disease. The suggestion was made during hypnosis that the skin disease would disappear and that the skin would return to normal. Psychotherapy was later utilized in addition to hypnosis in an effort to improve the skin conditions of the patients involved. In this investigation emotional factors were important in a wide range of common skin disorders. In some instances the skin disease responded completely to psychiatric treatment and hypnotism. One boy, twelve years of age, who had had eczema and asthma from the age of two, was completely cured of both in about six sessions. He was still clear of symptoms two and one-half years later. In another patient who had had a particular skin disease for ten years the disorder cleared up rapidly under hypnosis and psychotherapy, and there had been no recurrence of the skin disease two years afterwards. Dr. Gordon found that the psychic factor was important in estimated degrees of 50 to 100 per cent.

The foregoing studies and descriptions indicate that in many skin diseases there are emotional relationships. It should be obvious that the curing of a skin disease might well have a constructive effect upon the mental health of the patient. It is not always so obvious that by working through the mind of the patient the skin disease itself may be improved.

Burns

Burns are one form of injury to the skin that can create extensive damage, scarring and death. During childhood and old age in particular, burns are a leading accident hazard.

A severe burn to the body surface, amounting to only 8 per cent of the total, can cause severe shock to a child under the age of five years. A burn that affects as much as 12 per cent of the body surface will probably cause shock and threaten death in any child.

The small burn can be covered, kept clean, and treated with a bland ointment. The more severe burn must be carefully appraised by the physician. It is often difficult to estimate accurately the extent of the damage done by a severe burn, and hospitalization is the safest procedure.

Burns must be considered from the viewpoints of shock, loss of body fluid and the shifting of body electrolytes. Red blood cells may be destroyed in severe burns, much protein may be lost from the body tissues, and there may be extensive destruction of skin and the tissues underneath.

The most immediate hazard in severe burn is that of shock. Giving plasma or whole blood by transfusion may be a lifesaving necessity. The relief of pain also helps to combat shock, so that morphine or other drugs may be prescribed by the physician. Antibiotics given internally may be important in the prevention of secondary infections, which constitute a hazard.

Emergency treatment of burns is perhaps best achieved by immediate application of ice water or other comparable cold products. The primary effect of this first aid treatment is the prompt relief of pain.

Besides making the victim more comfortable this can also serve to reduce the amount of shock, since pain aggravates this condition.

The administration of proteins (or amino acids) is essential in severe burns since there has been considerable loss of these nutritional essentials both from the burn itself and also in the oozing of fluid from the tissues after the burn has been treated.

Skin grafting is necessary in most cases of bad burns. The surgeon can graft onto the injured surface of the body large sheets of split-thickness skin from donors or from skin banks with excellent results. In general, the small, pinpoint skin grafts are not as successful as the larger ones.

From the foregoing it should be plain that the badly burned patient needs medical and surgical treatment in a hospital. It is easy to underestimate the seriousness of a burn, especially in children. Burns are a complex problem in the physiology of the body and should be treated by experts. Burns should not be treated with ointments and salves by the person rendering first aid, for this material often has to be removed by the surgeon before the patient can be treated properly in the hospital. The best procedure is to call a physician and let him treat the patient.

Skin Banks

Postmortem skin banks have been urged to meet the needs of badly burned persons and to make it possible to secure skin donations from living persons at convenient times for the latter. The first skin bank was established at the Barnes Hospital in St. Louis.

Many live donors are needed to supply the same amount of skin that could be obtained from a recently deceased person. Although skin grafts taken after death do not survive indefinitely, they may last for twenty to thirty days and thus provide a temporary biological covering that may be lifesaving for the patient.

Human skin can be preserved in usable condition for about three weeks at ordinary refrigerator temperatures. Skin can be stored for several months if special techniques are used.

The banking of skin on a large scale would be extremely valuable in the saving of lives in the event of a mass burn catastrophe such as in an atomic bombing.

Skin Testing for Allergies

Skin testing is often done by the allergist in a search for pollens and foods to which the patient may be sensitive. Skin tests are not infallible, however. A positive reaction reveals a person who may or may not have active clinical or allergic symptoms. Sensitization may be a potential factor or may have existed in the past without present inconvenience.

Skin testing for allergies should be regarded as a method for getting supplementary evidence rather than for reaching definite conclusions without additional evidence of disease. It has been known for some time that skin tests for food allergies have limited value, because sometimes the skin test is negative despite a proved sensitivity to the food involved. In some instances a positive reaction to the skin test may occur without any concrete evidence of a definite food allergy. Reactions to foods may become negative after a person has avoided the food to which he is allergic. On the other hand, the patient may acquire new sensitizations to food that he commonly eats. In general, skin tests for food allergies are more revealing during childhood than in adult life.

Skin tests are sometimes used for their diagnostic values in inflammation of the skin due to work exposure to various chemical compounds. The patch test technique of skin testing consists in the application of a small amount of diluted material which is suspected of damaging the skin. The small amount of test material is covered with a small piece of gauze which is then covered with cellophane and sealed to the skin by adhesive tape. If the patient is sensitive to adhesive tape, the test materials can be held in place with a cotton or elastic bandage. The patch test materials are usually left in place for twenty-four to forty-eight hours before removal, although sometimes the materials are not taken off until after seventy-two hours. It is possible to use an open patch test by the application, for a few seconds or minutes, of the suspected material. The reaction can then be noted at the testing site for several days.

A positive reaction as a result of the skin test may be caused by the primary irritation or sensitization on the part of the person involved. If there is redness, swelling, welt production, blisters and sloughing off of skin, it is apparent that the person has a positive reaction to the test. When no reactions occur, the skin test is judged to be negative.

This type of skin testing cannot be used if the patient suffers from a generalized skin disease. The use of skin irritants such as kerosene, gasoline and strong solutions of acids, vapors and solvents must be avoided.

When properly used, the patch test can be of considerable diagnostic value in the search for substances that are causing occupational dermatitis.

Moles and Melanomas

The average adult has from 15 to 20 moles on his skin. One medical investigator has reported that only about two out of every one million and a half moles are found to be malignant melanomas, a most feared type of skin cancer.

It is, therefore, not the average mole or nevus that a person needs to be concerned about. It is when the mole changes size, becomes elevated, ulcerates, bleeds, deepens in color or shows other definite signs of alteration that a person should consult a physician or surgeon.

Treatment for a mole undergoing suspicious changes is complete surgical removal under local anesthesia by a well-qualified surgeon. Both moles and melanomas are reported to be highly radioresistant; so they should not be treated by radium, X-ray, or radioisotopes. Complete surgical removal remains the treatment of choice. This problem has also been discussed in the section on skin cancer.

Skin Conditions That Need Medical Attention

The Council on Pharmacy and Chemistry of the American Medical Association authorized the publication on February 25, 1955, of the following list of skin conditions that should receive professional medical attention.

1. Injuries to the skin of the scalp, eye, ear and anogenital region of the body.
2. Puncture wounds from nails, glass, slivers, steel wool, thorns, briars, light bulbs and similar materials.
3. Scratches and cuts from contaminated materials.
4. All injuries that cause persistent bleeding.
5. Injuries that have been healing, but begin to ooze or bleed, or show signs of irritation.
6. Burns from chemicals such as acids, alkalies and solvents.
7. Sunburn that has not been relieved by the application of milk of magnesia or calamine lotion without phenol.
8. Bites, when ticks or spiders are suspected as the cause.
9. All animal bites and especially human ones.
10. Irritations and rashes that itch and burn.
11. Skin conditions that show redness and swelling.
12. Suspected infections of the skin.
13. Fungus infections of the skin (no application of medicines should be made until laboratory tests and a proper diagnosis have been made).

The Council observes that: "Little cuts, scratches, and burns should be bandaged with sterile gauze. An ice cube or cold cloth pressed over them will relieve pain. Soap, household cleaning agents, wax, and cosmetics should not be allowed to contaminate them. Bandages should be changed as necessary and the injury kept dry until healing takes place, usually five days to a week. Bandaids may be used providing they allow aeration and are not medicated."

Skin Disease Emergencies

Skin specialists report that there is seldom an emergency in the practice of dermatology in which the life of the patient is at stake. Some diseases can be regarded as semi-emergencies, however, in which much better results can be secured if early diagnosis and treatment are obtained.

Dr. Paul A. O'Leary of Rochester, Minnesota, has described six skin conditions which should be regarded as approximating emergencies which should have immediate treatment. These semi-emergencies are as follows:

1. ACUTE DERMATITIS, in which there is a blistering eruption. Emergency care is needed to relieve the intense itching and to prevent hypersensitization to the offending agent.

2. LUPUS ERYTHEMATOSUS is a disease affecting the entire body and is manifested in skin symptoms and signs, although these may sometimes be rather slight and insignificant even when the disease has progressed to a severe extent. The patient's life may be at stake when this disease has progressed to a considerable extent.

3. URTICARIA in which there is edema or swelling of the throat or tongue may constitute a real emergency. The common name for urticaria is hives. This skin dis-

order, in which there is an eruption of itching wheals, is usually of internal origin from the consumption of foods to which the person is allergic. Ordinarily the patient is uncomfortable and somewhat below par, but his life is not in danger. It is different, however, when there is severe swelling of structures such as the throat or tongue, because this edema may block the air passage and cause asphyxiation. The antihistamine drugs have reduced this danger considerably, although tracheotomy (surgical opening of an airway into the throat below the blocked or swollen area) is sometimes necessary to save a life in this emergency.

4. INFECTIONS OF THE SKIN such as erysipelas, furuncles (boils), carbuncles and impetigo. The use of antibiotics causes a rapid regression of these infections, but when the patient has not sought medical care, there may be an emergency need for such antibiotics, since these conditions are sometimes severe.

5. HERPES ZOSTER, a painful disease in which blisters erupt on the skin, becomes an emergency when the tissues of the eye are involved. The involvement of the cornea of the eye by blisters may result in loss of vision; hence, medical care is a prompt necessity when the eye is involved.

6. ECZEMA (stasis dermatitis) is an emergency condition when it involves the lower parts of the legs and is associated with varicose veins, blood clots or any other condition that impairs the circulation in the legs. Treatment is directed primarily toward the involved limb.

Questions

1. What are some of the psychologic effects in a severe case of acne?
2. Do the advantages of sunbathing outweigh the possible hazards of this practice?
3. Why is it important to have a proper diagnosis of an inflammation of the skin?
4. Why is it difficult for the physician to cure some skin disorders?
5. In the application of ointments to the skin for an inflammation who has the greater responsibility: the physician or you? Why?

For Further Reading

1. Lawrence, Herbert: *The Care of Your Skin*. Boston, Little, Brown and Company, 1955.
2. Sauer, Gordon C.: *Manual of Skin Diseases*. Philadelphia, J. B. Lippincott Company, 1959.

For Advanced Reading

Rook, Arthur: *Progress in Biological Sciences in Relation to Dermatology*. New York, Cambridge University Press, 1960.

12

ACCIDENTS AND FIRST AID

FROM 90,000 to 100,000 persons lose their lives in accidents each year in the United States. In addition to this number of deaths, almost 10,000,000 people are injured in accidents each year. Of this great number of people who are injured annually, more than 300,000 may be permanently disabled.

In each year the cost of accidental deaths and injuries in terms of wages, medical expense, insurance cost and property damage may amount to approximately ten billion dollars or more. In 1958 such accidents cost the nation 12 billion, 100 million dollars, according to the National Safety Council. It can be seen that accidents have emerged as a major public health problem in this country.

Injuries happen from many different causes and in many different places, but *every single one of them could have been prevented,* but in order to prevent accidents we must know their causes. The National Office of Vital Statistics and the National Safety Council keep accurate records of accidents in the United States and summarize these data each year.

> "One of the definite mental blocks in the unceasing drive to reduce injuries to our workers is the use of the word accident when we mean injury."
> **Dr. Arthur Secord, 1959**

From these accurate records we know that injuries are caused by a multiplicity of factors. Deaths are caused from traffic crashes, falls, drownings, burns, railway collisions, firearms, agricultural and forestry mishaps, poison gas, air transport accidents, mechanical suffocation, poisoning, falling roofs and other mishaps in mines and quarries, contact with piercing instruments, lightning, cold, heat, cataclysm, and animals. Many other causes may also be involved in individual accidents.

The National Safety Council classifies the deaths from accidents into four main groups, as follows: (1) motor vehicle accidents, (2) home accidents, (3) occupational accidents and (4) public nonvehicle accidents.

Of these four categories of accidental deaths, the incidence of those in the home and on the highway lead all others by a large margin.

Traffic Accidents

Each year between 35,000 and 40,000 persons are killed, and well over one million persons are injured, in traffic accidents. On December 22, 1951, the one millionth death from traffic accidents in the United States occurred. The first death from an automobile in this country had occurred fifty-two years previously on September 13, 1899, when a New York real estate dealer stepped off a trolley car to assist a woman who was boarding the vehicle. This courteous gesture cost the man his life, for he was struck by a passing automobile and killed.

Many persons do not realize that these one million deaths from traffic accidents represent a loss of life greater than that from all the wars that this country has fought since its beginning.

There are some people who seriously question whether it is possible to reduce traffic accidents any more than we have done to date. There is both theoretical and practical evidence, however, that the death toll and injury rate from highway accidents can be substantially reduced. Theoretically, every accident is preventable. Practical evidence also indicates that when we give further attention to this problem, more lives will be saved. For example, in the first five years after the initial President's Highway Safety Conference, the national traffic death rate was reduced about 35 per cent.

Most drivers who are involved in fatal accidents on the highway are normal people who have been careless enough to take a chance. An analysis of 186 deaths that occurred over a New Year's weekend showed that drunken driving was responsible for only seven of the deaths, and mechanical failure such as defective lights or poor brakes and blowouts caused only five of the deaths; reckless driving and careless pedestrians were involved in the great majority. More than half of the deaths involved too much speed, taking a chance in passing, following a car too closely and similar driving behavior. In other words, most accidents can be prevented by a little more caution, a little more skill and a little more common sense.

> **TEEN-AGE DRIVERS**
> ". . . a survey covering 30 high schools and 20,000 students . . . shows that with proper guidance our teen-age drivers can avoid accidents. . . . Over a three-year period all teen-age drivers have about a 90 per cent chance of a crack-up. . . . Thirty-four per cent of the senior boys (alone) were involved in accidents."
> **James Drought, 1960**

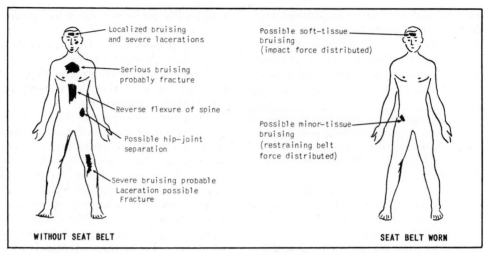

Localized bruising
and severe lacerations

Serious bruising
probably fracture

Reverse flexure of spine

Possible hip—joint
separation

Severe bruising probable
Laceration possible
Fracture

Possible soft—tissue
bruising
(impact force distributed)

Possible minor—tissue
bruising
(restraining belt
force distributed)

WITHOUT SEAT BELT   **SEAT BELT WORN**

Figure 7.   Sites of commonest auto-crash injuries. (Courtesy of Ford Motor Company.)

Crash Studies

Important fundamental research has been conducted in various states and universities within recent years on the effects of automobile accidents on the human body. In Indiana it was found that many accidents result in death of the drivers even though the force of the impact sustained by the body may be well within the limit of survival.

More than 60 per cent of all fatal injuries in the Indiana accidents were due to head or neck fractures. Crash injury research at Cornell University Medical College has shown that the head has terrific momentum when it strikes a dangerous object at 40 to 50 miles an hour. When the head hits an unyielding surface at this speed, the head itself must yield, and crushing injuries of the skull and brain cannot be avoided under such circumstances. On the other hand, if the head strikes a light, fairly strong metal surface which will dent and bend and absorb some of the energy of the blow, then the danger of skull fracture and concussion is somewhat reduced. The Cornell studies suggest that the future construction of automobiles may take into account such findings as those which are emerging from head-impact investigations.

The Indiana studies also reveal that the driver has a better chance of surviving an accident than the person who sits beside him in the front seat. The steering wheel gives some protection to the driver. People in the back seat are exposed to the same crash force, but get some protection from the back of the front seat. Back seat riders frequently survive accidents which are fatal for those in the front seat.

Many injuries and deaths are caused because accessories are mounted inside the automobile, which increase the injury hazard. A safety belt would save lives and prevent many injuries, according to research, but whether such equipment will ever be brought into general use is questionable.

The crash studies at Cornell resulted in four main conclusions: (1) To reduce injuries and deaths from traffic accidents the automobile should be constructed in such a manner that the occupants are not thrown out of the car in an accidental crash. (2) The interior of an automobile must be of sufficient strength to be capable of absorbing at least some of the energy of the crash. (3) The driver or passengers should be immobilized within the automobile in such a way that they are not thrown against dangerous parts of the car during a crash. (4) Some means must be found of transmitting force in an accident to the strongest part of the body.

Seat Belts

Seat belts reduce the frequency and severity of accidental injuries sustained by automobile drivers and passengers.

Studies by the Automotive Crash Injury Research team at Cornell University have shown that in a group of accidents in which the passengers were not wearing seat belts the frequency of injury was approximately 76 per cent. In other words, three out of every four persons in the automobile were injured. In contrast, the frequency of injury in accidents where the passengers were wearing seat belts was only 30 per cent.

Seat belts protect the passengers by reducing the violence of impact when the car strikes something solid. When the passenger is thrown forward from his seat against the dashboard it is the violence of the reduction in speed that occurs when the passenger strikes a hard surface that produces injury. The passenger wearing a seat belt is not exposed to such violence when the car stops. Even if the body does strike some hard part of the car the blow is not nearly so violent because the force has been partially broken by the seat belt.

Seat belts keep people inside automobiles during crashes and this increases the passenger's chance of living and escaping injury. In the Cornell studies it was found that approximately 13 per cent of car occupants who were thrown out were killed, whereas slightly less than 3 per cent of those who were within the cars were killed. The risk of death for those thrown from a car is about five times greater than that of those remaining in the car.

Some people worry about being trapped in an automobile by a seat belt in an accident when the car catches fire. Actually, even in this situation the seat belt is apt to be more protective than people realize. There is less chance that the person retained in his seat with a seat belt will be knocked unconscious. Retaining consciousness, he can easily divest himself of the seat belt under ordinary circumstances.

It is especially important to have seat belts for children in an automobile for they can be thrown forward even by sudden stops in which no accidents occur.

Seat belts can now be obtained at a cost of about fifteen dollars. This covers both the cost of the belt and the installation. Seat belts should meet the standards set by the Society of Automotive Engineers, which cover breaking strength, ease of releasing the buckle and resistance to wear and tear.

On October 30, 1958, the American Public Health Association passed a resolution urging that all government automobiles be equipped with seat belts and that every effort be made to educate the general public to a wider use of seat belts because: "The effectiveness of seat belts in minimizing the degree of injury and the number of deaths resulting from traffic accidents has been demonstrated."

Nearly 50 per cent of all deaths from automobile accidents occur at travel speeds below 40 miles per hour and approximately 65 per cent of such deaths occur within 25 miles of the driver's residence. This kind of information suggests that seat belts should be worn at all times, even in neighborhood driving.

Traffic Speeds and Automobile Accidents

A number of states and research centers have conducted investigations that reveal that excessive speed is a main cause of fatal accidents on the highway. Most people do not travel at high speeds, but those who do endanger the lives of others and, of course, increase their own chances of being killed.

Speed studies in Michigan have shown that approximately 6 per cent of highway drivers travel at a speed under 35 miles an hour. Approximately 57 per cent of the drivers operate their automobiles at speeds between 35 and 50 miles an hour. Some 37

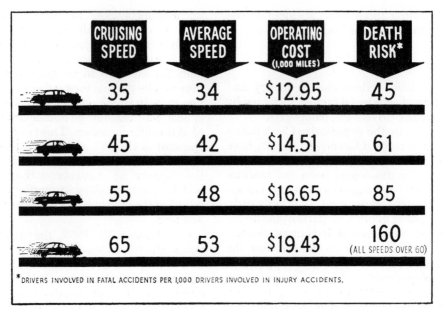

CRUISING SPEED	AVERAGE SPEED	OPERATING COST (1,000 MILES)	DEATH RISK*
35	34	$12.95	45
45	42	$14.51	61
55	48	$16.65	85
65	53	$19.43	160 (ALL SPEEDS OVER 60)

*DRIVERS INVOLVED IN FATAL ACCIDENTS PER 1,000 DRIVERS INVOLVED IN INJURY ACCIDENTS.

Figure 8.   Mathematics proves folly of fast driving. (Courtesy of National Safety Council.)

per cent of the drivers travel at a rate above 50 miles an hour. The average speed for all drivers is approximately 51 miles an hour. Over a ten-year span the Michigan authorities found that approximately the same rate of speed prevailed each year.

In a single year in which 516 drivers were involved in fatal accidents, 53 per cent were guilty of excessive speed. When drivers were traveling under 50 miles an hour, less than 2 per cent of the accidents that resulted throughout the state of Michigan caused deaths. On the other hand, when drivers were driving at more than 50 miles an hour, nearly 6 per cent of all accidents resulted in deaths.

The significance of high speeds can be better appreciated when there is understanding of reaction times of automobile drivers. In Ohio the reaction times of 1000 drivers were studied. The average reaction time for men was 0.57 second, compared to 0.62 second for women.

Few people realize the long distance that a car may travel in the interval before the brakes are applied. For example, a car traveling at 60 miles an hour and driven by a person with average reaction time of nearly 0.57 second will travel about 60 feet or more before the driver can even apply brake pressure. If the car has good brakes and the pavement is dry, the car will travel approximately 367 feet before it can be brought to a standstill. This distance is greater than the entire length of a football field. Obviously, when the car is traveling at a slower speed, it can be brought safely to a stop in a much shorter distance.

The Ohio studies also revealed that reaction times are not much different in the young and the old. The average reaction time for drivers under the age of twenty years was 0.58 second, whereas that for persons over sixty years of age was 0.63 second. This is a difference of only 0.05 second.

The Michigan State Highway Department began using radar in 1950 to check vehicle speeds. Data gathered by the radar speed meter has been used by engineers to set up control regulations and techniques in connection with signs, signals, marking and highway design. The radar speed meter gives the true speed of the vehicle toward which it is directed and makes a graphic record of the speed of every passing vehicle.

The Drinking Driver

It has long been established that when a person drives an automobile after drinking alcohol, his chances of having an accident are greatly increased. Statistics reveal that about one out of every six drivers who are involved in a *fatal* accident has been drinking. About one out of every four adult pedestrians *killed* in traffic accidents has been drinking.

When the concentration of alcohol in the blood is 0.15 per cent and over, the chances of having an accident while driving an automobile are fifty-five times greater than when no alcohol is in the blood stream.

In the past many persons thought that blood tests which proved a driver was intoxicated could not be used against him in court because, in a sense, he would be testifying against himself. This is no longer the case, however.

As early as 1946 the United States Court of Appeals for the District of Columbia had ruled that the prohibition of compelling a man to testify against himself did not exclude the use of his body as evidence. The Court ruled that "his body may be examined either in or out of Court, with or without his consent." On the basis of this decision the police department officials of Washington, D.C., began to take blood samples whenever they suspected a person of being intoxicated, provided, of course, he was involved in an automobile accident or was guilty of an infraction of some traffic law.

When such chemical tests were taken on 277 drivers, 91 per cent were convicted. Prior to the use of chemical tests the conviction rate in cases of this kind was about 65 per cent.

On June 9, 1952, the United States Supreme Court refused to hear an appeal on the ruling of the Colorado State Supreme Court which had upheld the legality of a blood alcohol test done on an unconscious driver.

This case involved a driver who was alleged to be responsible for a head-on collision in which three persons were killed. The driver was taken in an unconscious condition to a hospital where a state patrolman ordered blood samples to be taken. These blood samples were analyzed, and it was found that this driver was intoxicated. Legal counsel for the driver attempted to rule out this evidence at the trial that ensued, but the court held that this important information could be submitted in the case.

The decision of the United States Supreme Court not to hear the appeal from the ruling of the Colorado Court amounted to constitutional approval of blood alcohol tests. In other words, the police have a legal right to do a blood test on any person breaking a law on the public highway if it is suspected that he is intoxicated.

Dangerous Drivers

Drivers who have accidents often have unstable, aggressive or antisocial personalities.

In Detroit a psychiatric clinic is maintained where driver behavior is evaluated. Although it can be assumed that only drivers suspected of being emotionally disturbed or mentally ill would be referred to such a clinic, it is interesting to observe that of 812 traffic offenders studied in the Detroit Psychiatric Clinic, 244 were found to be feeble minded or of inferior intelligence, 101 were emotionally unstable, 18 had compulsive disorders, and 7 were in a state of senile deterioration. It should be obvious that such drivers are a hazard on the public streets and highways.

A University of Colorado School of Medicine research team found the following characteristics in drivers who had had accidents:

1. Less capacity for managing or controlling hostility.

2. Excessive self-centeredness and indifference to the rights of others.

3. Excessive preoccupation with fantasy satisfactions.

4. Fearfulness of loss of life and support and resentment toward persons responsible for depriving them.

5. Less ability to tolerate tension and a need for immediate discharge of their feelings.

Dr. Arnold R. Friesen and Dr. Purcell G. Schube, of Pasadena, California, feel that accident prone drivers should be recognized as belonging in the same categories as those who show egocentricity, aggressiveness, antisocial attitudes, irresponsibility, rebellion, and often low mentality. These two physicians feel that these drivers should be considered as sick people. "A car in the hands of such a driver is as much a weapon as a gun or a club. It can be used, consciously or unconsciously, to kill, maim, mutilate, destroy, eliminate or declare war on an enemy, real or imaginary. It can be used also for suicide, . . ." maintain these two physicians.

Greater attention is needed by the police force and the court on the problem of psychiatric aspects of accidents.

Mechanical Defects and Traffic Accidents

Some years ago a study of traffic accidents on a national scale was made by a committee especially appointed for this purpose by Congress. This investigation revealed that three different factors are generally involved in an accident. If one driver makes a mistake, but all other drivers do not, there may not be an accident, because the faulty driver will be protected by the actions of others. On the other hand, if one driver makes a mistake and then, in addition, has some mechanical defect in his car such as faulty brakes, the chances of having an accident are greatly increased. Furthermore, if another driver acts in a careless manner, then the *accumulation of forces* may be sufficient to cause an accident.

In an early study the Interstate Commerce Commission found that nearly 7 per cent of all traffic accidents involved some mechanical defect in the car. Three main types of defect or failure were revealed in this study. Faulty brakes, defective tires and engine failure led all other causes of accidents when the condition of the automobile was involved. It was found that faulty brakes were three times as important as tires in causing accidents.

Over a six-week period, the police officials of the United States, Canada and Honolulu examined 2,860,346 automobiles and found that one out of every three was being operated with some obvious and hazardous mechanical defect.

In Kansas the highway officials inspected 178,998 automobiles and found 33 per cent defective. These defects were corrected as a result of the checkup. In this study 13,527 cars had defective brakes. In 9866 automobiles the horns were not operating. Windshield wipers were out of commission on 13,060 automobiles, headlight beams were out on 12,105, tires were unsafe on 4564, 18,560 had taillights that were not working and 23,346 had stop lights that were out.

Kansas, incidentally, achieved one of the finest reports in the nation in this study, checking approximately 80,000 more cars than any other state in the union.

A Good Driver's Code

Three physicians from Denver, Colorado, have proposed a code for good driving. Dr. Murray E. Gibbens, Dr. William V. Smith, and Dr. Ward B. Studt believe that if each candidate for a driver's license were required to pledge himself to drive a car by such a code as the following, there would be fewer poor drivers. A condensed version of the proposed code follows:

1. I will keep my car in good mechanical condition at all times. . . .

2. I will never drive after drinking any alcoholic beverage, or after using any type of sedative drugs. . . .

3. I will obey the traffic regulations and speed laws of my city and state. . . .

4. I will never drive when sleepy or exhausted. . . .

5. I will keep alert to driving and traffic conditions. I will concentrate on the road and watch for obstructions . . . at high speeds it is necessary to watch the road for as much as a half-mile ahead. . . .

6. I will be courteous to other drivers and pedestrians. I will carefully note all intersections and give the right of way. . . .

7. I will control my temper at all times, I will not drive if I am angry or emotionally upset. . . .

8. I will always carefully signal my intentions to stop, slow, or turn, by both hand signals and electric signals. I will not turn suddenly, or change traffic lanes, without first checking my rear-view mirrors and signaling my intentions.

9. I will avoid driving close to the car in front of me, so that I may have plenty of time to stop. . . .

10. I will avoid cutting back into the driving lane too soon after passing. . . .

11. I will avoid racing, excessive speed, or show off driving at all times. . . .

12. I will avoid overdriving my headlights at night and will dim my lights for approaching traffic. . . .

13. I will avoid driving too slow in passing lanes or in fast-traffic lanes. . . .

14. I will carefully watch the other driver and his car and try to anticipate his actions or change of course or speed. . . .

15. I will not allow other drivers to use my car unless they also subscribe to these rules of driving.

The National Traffic Safety Program

In recent years national meetings of highway and traffic experts have established a broad national program for safety on the highways. This national traffic safety program has eight aspects, as follows:

1. *A better and more accurate system of keeping accident records* is needed in many cities and states. Such statistical data are used for the prevention of accidents on a limited scale in many parts of the country. When better records are kept and used in a preventive manner, then fewer accidents should occur.

2. *Uniformity of state and local traffic laws and ordinances is needed* throughout the nation. The Uniform Vehicle Code and the Model Traffic Ordinance are two standardized legal approaches to the reduction of traffic accidents. When people encounter the same driving regulations in various cities and states, there should be better communication among drivers through hand signals, road signs, and so on. This should make for greater safety.

3. *Highways should be constructed along sound engineering principles* for the reduction of accidents. Although this may be a very expensive process, it appears to be justified for economic reasons in terms of better transportation facilities as well as for humanitarian reasons in terms of the saving of human lives.

4. *Better enforcement of traffic laws is needed* throughout the United States. Improvements in traffic court procedures are essential as well as better training of traffic officers in courteous and sensible law enforcement on the highways.

5. *Schools need to do a more effective job in traffic safety education.* The elementary schools have done a magnificent job in the operation of safety patrols, but on the high school and college levels not enough work in this field has been done.

6. *Better leadership is needed among public officials* for the adoption of sound policies and procedures on traffic matters. Special emphasis needs to be given to driver licensing, vehicle inspection, and other regulatory measures.

7. *A continuous program of public information* on the activities of official and nonofficial agencies in the field of traffic safety is needed. More funds and more highly trained personnel are needed for this type of work.

8. *More community organizations are needed* from the general public for the support of programs in traffic safety. Such agencies should be on the local, state and national levels.

It is not generally known that the Federal Bureau of Investigation has maintained a traffic education program for police officials since 1935. One part of the program has been the subject of accident investigation. Instruction in this phase of traffic accidents includes instruction in such fundamental procedures as examination of the victim's body, the preservation of evidence, examination of the suspect car, photographing and drawing of the accident scene, and interviews. Other training is concerned with intoxication tests and problems created by the drinking driver. Advanced police training schools are also sponsored by the Bureau in the field of accident prevention.

The Home Accident Problem

Although accidents in the home are of such significance as to constitute a national public health problem, prevention of injuries and deaths in the home from accidents is primarily a problem for individual families and local groups.

Public health authorities, however, can make substantial contributions to the solution of the problem by conducting research and investigations of hazards and behavior that injure and destroy occupants of the home.

Each year between 25,000 and 30,000 people die from accidents in the home. An additional four to five million people receive injuries that are not fatal, although many of them result in permanent disability.

There are six leading causes of accidental deaths in the home: falls, asphyxiation, burns, poisons, suffocation and firearms.

Although suffocation is listed as one of the leading causes of death from accidents in the home, there is serious doubt as to whether many cases should be classified in this category. For example, research has shown that many infants found dead in their cribs have not died of suffocation even though they may be found in a position that suggests this as a cause of death. Rather, autopsies have shown that many such infants had been handicapped by defective development of the respiratory system. In such cases death was only a matter of time rather than a consequence

of suffocation by bed-clothes or sleeping position.

Slightly more than 1,000 persons are accidentally killed by firearms in the home each year. This is about half the total number of deaths in the United States from this cause. The best ways of preventing deaths and injuries from firearms is through the careful instruction of both children and adults in the safe handling of guns, the removal of guns from the reach of children and the careful handling of guns in general.

Falls

Nearly 12,000 persons die from falls *within the home* each year in the United States. Falls lead all other causes of head injuries that are serious enough to call for hospital admissions. A study made at the Detroit Receiving Hospital of the causes of head injuries to 892 persons who were brought consecutively to the hospital showed that falls lead all other causes. The statistics of this investigation are shown in an accompanying table.

The National Office of Vital Statistics has shown that deaths from falls occur overwhelmingly in the older population. For example, between the ages of five and fourteen only 1 death a year can be expected in every 100,000 persons; during that same year deaths from falls of people over the age of 85 can be expected to range between 500 and 1000 in every 100,000 persons. Deaths from falls begin to be more prominent after the age of 55 and much more so after the age of 65.

Many factors are involved in falling. Often with an old person who has fallen and suffered a fatal hazard, some other contributing cause, more important than the fall itself, is the cause of death. A slight stroke, for example, may cause a person to fall and die, but unless an autopsy were performed the cause of death might be attributed only to the fall.

Falls are especially hazardous for the very young and the very old. The waxing of floors and the use of nongripping rugs are especially hazardous. Many other factors may be involved, such as careless disposal of toys and other objects on floors and stairways. Only good housekeeping and a sensitivity to accident hazards can be expected to reduce the number of injuries and deaths from falls in the home.

Burns

Nearly 6,000 people die each year from burns received in the home. Most of these burns occur to children under the age of four and to adults over the age of sixty-five. It is estimated that burns cause the death of a child every four hours in the United States. Open fires, boiling water, hot cooking oils and cigarette lighters account for many injuries and deaths from burns. Especially to protect children, parents should turn pot handles inward on the stove and should keep matches and cigarette lighters well out of reach of children. In older persons it is important not to smoke in bed, for many a death from burns in the adult age group results from falling asleep while smoking.

EMERGENCY TREATMENT OF BURNS. Dr. Alex G. Shulman of Los Angeles has reported an effective new treatment for burns in a group of 150 patients. This new

FATAL HOME ACCIDENTS IN SAN JOSE, CALIFORNIA OVER A 12-YEAR PERIOD

Rank	Type of Accident	Total
1	Falls	118
2	Asphyxiation	21
3	Burns	17
4	Poisoning	17
5	Drowning	7
6	Firearms	7
7	All others	6
	Total	192

From: Bissell, Dwight Montgomery and Robert S. McInnes. Accident Control: A local health department's experience in development and evaluation of a home accident program, Am. J. Pub. Health, 49:1646–52 (No. 12), Dec. 1959.

HEAD INJURIES IN 892 PERSONS ADMITTED TO THE DETROIT RECEIVING HOSPITAL

Rank	Source of Injury	Number
1	Falls	323
2	Automobile accidents	312
3	Blunt blows to head	252
4	Gunshot wounds	5
	Total	892

From Hilst, W. D. and Aage Nielsen: The treatment of acute craniocerebral injuries. Am. J. Surg., 99:702–06, (No. 5), May, 1960.

method of rendering first aid for serious burns is the immediate immersion of the burned area in a large container of cold water to which ice cubes and a disinfectant such as hexachlorophene (pHisoHex) are added.

Dr. Shulman treated burns of all degrees in which less than 20 per cent of the body surface was affected, by plunging the burned areas into baths of ice water. When ice water was not immediately available he used ice cold compresses as promptly as possible. Relief of pain was the most immediate effect. In almost every instance the burned person expressed profound relief and gratitude because of the relief from pain. No infections were encountered in any of the patients who received this treatment within one hour of being burned. Although pain usually lasts about 24 hours or more in a first degree burn, the relief in these patients was immediate and pain was almost totally absent by the time the patient left the doctor's office.

Not only was there prompt relief of pain, but the burns appeared to heal more promptly and with less tissue destruction than under other kinds of treatment. Dr. Shulman found that redness and blistering from burns was also visibly reduced and that in general there was more rapid healing.

It is suggested that immersion in ice water replace other first aid practices in the immediate treatment of burns.

Poisonings

Household poisonings constitute a special hazard for children. A number of studies have shown that a great variety of poisonous substances are available in most homes. In one investigation of 221 cases of poisoning of children it was found that fifty-nine different poisons were involved.

Heading the list were kerosene, arsenic and oil of eucalyptus. A smaller number of poisonings involved the use of phenolphthalein, pine oil, barbiturates, salicylates, and many other substances.

Poisonings in the home are commonly associated with such substances as kitchen drain cleaners, insecticides, rat poisons,

	CLASS A FIRES Wood, paper, trash	CLASS B FIRES Flammable liquids	CLASS C FIRES Electrical equipment	USUAL OPERATION	RANGE	SERVICE BY
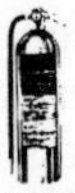 STORED PRESSURE	YES	NO	NO	Squeeze handle or turn valve	30'-40'	Check air pressure
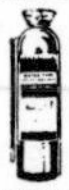 CARTRIDGE OPERATED	YES	NO	NO	Turn upside down and bump	30'-40'	Weigh gas cartridge Add water if required
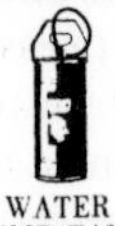 WATER PUMP TANK	YES	NO	NO	Pump handle	30'-40'	Discharge and fill with water annually
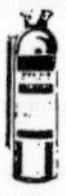 SODA ACID	YES	NO	NO	Turn upside down	30'-40'	Discharge annually Recharge
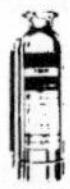 FOAM	NO But will control small fires	YES	NO	Turn upside down	30'-35'	Discharge annually Recharge
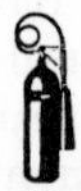 CO_2	NO But will control small surface fires	YES	YES	Rupture cartridge-squeeze release	2'-4'	Weigh semi-annually
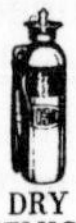 DRY CHEMICAL	NO But will control small surface fires	YES	YES	Rupture cartridge-squeeze release	6'-12'	Weigh gas cartridge Check dry powder

Figure 9. Types of fire extinguishers. (*Action for Safety,* *13*:3, May, 1960.)

drugs and so on. Spoiled foods are also a source of illness, although, in most cases, food infections involving disease-producing microorganisms rather than food poisonings from toxic chemicals are the consequence of the consumption of such products.

Tablets containing strychnine cause many fatal poisonings among children. These tablets are sometimes sugar coated and look like candy. Children have been known to eat as many as fifty of these pills and go into convulsions before parents realize that something is wrong. In a study of 158 deaths that occurred from poisonings in the home in the state of New York, it was found that almost half of all the fatalities were due to strychnine. The cases of strychnine poisoning were due to the use of cathartic and "tonic" pills that contained this drug.

Poisonings from kerosene and gasoline are common among children. When a child has consumed either of these substances, vomiting, diarrhea and abdominal cramps usually begin within a few minutes. Convulsions and coma follow, often within a short time. On the average, about 5 to 10 per cent of the persons poisoned with kerosene die, usually in less than twenty-four hours. The patient who is still alive after twenty-four hours is likely to recover completely and promptly. The cause of death is apparently a type of pneumonia in the sense that the lungs become filled with fluid. Children have recovered from drinking as much as 125 cc. of kerosene, although deaths have occurred from the ingestion of as little as 30 cc. of the product.

Each week about two children in the United States die from aspirin poisoning. Many other children are saved by medical treatment after swallowing great numbers of aspirin tablets. Although aspirin is frequently used to lower fevers in persons suffering from communicable diseases, an overdose, as in a poisoned child, causes a very high fever. Blood vessels are also damaged, so that the child may suffer from nosebleeds and internal hemorrhage. Difficult breathing, vomiting and coma may also occur, depending upon the amount of aspirin swallowed.

Aspirin has a valuable function to perform in the treatment of minor ailments, but small children should not be able to get to the aspirin bottle. When aspirin poisoning does occur, a physician should be notified at once and the child should be rushed to the emergency hospital. As with all poisonings, the container should be taken along so that the physician may make a rapid and correct identification of the poisonous materials.

Some children have died from eating a certain type of black shoe dye which contains nitrobenzene. This is a powerful poison. It is readily absorbed through the skin as well as by inhalation. When a child eats the shoe dye, there is especial danger to life.

Most children will survive poisonings if the physician is called promptly and first aid measures are given. In the study previously reported, in which 221 children were hospitalized for accidental poisonings, only 1 per cent of the children died, although the time between the poisoning and medical treatment ranged from about one-half hour to a full hour. If a physician is called promptly, there should be better than a 99 per cent chance that the child will survive the poisoning.

The best first-aid measure is to get the child to vomit. This can cause a substantial removal of poison from the stomach. Another effective protective measure is to give the victim milk or raw eggs. This slows down the absorption of the poison in the stomach. When the doctor is called, he should be informed of the type of poison involved, if it is known.

The best protection against poisoning in the home is to keep all substances containing poisons out of the reach of children and to mark them carefully so that adults and older children will recognize that poison is contained in them.

A number of "poison centers" have

been established in some of the leading cities in the United States. By calling these centers, the physicians in any part of the United States can get accurate information as to the poisonous ingredients of a great many products. He can also get the advice of a specialist as to how to treat the poisoned patient.

First Aid

Many people hesitate to render first aid when it is needed because of a sense of incompetence. This hesitation, perhaps a natural one, can cost a human life.

It may be helpful to the average person to realize that *there are only two emergency situations that demand instant action.* These two emergencies are (1) *serious bleeding* and (2) *stoppage of breathing.* In all other emergencies there is at least a little time in which to act, but in these two situations *a decision must be made immediately and first aid begun at once, or a life may be lost.*

Serious Bleeding

The loss of one quart of blood in an adult and a smaller amount in a child can have serious consequences. If a large blood vessel has been cut, this amount of blood can be lost *within one minute or less.*

This does not leave much time for reflection. External bleeding should be obvious when an injured person is inspected. If bleeding is extensive, it can be controlled by immediate application of pressure *directly over the wound* or at a so-called pressure point. In most cases it is much simpler to apply pressure immediately over the bleeding point. Many per-

sons who have received training in first aid may find it difficult to remember just where the pressure points are located, or may find it difficult to find the particular blood vessels at the recommended pressure points because of the size or weight of the injured person or their own lack of memory.

It is, therefore, advisable to think first of the application of pressure immediately on the bleeding point. This is best done by the application of a compress. A compress is simply a thick wad of cloth. A compress can be made by folding a towel, handkerchief or other cloth into an appropriate square and then putting this directly over the wound. The compress should then be bound into place as firmly as possible. Use a clean cloth if you have one at hand, but don't worry about using a cloth that is not clean if that is all you have. The important thing is to stop the bleeding; infection can be countered by the physician. If the compress becomes soaked with blood, it should not be removed. This may start further serious bleeding. *Another compress* can be added over the first one and bound in place.

If a tourniquet is applied, it should be placed near the wound, but not immediately adjoining it. The tourniquet should be applied tightly enough to stop bleeding and should not be released except by a physician. There is a mistaken belief that all tourniquets should be released every ten or fifteen minutes in order to prevent gangrene. This is not so. Battleground experiences with tourniquets have shown that they may be left in place for four or five hours without injury. It is well, however, to make a written record of the time the tourniquet was applied so that the physician may be properly guided. This record should be on the patient in such a manner that it can be readily seen. Tourniquets should be made of materials that are at least 1 or 2 inches wide in order to prevent damage to tissue. Wire or string, for example, may do more harm than

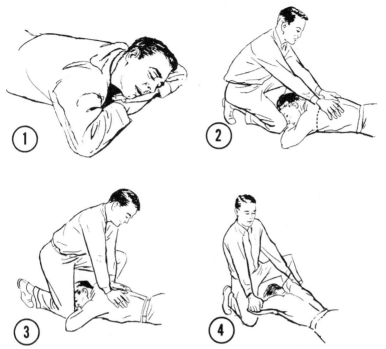

Figure 10. Artificial respiration. The back-pressure, arm-lift method.

1. Place the victim face-down, bend his elbows and place his hands one upon the other, turn his head slightly to one side and extend it as far as possible, making sure that the chin is jutting out.
2. Kneel at the head of the victim. Place your hands on the flat of the victim's back so that the palms lie just below an imaginary line running between the armpits.
3. Rock forward until the arms are approximately vertical and allow the weight of the upper part of your body to exert steady, even pressure downward upon the hands.
4. Immediately draw the victim's arms upward and toward you, applying enough lift to feel resistance and tension at his shoulders. Then lower the arms to the ground. Repeat this cycle about 12 times per minute, checking the mouth frequently for obstruction.

(American National Red Cross.)

good, and should not be used for a tourniquet.

Cessation of Breathing

If a person has stopped breathing, it should be apparent that he does not have long to live unless he is able to begin respiration again. The heart continues to beat for only a short time after breathing has stopped, so that first aid in the form of resuscitation must be started as rapidly as possible.

Artificial Respiration

In the last decade a number of different procedures for giving artificial respiration have created some confusion in the public mind as to their use and effectiveness. Most notable among the methods of artificial respiration are the arm-lift, back-pressure and the mouth-to-mouth techniques.

Mouth-to-Mouth Artificial Respiration

Careful tests have shown that the mouth-to-mouth technique of artificial

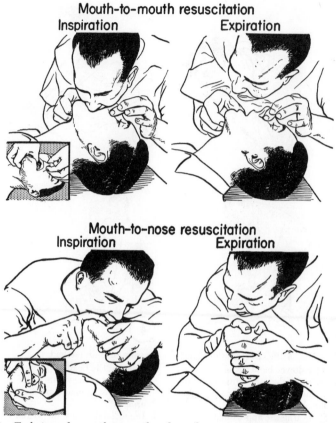

Mouth-to-mouth resuscitation
Inspiration   Expiration

Mouth-to-nose resuscitation
Inspiration   Expiration

Figure 11. Techniques for mouth-to-mouth and mouth-to-nose resuscitation. (Gordon, Archer S., et al.: Mouth-to-mouth versus manual artificial respiration for children and adults. J.A.M.A., *167*:326, 1958.)

respiration is the most effective method of rendering resuscitation when a person has stopped breathing from any cause.

There are several objections to this form of artificial respiration which make it wise for a person to learn more than one technique for resuscitation. A major objection to mouth-to-mouth breathing is that many people will have a natural hesitancy to enter into the intimate relationship that this method involves. This is to be expected especially among strangers and adults. Compounding this natural hesitancy for putting one's mouth to the mouth of another is the fear of possible infection with some contagious disease. Widespread national publicity was given

during 1960 to the New York City patrolman who used this method of artificial respiration only to discover later that the person he had tried to save had died of spinal meningitis. Fortunately, in this instance, the officer did not develop the disease. Other exposures have been reported, however.

Another disadvantage of mouth-to-mouth breathing is the reluctance of people to engage in training programs for the development of needed skills. Probably the natural hesitancy to engage in personal contact is the major cause of the deficiency of enrollments for learning the technique.

Attempts have been made to circumvent the objectionable parts of mouth-to-mouth breathing by the development of a mouth-to-mask resuscitator and by the production of artificial training devices.

The disadvantage of any mouth-to-mask device is that the average person would not have at his immediate disposal any such mechanical aid under ordinary circumstances when it might be necessary to render artificial respiration.

Attention has been called to the dangers of artificial airways when they are used by people who do not understand the anatomy and physiology of the air passageways, as well as the techniques of inserting such airways.

Sometimes the tongue has been pushed back into the throat so that blocking of the normal breathing route has resulted. Sometimes airways have been forced into the mouth when the jaws were closed with resultant injury to gums and teeth.

Some physicians maintain that an artificial airway device is not necessary because the same results can be achieved by putting the head in a proper position and elevating the jaw. If the mouth-to-mouth method of artificial respiration is used, the proper position of the head is one of hyperextension. The neck, too, is hyperextended. After this positioning of the head, there should be a forward movement of displacement of the lower jaw. This arrangement permits air to pass freely into and out of the victim's airway.

Arm-lift, Back-pressure Method

The arm-lift, back-pressure method of artificial respiration proved to be of much greater value than the old and widely known Schafer prone-pressure method. Actual measurement of the amount of air that goes in and out of the lungs during these two methods has shown that 1056 cubic centimeters of air are exchanged with the arm-lift, back-pressure method, in contrast to 485 cubic centimeters of air with the Schafer method. This method of artificial respiration should be demon-

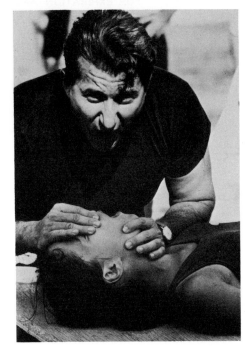

Figure 12. The beginning of mouth-to-mouth resuscitation as demonstrated by Dr. Theodore R. Struhl of the American Red Cross, and his daughter Wendy. Note closure of the nostrils and holding of chin to maintain open airway through the mouth and throat as air will be blown into the lungs. (Courtesy of Physician's News Service, Inc., and Frank Zagarino.)

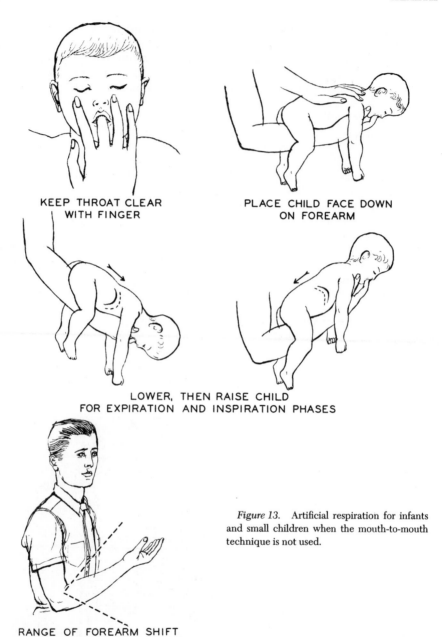

KEEP THROAT CLEAR
WITH FINGER

PLACE CHILD FACE DOWN
ON FOREARM

LOWER, THEN RAISE CHILD
FOR EXPIRATION AND INSPIRATION PHASES

RANGE OF FOREARM SHIFT

Figure 13. Artificial respiration for infants
and small children when the mouth-to-mouth
technique is not used.

strated by the instructor and practiced by
the individual, if confidence in its application is to be gained. The basic procedure
involves the placing of the patient face
downward and then alternation of a lifting

of the victim's arms and application of
pressure on the back of the chest.

A method of artificial respiration for
infants and small children is illustrated
above.

Questions

1. Why do some authorities believe accidents outrank heart disease and cancer as a leading health problem in the United States?

2. Why do most accidents in the home occur to children and old people?

3. Is an accident-prone person one who is bound to have more accidents because of his personality, or is he one who happens to work or live in an environment in which more accidents can be expected?

4. Can *all* accidents be prevented?

5. What can a community do to reduce home accidents?

6. What are the two greatest emergencies in the field of first aid? Why is it that on-the-spot aid must be given immediately?

7. What are the arguments for and against the use of seat belts in automobiles.

8. In a training program, how would you overcome the reluctance of some people to use mouth-to-mouth breathing?

For Further Reading

1. Dreisbach, Robert H.: *Handbook of Poisoning: Diagnosis and Treatment.* Los Altos, California, Lange Medical Publications, 1959.

2. Florio, A. E., and Stafford, G. T.: *Safety Education.* New York, McGraw-Hill Book Company, 1956.

3. Garland, T. O.: *Artificial Respiration.* New York, Macmillan Company, 1955.

4. Henderson, John: *The Complete Book of First Aid.* New York, Bantam Books, 1955.

5. National Safety Council: *Accident Facts.* Chicago, The Council, Annual Report.

6. Schulzinger, Morris S.: *The Accident Syndrome.* Springfield, Ill., Charles C Thomas, 1956.

For Advanced Reading

1. Astock, Herbert J., and Elkow, J. Duke: *Education for Safe Living.* Englewood Cliffs, New Jersey, Prentice-Hall, Inc., 1957.

2. Hyman, Albert Salisbury: *The Acute Medical Syndromes and Emergencies.* New York, Landsberger, 1959.

3. Kulowski, Jacob: *Crash Injuries: The Integrated Medical Aspects of Automobile Injuries and Deaths.* Springfield, Ill., Charles C Thomas, 1956.

Recommended Films

1. *Safety Through Seat Belts.* 16 mm., black and white, sound, showing time 13½ minutes, 1960. Communicable Disease Center, Audio-visual, Atlanta 22, Georgia.

2. *Accidents Don't Just Happen.* 16 mm., color, sound, showing time 13½ minutes, 1958. Communicable Disease Center, as above (rental) and Creative Arts Studio, Inc., (purchase), Washington, D.C.

13

SAFETY IN SPORTS

MANY college students engage in a variety of physical sports with an intensity and vigor that will be equaled at no other time of life.

Participation in college sports and comparable activities may bring many personal rewards in terms of psychologic satisfaction, social adjustment, inner discipline, improvements in physical qualities such as coordination and endurance, and other favorable results.

Engaging in sports may be hazardous also, because speed, force, violence of physical effort, and emotional concentration heighten the possibility of injury in body contact and physical interaction.

Knowledge of accident hazards that are most commonplace in sports may alert the participant to the often unrecognized possibility of their occurrence. Understanding the ways in which these accidents can be prevented should increase the pleasure of engaging in sports and may save a participant serious injury or even death.

> "The first right of the athlete is good coaching ... good equipment is second ... the third right of the player is good medical care."
> Dr. Thomas P. Quigley, 1957

Not all of the sports that appeal to the college-age person will be discussed in this chapter, but enough will be considered so that the nature of most sports injuries will be apparent and the general pattern of their prevention should become obvious.

Types of Injuries

The types of injuries sustained in sports have been studied by Dr. Augustus Thorndike of Harvard University. Dr. Thorndike found over a period of 20 years that sprains and muscle contusions led all other kinds of injuries from athletics. A more complete indication, from the Harvard study, of the kinds of injuries sustained in athletics is supplied in the following table:

Rank	Injury	Totals
1.	Sprain	1612
2.	Muscle contusion	1016
3.	Strain	885
4.	Fracture and dislocation	738
5.	Simple contusion	570
6.	Inflammation and infection	546
7.	Miscellaneous	512
8.	Joint contusion	430
9.	Laceration and abrasion	415
10.	Internal injury	366
	Total	7090

Exclusion from Athletics Because of Injuries

Dr. Thorndike believes that certain ath-

letes who have been injured in sports should thereafter be excluded from participation. He believes that no student athlete who has suffered three brain concussions of moderate intensity or one concussion that has involved laceration of the brain should be permitted to engage in body contact sports. He feels that contact sports should be restricted for anyone who has had the removal of the spleen or a kidney or who has had such extensive surgery as to leave a large abdominal scar. Dr. Thorndike would not restrict these athletes from participating in other selected sports but would exclude them from body contact activities.

The loss of an eye should also lead to a restriction of athletic participation according to this physician because of the great importance of vision and the possibility that an injury to the remaining eye might cause blindness. Some physicians believe that the loss of any paired organ of the body should result in restriction from many sports.

Fatal Injuries in Sports

Dr. Thomas A. Gonzalez of New York City reported a study of deaths from sports injuries that occurred in that city during a period of thirty-two years. Dr. Gonzalez found that 104 persons had died while participating in various sports during this time. The results of this investigation are summarized in the following table:

Rank	Sport	Number of Cases
1.	Baseball	43
2.	Football	22
3.	Boxing	21
4.	Basketball	7
5.	Handball	3
6.	Soccer	2
7.	Wrestling	2
8.	Cricket	1
9.	Golf	1
10.	Polo	1
11.	Relay races	1
	Total	104

Injuries in Different Sports

In most studies of college sports, differences will be found in the accident hazard of specific activities. In some sports accidents and injuries will be more numerous simply because larger numbers of persons are participating rather than because of greater inherent dangers. A sport that yields few injuries may also provide the more severe ones, but in general an activity that injures the greater number of students will be looked upon as the larger problem from the medical viewpoint. The exception to this will occur only when severe injuries or fatalities appear to characterize a sport, even though it may have far fewer casualties.

At Yale University, Dr. Henry M. Parrish classified injuries in sports over a period of four years as part of a much larger study of accidental deaths among college students. The number of injuries occurring in various sports during this period of four years is indicated in the following table:

Rank	Sport	Injuries
1.	Football	2,019
2.	Basketball	630
3.	Soccer	318
4.	Hockey	310
5.	Skiing	281
6.	Baseball	261
7.	Wrestling	242
8.	Squash	223
9.	Lacrosse	219
10.	Track	169
11.	Crew	169
12.	Swimming	92
13.	Tennis	84
14.	Handball	66
15.	Softball	58
16.	Boxing	53
17.	Rugby	42
18.	Fencing	27
19.	Golf	23
20.	Polo	17
21.	Ju-jitsu	14
22.	Volleyball	12
23.	Ping-pong	9
24.	Bowling	5

From such studies as the foregoing we can see at once that major college sports such as football and basketball have more injuries than milder activities such as ping-pong and bowling. Vigorous sports such as boxing and ju-jitsu, which ranked 16th and 21st respectively in the Yale study, also produced far fewer injuries. Pertinent questions about these sports would concern the number of persons participating in these activities (as opposed to the number of accidents) and the severity of the accidents that did occur.

Football

There were 108 deaths associated with the playing of football in the United States during the five-year period from 1955 to 1959. Not all of these deaths were directly attributed to the game itself. Twenty-seven of the deaths were caused by heat stroke, heart failure or other conditions during football practice or a football game. Eighty-one of the deaths were directly associated with the game. Tackling was responsible for more than one fourth of the fatalities.

Fifty-one of the eighty-one deaths that were directly due to football were among high school players. Slightly less than 2 high school players out of every 100,000 engaged in the game were fatally injured over this five-year period. The rate was slightly higher for college football, but approximately the same.

On the basis of the foregoing figures football cannot be considered a hazardous sport from the viewpoint of probable death. Thousands of college students of football-playing age will be injured or killed in motor vehicles and normal activities for every fatality in football. This same statement can be applied to every sporting activity. Deaths in sports, when they do occur, result from circumstances that are not typical of the activities. Football injuries are a different matter.

According to Dr. Thomas F. Dowd, physician for the Philadelphia Eagles Football Club, severe injuries to the knee are the greatest problem in football. In complete tears of the ligaments of the knee, there is a need for prompt surgery if permanent damage is to be prevented and the player is to be rehabilitated. In a number of professional football players prompt surgery for knee injuries has enabled the player to return to football with complete efficiency of the joint. The player who has torn the inside knee ligament is apt to hear a distinct "pop" at the time of the injury. Although there may be little pain, there is great instability of the joint.

THE KNEE

"Ligamentous injuries to the knee are among the most common of the permanently incapacitating injuries received in football."

Dr. James Daly, 1958

Dr. Thomas B. Quigley of Harvard University has reported that the five most common knee injuries that occur in athletes are contusion and ligament sprain, meniscus injury, ligament rupture, fracture, and epiphyseal displacement. Injury to the soft tissue around the knee may be painful and temporarily disabling but contusions and sprains of this kind are often not so serious as to preclude a return to function within a short while. For severe injuries of this kind, ice packs should be applied at once to reduce hemorrhage into the surrounding tissues. Elevation and compression also help to reduce swelling. Rest is then necessary for healing. Heat should not be applied until after a period of 24 hours.

The rupture of a ligament needs prompt medical and surgical treatment. Pain and muscle spasm is apt to occur from this kind of injury after about 15 to 20 minutes.

Surgery is usually necessary for meniscus injuries.

Epiphyseal injury occurs seldom and usually in the femur. After manipulation under general anesthesia, it is usually necessary that the knee be placed in a cast for at least eight weeks.

Surgery on the knee because of football injuries can be very successful, as is shown in Figure 14 on page 159 of the results obtained by Dr. Don H. O'Donoghue, although the final outcome is significantly related to the amount of damage done to the knee.

Accident insurance figures from the Security Life and Accident Company of Denver indicate that a football player has about one chance in 38 of having one or more teeth chipped, broken or knocked out if he does not wear a mouth guard, but that if he uses this protection he has only one chance in 3,600 of receiving a serious dental injury.

According to Dr. Leonard S. Morvay, an oral surgeon of Newark, New Jersey, football is responsible for most athletic dental injuries. Football accounts for about twice as many injuries to the teeth as basketball and about four times as many as wrestling.

Dental injuries do not always result in the loss of a tooth. If a tooth is loose following an injury, the player should see a dentist as quickly as possible and should take only liquid foods if his visit to the dentist is delayed. Dr. Morvay reports that "even teeth that have been hanging on by a thread may tighten and become permanently stabilized within a week or ten days after treatment."

Any tooth that has been knocked out should be wrapped in clean cloth or sterile gauze and should be taken to the dentist. If the player gets to the dentist promptly there may be success in replanting the tooth. In most cases this cannot be done if there is a delay of more than two or three hours following the dislodgment of the

---

INJURIES

"In the foreseeable future, with the increased use of softer, but amply protective padding, a significant decline in football injuries can be envisaged ... A wider use ... of closing-cell foam plastics ... is advocated.

Dr. Alexius Rachun and
Frank J. Kavanagh, 1959

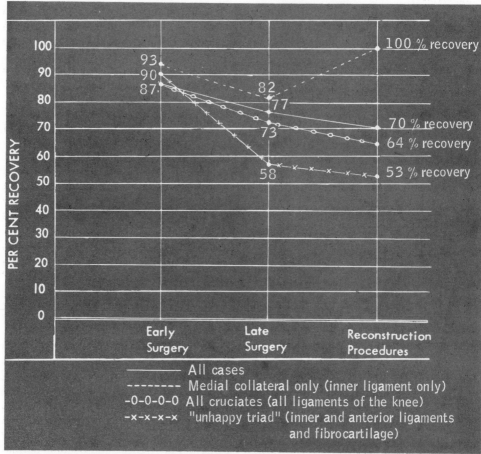

Figure 14. Final results of surgery on the knee for athletic injuries. (O'Donoghue, Don H.: Injuries to the knee. Am. J. Surg., 98:463–76, Sept., 1959.)

tooth. Replaced teeth seldom last permanently but they may survive for 10 to 15 years according to Dr. Morvay.

Baseball

Baseball ranked first in the number of deaths from sports injuries that occurred in New York City over a period of thirty-two years and baseball injuries ranked sixth at Yale University over a period of four years. The general conclusion is that fatal injuries do not often occur in this sport. There have been no deaths due to baseball in the major leagues since 1920. It is estimated that, although more than two million boys participate on baseball teams each year, there are few fatal injuries.

Some physicians have maintained that little league baseball can prove harmful to the health of participating boys. These physicians believe that the sport may stimulate the child excessively and that there is a greater risk of injury during periods of rapid growth, especially in respect to dislocations of joints and bone injuries. The primary objections of these physicians are centered around the strong desires of some adults and communities for winning teams.

A SIMPLE TEST FOR LITTLE LEAGUERS

"A simple test for parents: can he laugh while he plays? If he can, don't worry."

John Kord Lagemann, 1958

Creighton J. Hale has reported that pre-high school children benefit from athletic experience. His studies indicate that participation in little league baseball and other such sports does not cause behavior difficulties, disturbances of social adaptations, unsatisfactory character traits or psychoneurotic reactions. On the contrary, he has found that children who participate in competitive athletics have social status and prestige with their peers and show many signs of good adjustment and desirable personality.

One of the most dangerous injuries in baseball occurs when a ball strikes the head. In recent years the use of a protective baseball helmet has become widespread and this should be mandatory equipment for every batter. In 1959 a new type of baseball helmet was developed which keeps the pitched ball from coming into contact with the head and prevents the force of the blow from being communicated to the brain.

When it is realized that most big league pitchers can throw a baseball at a velocity of 90 to 100 miles an hour and that some little league or middle league pitchers can throw at a velocity up to 70 miles an hour, it can be seen that serious head injury may occur if the ball strikes an unprotected head.

Baseball catchers are more apt to be injured than any other player, according to major league reports. Catchers are especially apt to be injured if the ball strikes the ends or backs of the fingers. This frequently happens, because the catcher does not have time to move his hands for a ball that has been tipped by the bat. Keeping the fingers of the ungloved hand closed is about the only protection the catcher has against this hazard. The catcher also uses the muscles of the thigh to an abnormal extent because of his catching stance. Although the catcher is well insulated against injuries by a mask, fist protector and leg guards, the 100 mile an hour baseball thrown by some pitchers occasionally breaks through this armament to injure the catcher.

Chronic inflammation and irritation of the elbow and shoulder are frequent disabling injuries for baseball players. Sometimes the general health of the player is at fault rather than any direct injury to the elbow or shoulder. Physicians sometimes report that infected teeth or infected tonsils are associated with the inflamed joints. Bone deposits in the shoulders of baseball players sometimes occur because of the excessive use of the shoulder. These bony deposits may produce irritation of joint membranes and other portions of the shoulder. Pain and discomfort after hard throwing may be disabling.

Elvera Skubic reported a study of 100 baseball players between the ages of eight and fifteen and found that this group had suffered 244 injuries from the sport. The most serious injuries included 69 sprains and 5 broken bones. Of the 100 boys, 27 had not been injured at any time during the baseball season.

More complete information on this study is given in the table on the next page.

Basketball

Dr. Simon Ball, physician for the Philadelphia Warriors, believes that a basketball player reaches the peak of his skill and ability about the age of 27 and that he can maintain this plateau of ability for about two years, after which he declines as a

NUMBER AND TYPE OF INJURIES TO EACH PART OF THE BODY (100 SUBJECTS)

Part Injured	No.	Sprain	Bruise	Break	Cut
Finger	46	32	11	0	3
Arm	29	6	19	0	4
Upper leg	24	2	18	0	4
Head	19	0	19	0	0
Lower leg	19	2	14	0	3
Ankle	18	12	5	0	1
Back	17	4	13	0	0
Shoulder	16	1	15	0	0
Hip	11	2	4	3	2
Knee	11	3	6	1	1
Foot	9	1	6	0	2
Face	6	0	3	0	3
Stomach	5	0	5	0	0
Chest	4	0	4	0	0
Toe	4	0	2	1	1
Wrist	4	4	0	0	0
Elbow	1	0	1	0	0
Hand	1	0	1	0	0
Total	**244**	**69**	**146**	**5**	**24**

From: Skubic, Elvera: Studies of Little League and Middle League Baseball. Research Quarterly, 27:97–110, March, 1956.

player. Dr. Ball reports that there have been professional players who stayed with the game until the age of 33 to 35 but that this is a rare occurrence.

The most serious injury in basketball is one that results in damage to the knee. According to this physician, although ankle injuries occur more frequently than those of the knee, the severity of the damage is usually less significant. Rupture of the Achilles tendon presents a serious problem for a few players. Hemorrhage in the quadriceps muscles often occurs among basketball players and this injury is usually due to a direct or indirect blow to the muscles of the leg.

An opponent's elbow is a hazard in basketball and is a cause of numerous fractures of the nasal bone. Eye injuries occur frequently but are rarely incapacitating. Dislocations, lacerations, and contusions occur frequently among basketball players but are usually not too serious.

An indication of the kinds of injuries that may be sustained by a basketball player is given in the injury history of George Mikan, a professional player who was in basketball for twelve years. During his professional experience, Mikan had five teeth knocked out, dislocated his right ring finger and fractured his right wrist. In amateur basketball he had previously broken his right leg and in professional basketball he fractured his leg. In addition, he suffered a tear of the periosteum of a leg bone with subsequent growth of a bony spur because of this injury. When Mikan's amateur and professional injury experience is combined, it is found that he had fractured, at one time or another, both ankles and both wrists.

Soccer

The greatest hazard in soccer is head injury. Because soccer prohibits much body contact, the kinds of injuries received are not comparable to those in American football.

The commonest head injuries received in soccer are the cuts and tears that occur when the ball strikes the head. This is especially true when the lacing of the ball strikes the head.

When two players drive for the ball simultaneously and come into contact, there may be head-against-head injuries. In kicking at the ball, a soccer player may accidentally strike the head of another player with his foot. A kicked ball travels with great velocity and has been known to cause concussions on striking the head of a player.

Fractures of the leg may also occur in soccer, usually of the tibia, fibula and ankle. Sprains occur, as in other vigorous sports, at the ankle, knee, shoulder, wrist and elbow, "in just about that order," according to Dr. Otto C. Kestler, Medical Consultant for the International League.

Swimming

The greatest hazard of swimming is drowning. In 1960 the National Office of Vital Statistics reported that ordinarily approximately 5,000 persons drown each year.

Many people think that one of the major hazards of swimming is stomach cramps. This is a fallacious belief as has been shown by a study at the Georgia Institute of Technology. Fred Lanoue, a national leader on safety in the water, has reported that in a group of 1,400 students who spent a total of about 30,000 hours in the water, only 63 cramps occurred during the entire year and that not one of these could be identified as "stomach cramps." In questioning 10,000 boys, this investigator could not find one person who had ever suffered from "stomach cramps" while swimming. Undoubtedly, many swimmers who have thought that they were suffering from "stomach cramps" were actually suffering from indigestion, heart failure, muscle cramps or some other problem.

When a swimmer does have a warning sign that he is going to have a muscle cramp he can eliminate practically all of the pain and can prevent the return of the muscle spasm by *stretching the affected muscle before it shortens.* The majority of swimming cramps occur in the calf of the leg. The correction of this condition is to straighten the knee and hook or turn the foot and toes up toward the face as vigorously as can be done. This stretching of the calf muscle usually alleviates the muscle spasm promptly.

Perhaps the greatest protection against drowning for both the swimmer and the non-swimmer is to learn the technique called drownproofing.

DROWNPROOFING. Drownproofing is a term and technique that originated with Frederick R. Lanoue, professor of physical education at the Georgia Institute of Technology. Drownproofing signifies the ability of a swimmer or non-swimmer to remain afloat for hours without the full use of the limbs and while fully dressed.

It is a technique for floating in the water that prevents fatigue and panic and is based on controlled breathing without waste of energy. No effort is made to keep the head out of the water except for the few seconds that a person needs to take a fresh breath of air. The swimmer puts his face down in the water and lets his arms and legs dangle freely. Every few seconds the drownproofer raises his head slowly and breathes out through his nose. When his mouth emerges from the water he then takes a new breath of air. While this is going on the arms and legs are thrust downward to help sustain buoyancy. Once the lungs are filled with fresh air the head is turned downward into the water and the arms and legs are permitted to relax again. Complete relaxation is maintained until it is time to breathe again.

Mr. Lanoue says that most drownings occur because most people do not understand the laws of floating bodies. Instead of struggling, a person in the water should take a deep breath and then let himself sink. He will come up again close to the surface and a gentle thrust with the hands or legs will raise the head above the water enough to get a fresh breath of air. The person should then relax and let himself sink again.

In experiments at Georgia Tech, 20 poor swimmers were bound at the wrists and ankles. Another 20 were bound at the ankles only and a final group of 20 swimmers were left unbound. By using the drownproofing technique, all the swimmers were able to bob up and down in the water for an average of four hours and forty-three minutes. Sixteen of the poor swimmers stayed afloat for eight hours. The basis for the drownproofing system is the fact that more than 99 per cent of human beings will float when the lungs are full of air.

EAR INFECTIONS. Ear infections from swimming are almost always restricted to

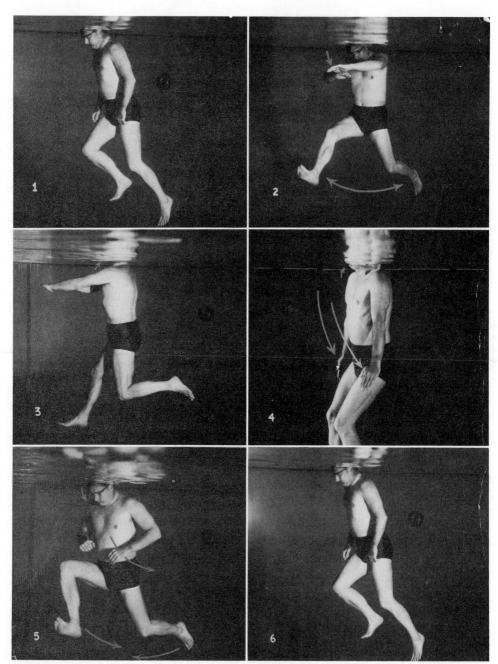

Figure 15.

Step 1. Relaxed, the downproofer floats face down with air-filled lungs to keep him near surface.

Step 3. The drownproofer exhales air through his nose while raising the head enough to get his chin out of water.

Step 5. When his lungs are full again, the drownproofer drops his face to a horizontal position under water and gives a slow arm thrust backward and downward.

Step 2. Getting ready to surface, the drownproofer begins a downward push with his hands and kicks his legs to lift the head above water.

Step 4. The instant his head is above water the drownproofer inhales air through the mouth while he makes a downward thrust with his arms to keep above water.

Step 6. The drownproofer now starts to repeat the cycle by holding his breath for 4 or 5 seconds and relaxing the head and limbs under water.

158   (Physician's News Service, Inc. Burk Uzzle from Leviton-Atlanta.)

the outer ear canal and result from the re-tention of moisture in that area, which causes a favorable situation for the growth of certain organisms. Anything that helps to keep the ear canal dry will help to pre-vent infection. A silicone preparation has been found to be especially helpful in pre-venting ear infections due to swimming. The wisdom of using protective measures is indicated by a study conducted by Wes-ley M. Staton who found that approxi-mately 8 per cent of regular swimmers may have infections of the ear, nose, and throat. This was in contrast to approxi-mately 2 per cent in a group of non-swim-mers.

Water Skiing

Dr. Robert L. Romano, Dr. Ernest M. Burgess and Dr. James A. Tupper, three Seattle physicians who are also water skiers, have reported that skiing on water is more hazardous than skiing on snow. These physicians report that injuries com-monly sustained in water skiing are frac-tures, dislocations, torn muscles, cuts, rope burns and damage to the ear, nose and throat. Drowning has also occurred.

The three physicians found four major causes of water skiing injuries as follows: (1) collision with docks or floating objects, (2) a fall into the water even though there is no contact with a solid object, (3) en-tanglement in the tow rope and (4) being struck by a boat including contact with the propeller.

Most of the broken bones suffered in water skiing result from errors in the judgment of speed when the water skier is being unloaded or returned to the dock.

Many severe injuries have resulted when water skiers simply fall into the water. The Seattle physicians reported four cases of dislocation of the knee by simple falling into the water. In one in-stance the knee was so badly injured, espe-cially close to its blood supply, that ampu-tation was necessary.

The tow rope is a greater hazard than many water skiers realize. The rope may entangle a finger, arm or leg and result in considerable tissue damage. This is espe-cially apt to happen when the water skier takes off from the dock or falls in the water.

A fall into the water often injures the ear drum or nose and throat.

Four safety measures have been pro-posed as follows:

1. Skiers should be given proper instructions in handling the rope on take-off to prevent a coil from catching a skier's extremity.

2. A bathing cap or ear plugs should be worn to pre-vent ear, nose, and throat complications.

3. There should be at least two persons in the boat, one to drive and one to watch the skier. One person cannot do both jobs adequately.

4. It should be mandatory that all skiers wear a light weight life belt.

Skin Diving

Skin diving as a sport has experienced great popularity in recent years. It is esti-mated that about 400 skin diving clubs, with about 6,000,000 members exist throughout the United States. The average age of the skin diver is about 20 years.

On the basis of experience in California over a period of two years, it can be ex-pected that about one person each month will lose his life in skin diving. There are many more non-fatal accidents associated with this sport.

PROTECTION

"Much of the danger can be removed, if prospec-tive divers will first assure themselves of adequate physical condition, information on the hazards involved, and proper training in the use of equip-ment."

Captain Albert R. Behnke, U.S.N. (M.C.), 1960

According to Dr. William T. Burns of Long Beach, California, there are five ma-jor health hazards to skin diving. These are as follows:

1. CAISSON DISEASE.   A popular name for this disorder is "bends." This disorder

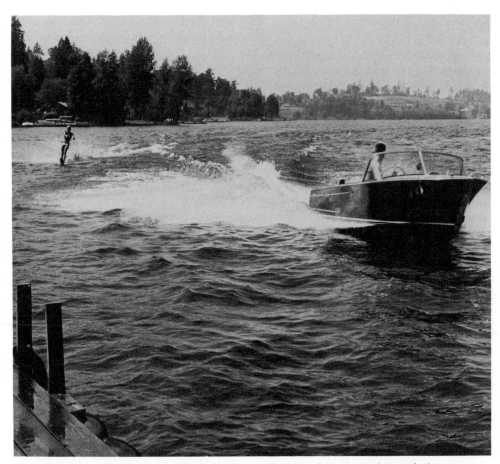

Figure 16.   Hazards of water skiing: A towboat with a crew of one is not safe enough. One crew
member is needed to steer the boat and look ahead, while another is needed to watch the skier in order
to protect him. (Courtesy of Physician's News Service, Inc.)

occurs when nitrogen bubbles form in the blood stream because of a rapid release of pressure. Nitrogen in the tissue surges into the blood stream when a diver surfaces too rapidly after being under water at depths of 40 feet or more.

The diver suffering from bends may begin to feel ill even before he reaches the surface of the water, but symptoms have been known to start as long as 15 hours later. Mild symptoms are itching and pain in the joints, tendons or muscles. More serious symptoms are dizziness, vomiting, visual disturbances and paralysis.

Treatment for caisson disease calls for the relief of pain, the treatment of shock and the use of a recompression chamber as quickly as possible. In the chamber the victim is put under pressure again and is then gradually brought back to atmospheric pressure over a period of hours. This gradual return may save the diver's life.

2. AIR EMBOLISM.   An air bubble in the blood may occur when a diver using an underwater breathing apparatus comes to the surface holding his breath. The com-

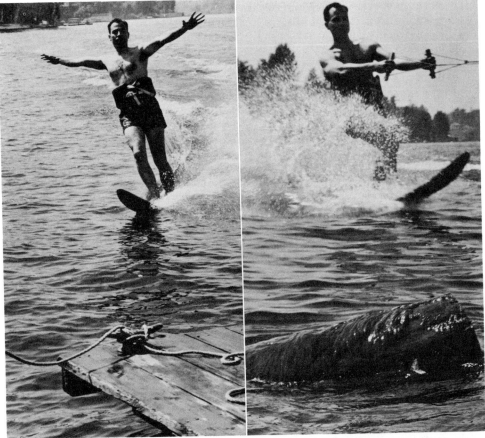

Figure 17   *Figure 18*

Figure 17.   Hazards in water skiing: A dangerous grandstand approach to the dock on completion of the pull.

Figure 18.   Hazards in water skiing: Floating or partially submerged objects in the water such as this log. (Courtesy of Physician's News Service, Inc.)

pressed air in his lungs must expand and this expansion may rupture a part of a lung and blood vessels and allow air bubbles to gain access to the blood. These may collect in the heart or elsewhere and cause serious illness or death. For the prevention of this complication, the skin diver should be expelling the air from his lungs as he rises to the surface.

3. Oxygen Poisoning. Dr. Burns points out that this complication can occur when a skin diver uses pure oxygen in his underwater breathing apparatus. Prevention can be achieved by avoiding the use of pure oxygen and by reducing the amount of pressure under which the latter is inhaled. Symptoms of oxygen poisoning include nausea, respiratory irritation, dizziness, emotional disturbance and convulsions.

4. Carbon Monoxide Poisoning. This complication occurs when the diver's breathing apparatus permits contamination of the air supply with exhaust fumes.

This can occur when gasoline driven compressors are not properly vented. Symptoms of poisoning include severe headache, fatigue, dizziness, faintness and loss of consciousness. Artificial respiration is imperative.

5. PSYCHOLOGIC HAZARDS.   The fifth hazard of skin diving occurring to Dr. Burns is psychologic. Unstable persons and those who are afraid of the water should not participate in skin diving.

Diving experts of the United States Navy have recommended that amateur skin divers should not go below a depth of sixty feet and should not stay at even this depth for a period of more than two hours.

Captain Albert R. Behnke, an expert in deep sea diving, suggests that amateur skin divers can reduce the hazards of their sport by a few fundamental rules. He believes that training in the use of equipment is the most important preventive measure that the skin diver can take. This expert says that even divers who are experienced will have trouble with valves, will run out of gas, will get cold or dizzy or will come up to the surface too quickly.

The importance of maintaining a calm temperament in skin diving is illustrated by the fact that when a diver becomes panicky, he breathes too fast and may use up his air supply in a much shorter time than usual.

Captain Behnke believes that skin divers should operate in groups or clubs and that each group should have a portable recompression chamber which they can establish for immediate emergency treatment if a diver suffers from bends.

SHARKS

"Skin divers who hunt or provoke sharks are flirting with death or severe mutilation . . . Deaths result in thirty to forty per cent of all cases of shark attack . . ."

Shark Research Panel,
American Institute of Biological Sciences, 1960

The hazard of sharks should be recognized by skin divers, especially along the coastline of the United States. Dr. Perry W. Gilbert of Cornell University says that the likelihood of a swimmer being attacked by a shark is less probable than being struck by lightning, but that a shark, provoked by skin divers, will almost certainly attack them.

Skin divers are safest if they dive in pairs, leave sharks alone and put speared fish in a boat rather than towing them or tying them around the waist. A shark usually circles several times before attacking and a skin diver should get into boat quickly if he sees a circling shark. If no boat is available, the releasing of air bubbles, shouting under water, or hitting the shark on the snout with a club may discourage him. A skin diver should never remain in the water with a bleeding wound.

Skiing

The National Ski Patrol has reported that there are nearly four million skiers in the United States and that more than one hundred thousand injuries occur during a single season. Most skiing accidents happen because of the inability to make turns, avoid obstacles or control speed.

The great hazard in skiing is sprain or fracture of the ankle. This fracture is most apt to occur in the person who is just learning to ski and his attempts to learn the "snow plow" or the "stem turn." In this effort the feet are turned inward and stress is placed on the ankles in such a manner that if the skier falls, the foot is bent inward and fracture occurs.

Other fractures of the leg may also occur, of course. Both of the large bones of the leg may be broken when skiers hit a "sitzmark," or hole which a previous fallen skier has failed to fill in with snow. This type of fracture is more apt to occur in skiers traveling fast.

The Ski Patrol reports that the knee is injured in about 25 per cent of ski injuries.

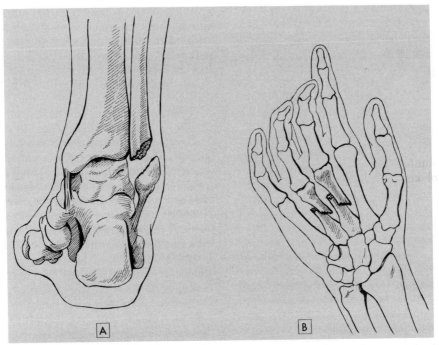

Figure 19. Two common fractures in skiing. A, The ski fracture, oblique fracture of lateral malleolus of fibula. B, Ski pole fracture, oblique fracture of third and fourth metacarpals. (Pfizer Spectrum, Feb., 1959.)

The "ski pole fracture" may result if the skier falls with his pole in his hand.

Five recommendations are given by physicians for the prevention of ski injuries, as follows:

1. The skier should be in adequate physical condition before he attempts to ski. Fatigue is apt to be a major cause of injuries late in the day.

2. Gradual warming up before taking off on skis.

3. Cessation of skiing, or reduction to small runs, when the skier is fatigued.

4. Proper adjustment of all equipment.

5. The use of modern safety-release bindings. The use of these modern bindings is exceedingly important because they permit the skier to kick or twist out of them without difficulty. It is estimated that the use of these bindings has reduced injuries to the lower part of the legs by more than one half. The binding must be properly adjusted and tested each day before skiing.

The value of physical conditioning in the prevention of ski injuries has been demonstrated. A ski club in Montana went through an entire season of skiing without a single accident after the members participated in a program of advanced physical conditioning. In Lake Placid, New York, fifty children of the North County School accumulated a total of 5,000 skiing hours with seven fractures and five sprains. After an advance conditioning program was adopted, the children went 5,000 skiing hours without an accident, although two boys who did not engage in the advanced physical conditioning program did suffer fractures of the leg.

In some ski resorts, hospitals have been established with medical personnel immediately available for prompt treatment of casualties.

At Mount Snow in Vermont, for example, where about 8,000 skiers come for weekends, medical aid is provided within 10 minutes after an accident has occurred.

SKIING INJURIES
PERCENTAGE DISTRIBUTION°

Type of Injury		Body Part Affected	
Sprains	46	Ankle	44
Fractures	29	Knee	19
Wounds	13	Leg	16
Dislocations	8	Face	6
Miscellaneous	4	Shoulder	5
	100		
		Hand and wrist	3
		Other parts	7
			100

°Rounded to nearest whole number.
From: What's New, No. 214, 1959.

The ski hospital is located about 150 yards from the ski lifts.

Volunteer members of the National Ski Patrol keep all trails under watch and bring injured skiers rapidly to medical service.

> **INJURY EXPECTANCY**
> "In any given skiing holiday of two-weeks duration, ten per cent of the skiing group will report an injury..."
>
> *Dr. John R. Moritz, 1959*

On some ski slopes there may be more than 2,000 persons skiing as long as 8 hours a day, and under these circumstances some injuries are almost certain to occur.

Under ordinary circumstances a physician sees an injured skier from three to ten hours after an accident. At Mount Snow physicians treat the injured person within 10 minutes or so. About 40 patients are treated each weekend at this ski resort.

Ice Hockey

Ice hockey players have been warned by physicians to wear protective helmets because of the hazard of being struck on the head by a flying puck. In Canada, where ice hockey is virtually the national game, physicians have reported serious injuries to players who were struck on the side of the head by hockey pucks. Since the puck may travel at a speed in excess of 120 feet per second, it can be seen that great force can be exerted by this flying object.

In some sections of the country ice hockey is a popular high school as well as college sport. Minneapolis has been reported as the "ice hockey capitol of the nation." In that city about 500 high school athletes engage in this sport. In Minneapolis high school experience, statistics show that proportionately there are more hockey than football injuries, but they are of a less serious nature.

Dr. Isadore M. Goldberg has reported that only once in 12 years had he treated a high school ice hockey player for a serious injury. This was a hemorrhage in the eye of a player who had been hit with a hockey stick. Dr. Goldberg, as medical director supervising high school athletics, reports that certain injuries are more apt to occur in ice hockey than in some other sports. Cuts on the face, especially in the area of the cheek bones, split lips, and cuts of the scalp are the commonest kinds of injuries in this sport.

The following rules for high school ice hockey have helped to control injuries in Minneapolis: the puck is to be kept low at all times, the stick is not to be raised higher than three feet off the ice, a player must not charge more than two steps and checking an opponent against the boards is prohibited.

Dr. Goldberg also reports that all ice hockey players must take part in an ice skating and conditioning program in the regular physical education classes before the season begins.

Boxing

Boxing is the controversial sport of the present college generation. Some physicians and physical educators defend the sport for its development of rugged individualism and self-reliance and make a sharp distinction between college boxing and professional boxing. Other physicians and educators condemn boxing in general and make no distinction between professional fighting and the college sport on the grounds that it is an activity that is inherently dangerous.

> **HAZARDOUS**
> "Prize fighting is one of the oldest and most hazardous of the trades, and the risks involved have changed little in thousands of years."
> *Dr. Frank R. Ferlaino, 1952*

Most of the opposition to boxing has stemmed from deaths that have occurred to fighters and which have been proven to have been related to head injuries. Actually, there are few deaths from this sport.

Annual surveys of *Ring* magazine indicate that during a five year period from 1955 to 1959 that 12 amateur fighters and 6 professional fighters were killed. Most of these deaths occurred during actual bouts rather than in sparring practice.

Boxing has become one of the controversial sports in amateur athletics. Injuries to professional or amateur boxers receive widespread publicity and the public clamor that has arisen from reading about these injuries has challenged the sport.

Public concern with boxing injuries has resulted in substantial improvements aimed at the prevention of injuries. The use of heavier gloves containing padding that cannot be shifted away from the knuckles, the substitution of calcium carbonate for resin on ring floors and the use of a more substantial cushion on the floor of the ring have all helped to protect the boxer. More effective mouth pieces have helped to decrease the shock of blows to the body.

Tests have shown that when a fighter is knocked down his head may strike the ring floor with the force of a ten pound weight dropped about 8 feet. This is a far greater force than is needed to fracture the base of the skull and is sufficient to cause injury to the brain, including laceration and hemorrhage. Improved cushions on the floor have helped greatly to reduce injury from the impact of knockdowns.

> **IN DANGER**
> "A fighter is most in danger after he has been stunned by a knockdown . . . surely the most important factor in preventing ring deaths is immediate action by the referee or ring physician at this time."
> *Dr. Charles Harris, 1954*

Robert E. Keefer of Los Angeles, who made a study of college boxing a few years ago, did not find many injuries occurring in this sport. His conclusion was that boxing does have certain definite educational values and may be included in college programs under certain safeguards, which he enumerated as follows:

1. A complete medical examination should be given before competition.
2. The doctor should be present at all bouts and within easy reach during practice.
3. Participants should be in good physical condition with sufficient instruction to enable them to "take care of themselves."
4. The boxing instructor should be of the highest caliber, with considerable experience in the sport.
5. National Intercollegiate Boxing Rules should be

NUMBER OF ACCIDENTAL DEATHS FROM BOXING United States, 1955–1959		
Year	*Amateur*	*Professional*
1955–59	12	6
1959	5	0
1958	3	1
1957	2	0
1956	2	2
1955	0	3

From: Annual surveys by *The Ring* magazine.

followed, and extreme care should be taken in the matching of contestants.

6. Equipment should be of the best obtainable, and each participant should be fully equipped.

In 1959 fourteen physicians who were honorary officers of the British Amateur Boxing Association strongly defended this sport. They reported that during thirty years of experience in the supervision of amateur boxing they had seen only one case of permanent damage to the brain and that they had found no progressive deterioration of the mind. In these same thirty years the physicians had seen no case of blindness due to boxing, and in fifty-seven brainwave recordings on amateur boxers who had severe concussion of the brain no abnormalities were revealed after one month.

These physicians stated that boxing injuries are eighth, not first, in their frequencies among sports. Their observations were based upon amateur boxing only and did not apply to professional fighting. Statistics on boxing injuries in New York State over a period of seven years are described in the accompanying table.

Another British physician has recently defended boxing as an amateur sport, although he believes that boxing should not be encouraged for those under the age of 16. He thinks that boxing develops a certain toughness and resilience that is good for the spirit.

In New York State a medical advisory board composed of nine physicians was established to protect the health of boxers. This group of physicians has recommended the following procedures to reduce the hazards of boxing. It should be noted that the group is concerned with professional boxing; nevertheless, their suggestions make good sense and are offered herewith:

1. A new type of protective mat for the ring is now mandatory in every boxing arena in New York State. This mat was developed after considerable research by the Cornell Aeronautical Laboratories and has reduced

injuries from knockdowns to insignificant and minor effects.

2. Substitution of eight-ounce gloves for the conventional four- and six-ounce gloves in all rings in New York State except for championship bouts.

3. A mandatory eight-count knockdown rule for all except championship bouts. Three successive knockdown counts in any one round now terminates the bout for all except championship bouts.

4. An automatic thirty day suspension rule for any boxer who has been knocked out or who has received some other injury.

5. A compulsory electroencephalogram for any boxer who has been knocked out or injured in such a way that a brainwave recording is considered justifiable. These recordings are evaluated by an outstanding neurosurgeon.

6. A resuscitator with oxygen equipment is now mandatory and available at all ringsides for every boxing bout.

7. A standard emergency medical kit is available for emergency use at the ringside.

8. Any boxer who loses six consecutive bouts or who sustains four consecutive knockouts is automatically suspended until a critical review of his medical and boxing record is made. Reinstatement of the boxer is permitted only if this review indicates that such action is justifiable.

9. There must be complete integration of the boxing record and physical and mental status of all boxers before bouts will be approved.

10. Two ringside physicians must be available for all boxing bouts in New York State.

11. Calcium carbonate has been approved as a substitute for resin at the ringside on an experimental basis.

12. Urine examinations before and after bouts are now compulsory to determine if there are any microscopic changes that might be suggestive of kidney damage.

13. The temperature of the boxer must be taken before and after bouts to determine if there are metabolic alterations.

14. All referees and judges must be examined by the official State Commission physician every six months.

Dr. Ira A. McCown of New York City has reported a study of injuries to 11,173 boxers in the State of New York over a seven-year period. Cuts and other damage to the soft tissues of the face led all other types of injuries.

Cuts on the face of the boxer where the

contest is permitted to continue, such as may occur in the professional ring, are best treated with effective coagulants such as thrombin or thromboplastic substances. This treatment helps to control bleeding. Ice compresses may also help by reduction of blood flow to the injured area.

A more complete account of the injuries occurring to the 11,173 boxers of Dr. McCown's study is given in the accompanying table.

Physicians at the University of Colorado have reported symptoms of physical, nervous and mental deterioration including headaches, tremors, loss of memory and inability to learn, in professional boxers several years after their retirement.

These medical investigators have made autopsy studies of the brains of former boxers and have found the most extensive damage in the cortex of the frontal lobes. They believe anatomical changes are caused by repeated concussions and that the damage is irreversible, causing premature aging that occurs among certain boxers.

The State Athletic Commission of Colorado now requires regular brain wave examinations of all professional boxers who fight in that state. The commission has established the following rules: (1) a professional boxer must have an electroencephalogram at least once a year, (2) in case of a knockout another electroencephalogram must be taken within two weeks and (3) frequent brain wave examinations may be required in the case of a boxer with recordings suggestive of a brain injury.

The first 24 compulsory brain wave recordings of professional boxers in Colorado revealed evidence of brain damage in nearly 40 per cent of the group. One boxer who was 21 years of age showed no neurologic or psychologic signs of injury, but brain wave recordings revealed brain damage. He was permanently suspended from boxing for his own good.

It must be strongly emphasized that there is a sharp distinction between professional and amateur boxing. College box-

MEDICAL AND STATISTICAL REPORT OF INJURIES AMONG PROFESSIONAL BOXERS IN NEW YORK STATE (A SEVEN YEAR STUDY—1952 THROUGH 1958)

Data	No. of Cases
Total number of participating boxers	11,173
Knockouts	325
Knockouts requiring hospitalization	10
Technical knockouts	789
Secondary to injury, fight stopped	557
Fight stopped as result of inability to defend self, fatigue, exhaustion, out-classed, etc.	232
Lacerations and contusions (trauma to the soft tissue)	1,010
Injuries to the eye	19
Corneal injuries	13
Detached retina	6
Fractures	38
Nasal bones	16
Metacarpals	14
Jaw	4
Phalanges	3
Ankle (external malleolus fibula)	1
Dislocations (shoulder joint, anterior)	4
Miscellaneous—"boxer's knuckle"	18
Retirements—poor records, neurological disorder, heart, disease, etc.	148
Total mortality	0

From: McCown, Ira A.: Boxing injuries. Am. J. Surg., 98:509–16, 1959.

ing coaches have taken national leadership in the development of protective standards and the requirement of protective equipment. These measures have been so effective in reducing injuries that the college sport has been judged to be safer than a number of other widely accepted college activities.

One of the most vigorous opponents of boxing as a sport has been Dr. Arthur H. Steinhaus. This scientist maintains that boxing should be discontinued as a sport for two primary reasons: (1) a man's head is not constructed to take the blows of boxing, and (2) boxing is not a true sport when measured by modern standards of sportsmanship.

The vigorous assault that Dr. Steinhaus makes against boxing can be summarized by his following statement:

First, there is no sport except boxing in which the primary purpose is to inflict bodily injury on an opponent, and in which victory goes to a man because he has successfully beaten his opponent into temporary unconsciousness.

Second, in no sport except boxing do spectators expect and even demand that bodily damage be inflicted.

Third, in every sport except boxing everyone feels badly when someone is injured, and the injured player is respected, even applauded by both sides.

Fourth, in every American sport except boxing there is provision for time out and for substitution when there is bodily injury. The injured contestant may leave the field without disgrace and without loss of self-respect.

Fifth, in no sport except boxing is a man's competence or courage judged by his readiness to continue in contest after suffering bodily injury.

Sixth, in every sport except boxing a bloody nose, a lacerated face, or temporary unconsciousness are recorded as accidents. In boxing these are produced on purpose and not reported as accidents. Thus boxing has a fictitiously low accident record.

Questions

1. When does justification for a sport come under challenge because of injuries?
2. What should be the penalty for an athlete who deliberately injures an opponent to get him out of the game?
3. Do the advantages of boxing outweigh the disadvantages of the activity?
4. Are accidents in sports inevitable?
5. Which is the most dangerous of all college sports?
6. Is participation in sports justified when the effects of minor injuries may last a lifetime?

For Further Reading

1. Seaton, Don Cash: *Physical Education Handbook.* New York, Prentice-Hall, 1959.
2. Thorndike, Augustus: *Athletic Injuries.* Philadelphia, Lea & Febiger, 1956.

For Advanced Reading

1. Lewin, Philip: *The Foot and Ankle.* Philadelphia, Lea & Febiger, 1959.
2. Lewin, Philip: *The Knee and Related Structures.* Philadelphia, Lea & Febiger, 1952.
3. Thorndike, Augustus: *Manual of Bandaging, Straping and Splinting.* Philadelphia, Lea & Febiger, 1959.

14

ALCOHOL

THE EXCESSIVE and unwise use of alcohol on college and university campuses has led one dean of men to describe drinking as the "number one social problem on the campus."

The excessive use of alcohol should not be confused with the temperate or moderate use of this beverage. Alcohol is used in moderation in many families in which it appears to do no harm.

When alcohol is taken in *excessive* amounts, however, the effects can be destructive out of all proportion to the amount consumed. The problem is not only that of measuring the influence of alcoholism on society, but includes problems that may arise from a single instance of intoxication.

A normally sober person, for example, may become intoxicated just once during his lifetime. If, on this occasion, he should drive an automobile and be involved in an accident in which death to another person occurs, the drinker may be found guilty of manslaughter and may possibly be sentenced to a number of years in a penitentiary. In such a dramatic case the impact of alcohol on the life of this one person could be devastating. The problem, therefore, is not solely one involving the alcoholic, for the average person may suffer from the unwise consumption of alcohol as well.

DECISION

"The decision as to the responsible use of alcoholic beverages requires a degree of maturity that the young person does not have. The proper age for such decision, to drink or not to drink, will remain an individual matter between parents, teachers, and the young people ... Young people need alcohol education in preparation for their adult responsibilities ..."

Joint Commission on Alcoholism of the Protestant Episcopal Church, 1958

An increasing number of studies have been made in recent years of the reasons for alcoholism. Some studies have suggested that it is family unity that may be an important factor in the prevention of this disorder. If this be the case, *the problem of alcoholism tends to be one of social relations within the family and community* rather than of alcohol alone.

The unwholesome effects of the excessive consumption of alcohol which are described in the next section probably represent an exaggerated view to most people, but *for the alcoholic* the social degradation encountered today is but a duplication of what discerning people have observed for thousands of years.

The fundamental problem of alcohol is its effect upon human behavior. When alcohol impairs human relations between the drinker and others in his family, work-group or community, then alcohol becomes a social and community problem.

"The Naked Truth Saloon"

In the February 24, 1886, issue of the *Boise Democrat* James Lawrence ran an advertisement concerning his saloon which he had named "The Naked Truth Saloon." The following is a transcript of this advertisement:

Friends and neighbors, having just opened a commodious shop for the sale of liquid fire, I embrace this opportunity of informing you that I have commenced the business of making drunkards, paupers and beggars for the sober, industrious, and respectable portion of the community to support.

I shall deal in family spirits which will incite men to deeds of riot, robbery, and blood shed, and by so doing, diminish the comfort, augment the expenses and endanger the welfare of the community.

I will, on short notice, for a small sum, and with great expectations, undertake to prepare victims for the asylums, poor farms, prisons, and gallows.

I will furnish an article that will increase accidents, multiply the number of distressing diseases, and render those who are harmless incurable.

I will deal in drugs which will deprive some of life, many of reason, most of their property, and all of their peace; which will cause fathers to become fiends, and wives widows, children to become orphans, and all mendicants.

I will cause many of the rising generation to grow up in ignorance and prove a burden and a nuisance to the nation. I will cause mothers to forget their offsprings, and cruelty to take the place of love.

I will sometimes corrupt the ministers of religion; defile the purity of the church and cause temporal, spiritual, and eternal death; and if any be so impertinent as to ask me why I have the audacity to bring such accumulated misery upon the people, my honest reply is, "Money." The spirit trade is lucrative and some professing Christians give their cheerful countenance to it.

From the United States government I have purchased the right to demolish the character, destroy the health, and shorten the lives, and ruin the souls of those who choose to honor me with their custom.

I pledge myself to do all that I have promised. Those who wish any of the evils above specified brought upon themselves or their dear friends, are requested to meet me at my bar where I will, for a few cents, furnish them with the certain means of doing so.

Lawrence's original advertisement was undoubtedly based upon his sense of humor plus the fact that he had observed damaging effects from the excessive consumption of alcohol. We know that the great majority of people who drink alcohol do so in moderation and that they do not suffer from the foregoing ailments of spirit and body. We know that approximately 75 per cent of the adult population in the United States will drink liquor on occasion. We know also that 75 per cent of our adult population does not fit the foregoing description. Nevertheless, there is much truth in this advertisement of 1886, and it reflects man's long experience with alcohol and the observations that he has made upon the destructive influences of this substance in respect to certain members of the population. *For the person who becomes an alcoholic, the description still fits.*

Drunkenness

Each year more than a million persons are arrested in the United States for drunkenness or for some violation of the law connected with liquor. The cost of maintaining drunken persons in jail is about twenty-five million dollars annually. In just one city, Washington, D.C., for a number of years 61 per cent of all jail commitments were for drunkenness. Of 7000 women passing through the District's jails each year, about 50 per cent were charged with drunkenness or disorderly conduct resulting from drinking. Among them were many women of education and good family.

In Los Angeles City some 70 per cent of the cases that pass through the local courts are concerned with alcohol violations. It is estimated that 40 per cent of the energy of the city police force goes to handling problems related to drinking.

In Los Angeles County it is estimated that two and a half million dollars is spent each year because of arrests of alcoholics and vagrants at the rate of approximately 10,000 a month, at the cost of about twenty dollars for each arrest.

In San Francisco a municipal judge stated publicly that his community was throwing away two hundred and fifty thousand dollars a year by tossing drunks in jail instead of diverting this money toward the treatment of alcoholics.

It is reasonably certain that the number of arrests for drunkenness does reflect the intensity of police activities along these lines as well as the amount of excessive drinking.

Alcohol, Crime and Violence

The consumption of alcohol has a close relationship to crime and violence. In a sense, this is to be expected because alcohol tends to remove the restraints of social standards, tends to impair judgment and to disturb the normal personality.

In one study of 246 cases of violent death during a single year in a community of about 600,000 persons, it was found that alcohol was involved in 27 per cent of the violent deaths. Of 78 suicides, alcohol was found to be an immediate precipitating factor in 19 per cent of the cases. Of 8 murders, 7 were done while the persons involved were heavily intoxicated. In practically all cases there was no premeditation or malicious intent.

Of 78 traffic deaths, those involving alcohol were due to the behavior of people who were not alcoholics but who had been drinking at a cocktail party, a tavern, a wedding or some celebration.

On a national scale it is estimated that 16 per cent of all murders are committed under the influence of alcohol. Often a murderer, on trial, will plead in his defense that he had been drinking, and therefore was not aware of what he was doing.

Sometimes legal defense may ask for a complete acquittal of the prisoner on the basis that he was so drunk that he did not know the difference between right and wrong. This amounts to putting the blame for the crime entirely upon alcohol. Generally, the courts resist such a plea. Getting drunk is held to be a voluntary act. Some judges have actually stated that there would be no safety for human life if a murderer could go free because he was inebriated at the time he committed a crime.

The chief psychiatrist of Sing Sing Prison made a two-year study of all new prisoners admitted to that penal institution and concluded that about 25 per cent of them had been sent to prison because of crimes that were traceable to the use of alcohol. In this study crimes of assault and violence were more numerous among alcoholics than among nonalcoholics.

Alcohol probably should be looked upon as a supplementary factor in crime and violence rather than a main cause of such antisocial behavior. It is immaterial, however, whether alcohol is a major or a minor factor in crime. That there is a definite association in some cases of violence is enough to warrant social attention to the problem.

Alcohol, Marriage and Divorce

The person who drinks excessively has a more difficult time getting married and a harder time staying married.

A study of 1000 persons arrested for drunkenness during a period of five weeks in eight towns in Connecticut showed that only 47 per cent of the drunkards in this group had ever been married in contrast to 80 per cent of a control group arrested for other infractions of the law. It was also found that only 23 per cent of the inebriates were married and living with their wives at the time of their arrest, compared to 73 per cent for the nondrinkers. Of the alcoholics who had been married, 25 per cent were separated, whereas in the other

group only 4 per cent had left their families. Of the inebriates who had married, 16 per cent were divorced compared to 1 per cent of the nondrinkers.

ABSTINENCE

"This stand against all drinking, even so-called moderate drinking is summed up in the words of Henry Ward Beecher who said: 'To speak about a moderate use of alcohol is like speaking of a moderate use of the plague.'"

U.S. News and World Report, 1958

Statistics on the cause or causes of divorce are misleading so far as the role of alcohol is concerned. Probably the majority of divorces are granted on the grounds of cruelty or desertion rather than on that of alcoholism. Either or both of these grounds, however, might be closely connected with the excessive consumption of alcohol.

Although various studies have indicated that alcoholics have a more difficult time holding on to their jobs and their wives and keeping their families intact, this is not always so. A recent study by two authorities at the Yale Center of Alcohol Studies covering 2023 males coming to community clinics for help with the problem of alcohol showed that this group possessed a high degree of social and occupational integration.

It was found that over 50 per cent of the alcoholics in this group were married and living with their wives and that 90 per cent had lived in the community for two years or more. In other words, there was a fairly high level of community and family stability despite the problems of alcoholism. Nearly two thirds of the group were employed, and 56 per cent had held steady jobs for at least three years despite their heavy drinking. Approximately 25 per cent of the alcoholics had held jobs for ten years or more.

The significance of this kind of study lies in the fact that it illustrates that family, industrial and community relationships can be maintained to a surprising degree by alcoholics.

Alcohol and Work

It has been estimated that there are nearly two million problem drinkers in industry and that about 30 out of every 1000 workers are alcoholics. On a national scale it has been estimated that an alcoholic loses about 22 to 25 days from work each year because of illness due to alcohol. There is tremendous variation, however, between industries and individual companies.

In Jackson, Mississippi, nine business and industrial concerns reported an annual loss of 5400 man hours and about nine thousand dollars because of absenteeism due to excessive consumption of alcohol. One company employing 750 workers stated that 7 per cent were problem drinkers. In this group of business organizations, 41 men had lost their jobs because of drinking.

The value of an effective program aimed at helping the alcoholic worker has been demonstrated by the Consolidated Edison Company of New York. This organization has a program of rehabilitation for the alcoholic that starts with a friendly talk with his supervisor. The worker is then put on probation after a warning and is referred to the medical department. Here a social worker and a psychologist assist the medical staff in rehabilitating the worker. Community facilities are used for this purpose. If drinking continues, the worker is suspended and a panel of fellow employees decides what shall be done about the individual case. In some instances the alcoholic is retired with a disability rating just as any other worker might be retired.

After three years of this program of trying to assist alcoholics, it was found that the losses associated with drinking decreased from $134,250 to $65,450. This was a reduction of approximately 49 per cent in costs due to alcoholism.

In another study of 1223 men arrested for drunkenness it was found that the alcoholics were out of work to a much greater extent than people who did not drink. It was also shown that there were fewer excessive drinkers who were members of professions, owners of businesses or managers of departments. Instead, the inebriates were found to gravitate toward unskilled labor and unskilled service jobs.

Always, however, one must be careful in interpreting such evidence as proof that the inability to secure superior types of work is due to alcohol. While it is perfectly reasonable to assume that there is such a connection, it could also be concluded that the same personality characteristics that make a person an alcoholic may also handicap him in his working relationships.

Alcohol and Traffic Accidents

Almost everyone recognizes that the chances of having an automobile accident are definitely increased when a person is intoxicated. Many people, however, do not realize how *much* the chance of having an accident is increased when a person has been drinking.

> **CHEMICAL BLOOD TESTS**
>
> "'I had only two beers. Naturally I acted a little upset when the police told me I was being arrested.' The speaker, a neatly dressed, mild-mannered man, was making his first appearance in court on a charge of driving under the influence of intoxicants. Arresting officers testified his automobile weaved, his breath was alcoholic and he staggered and was belligerent. His case is similar to thousands which judges and juries must decide every year . . ."
> *American Medical Association, 1960*

In Evanston, Illinois, a study was made in which a striking correlation between the concentration of alcohol in the blood stream and the chances of having an accident were established.

The results of this study are summarized in the table below.

It must not be assumed that drunken drivers are responsible for most of the accidents that occur on public highways. As a matter of fact, the normal, sober driver is responsible for the great majority of accidents, and carelessness is usually the factor that precipitates the accident. However, when a person does drive an automobile under the influence of alcohol, his particular chances of having an accident are tremendously increased. This means that he is also a much greater hazard to other people on the highway even though they have not been drinking.

The police are now within their legal rights when they insist that a person suspected of drunken driving submit to a blood test for intoxication.

In 1957 the United States Supreme Court upheld the decision of a lower court that taking a blood test was a legal procedure. This decision was based upon a case in which a New Mexico driver was involved in a collision with another automobile in which three persons from the latter car were killed. A pint whiskey bottle, almost empty, was found in the vehicle of the suspected drunken driver. Liquor was detected on his breath in the hospital emergency room to which he was taken for medical treatment. While the injured driver was still unconscious a physician took a sample of blood from him which laboratory tests showed to contain about 0.17 per cent alcohol. The driver was charged with involuntary manslaughter and he was convicted. Later he sought

freedom under the 14th amendment on the grounds that the involuntary blood test had deprived him of liberty without due process of law.

The Supreme Court ruled against him and upheld the right of the State to perform a blood test when it is suspected that the driver of an automobile is intoxicated.

In Oklahoma a woman driver who was judged to be intoxicated after she had been tested in a police station brought legal action for freedom on the grounds that the drunkometer test resulted in self-incrimination. The court ruled, however, that there was ample evidence to support the verdict of the jury that the woman was intoxicated.

There seems to be no doubt that the courts have established the legal standing of the blood test for intoxication.

Alcohol and Venereal Disease

Public health authorities have long observed that there is an association between alcohol and venereal disease. "Alcohol," once wrote Dr. Milton Rosenau, then professor of preventive medicine at Harvard, "is the bedfellow of syphilis and gonorrhea."

Alcohol itself, contrary to popular opinion, does not stimulate sexual desire, but it does weaken discretion, judgment and restraint. As a consequence, the proportion of cases of venereal disease that are linked with intoxication is high. Some investigators have estimated that from 75 to 90 per cent of all cases of venereal disease have been contracted under the influence of alcohol. It would be difficult to verify this statement, but it is common knowledge in the field of public health that there is a strong association between the two.

Skid Row

Most large cities contain a small section in which the most debilitated type of al-

Per Cent Alcohol in the Blood	Relative Chances of Accident
No alcohol...........................	1
Under 0.07 per cent..................	3
0.07 to 0.11 per cent................	5
0.11 to 0.15 per cent................	15
0.15 per cent and over	55

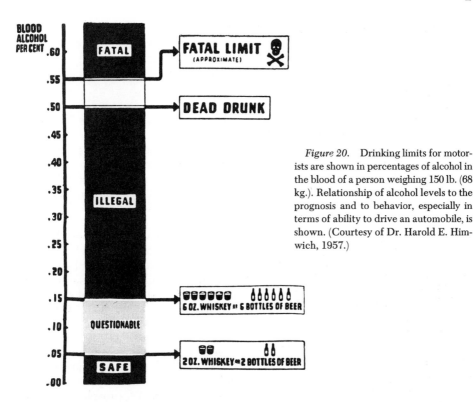

BLOOD
ALCOHOL
PER CENT

.60 — FATAL

→ **FATAL LIMIT** ☠
(APPROXIMATE)

.55

.50 — → **DEAD DRUNK**

.45

.40

.35

ILLEGAL

.30

.25

.20

.15 — → 🍺🍺🍺🍺🍺🍺 🍸🍸🍸🍸🍸🍸
6 OZ. WHISKEY = 6 BOTTLES OF BEER

.10 QUESTIONABLE

.05 — → 🍺🍺 🍸🍸
2 OZ. WHISKEY = 2 BOTTLES OF BEER

SAFE

.00

Figure 20. Drinking limits for motorists are shown in percentages of alcohol in the blood of a person weighing 150 lb. (68 kg.). Relationship of alcohol levels to the prognosis and to behavior, especially in terms of ability to drive an automobile, is shown. (Courtesy of Dr. Harold E. Himwich, 1957.)

coholic patient can be seen in company with others in the same general state of degeneration and social degradation. Usually this part of town is a business equivalent of the residential slum area, with a definite pattern of life for its inhabitants. The alcoholics on Skid Row invariably have profound personality disturbances, and their lives reflect complete resignation to the abandonment of family and social life of a more respected quality.

Dr. David J. Myerson of Boston studied the lives of 101 destitute and homeless men of the Skid Row section of that community. He found that the majority of these men were in their middle forties and that they came from all social and economic levels of our society. Over a period of ten years these 101 alcoholics had spent a group total of over 40,000 days in jails or public institutions. Forty-nine marriages had been dissolved, so that 49 wives and 76 children had become de-

pendent on city agencies or various charities for support. All but a small part of the group had been drinking for twenty years or more; thus the great majority had begun to drink in their twenties. Sporadic employment kept some of the men economically able for a time to support themselves in their alcoholic habits, but ultimately they had lost their jobs and had come to devote their full energies to the acquisition of alcohol on Skid Row by begging, borrowing or stealing.

Rehabilitation efforts with the foregoing group of 101 men were not a complete failure. Twelve men of the group were brought back to a normal life. Twenty men were able to remain sober for three years, but could not adjust themselves to anything except hospital life. For others there was no substantial progress. For the alcoholic, Skid Row is almost the last stop on his life journey.

The Problem of the Tavern

It is estimated that there are about 200,000 taverns in the United States. Many people consider the tavern the center of all the problems associated with alcohol. That this is an extreme view has been shown recently by a study in Dane County, Wisconsin. It was found in this investigation that 75 per cent of the men participating in the study, and 40 per cent of the women, patronized taverns at one time or another.

It is enlightening to discover from this study that a great many people look upon the tavern as a social center or as a poor man's club. This study revealed that many taverns were clean, orderly and well controlled. It appears that the bad reputation of taverns is often developed from the Skid Row tavern, in which there is a great deal of drunkenness, vagrancy, gambling, prostitution and brawling. Such taverns are usually located near the downtown areas in big cities.

If a large proportion of the American population looks upon the tavern as a social club, it would appear that there is something lacking in the community in terms of supplying opportunities for people to get together in small groups for conviviality and social festivities.

In connection with this problem it is interesting to review the results of a study made at the University of Rochester. In this investigation, 383 college women of various religious affiliations were questioned regarding their drinking habits. It was found that from 26 to 51 per cent of the different religious groups consumed alcohol. Of those who did drink, 54 per cent admitted drinking in bars and taverns.

It should be obvious that if the tavern is the center of the problem of alcohol in the United States, greater community attention should be given to this institution. On the other hand, it may well be that many people frequent bars and taverns not primarily to secure alcohol, but mostly for the social pleasure they derive from meeting others. If this is the case, the community has a problem in providing better facilities for such meetings.

Moderate Leadership Is Needed

If alcohol did not have a constructive function in our society, there would be less of a problem associated with its use. But alcohol has a position fundamental to many aspects of our modern industrial life. Used unwisely as a beverage, however, it has a destructive effect upon the person who drinks to excess, on his family and on the community in which he lives. Alcohol is a national problem because we need the product in many phases of our modern civilization, but we do not need the harmful effects that come from overindulgence in alcohol as a beverage.

It is unlikely that the problem of alcoholism will be conquered unless we are able to develop a coordinated community, state and national approach to its solution, based upon intelligent participation of government, industry (including the alcohol industry), medicine, psychiatry, schools, many social agencies, churches, voluntary health organizations and such effective groups as Alcoholics Anonymous. When these important segments of our social structure are brought together on this problem, under a leadership that is moderate in viewpoint, greater progress may be expected than has yet been achieved.

Effects of Alcohol on the Body

Unlike other foods, alcohol does not have to be digested before being absorbed by the body. Alcohol when drunk in a beverage is absorbed from the stomach and intestines; it passes directly into the blood stream, and the blood stream distributes it to all parts of the body.

Within a minute or two after being consumed, alcohol is present in the blood stream. Within a few minutes, therefore, varying with his degree of tolerance, alcohol can be producing characteristic effects upon a person.

The rate of absorption of alcohol into the blood, however, is not constant but decreasing. The first alcohol reaching the stomach is absorbed rapidly, but as more and more alcohol is taken in, the process is slowed down. An hour or more is required for the maximum concentration of alcohol to build up in the blood stream. Furthermore, passage of alcohol into the intestine is hindered by the presence of food in the stomach.

Concentration in the Blood

The percentage of concentration of alcohol in the blood does not rise in exact ratio to the amount of alcohol drunk; time is a factor. Immediately upon being taken into the body, alcohol starts being eliminated and oxidized. Furthermore, from a half hour to several hours are required for all the alcohol from a beverage to pass from the digestive system into the blood stream, depending upon the sort of drink (whether beer or whisky, for example) and on whether the stomach is empty or full of food, which delays absorption. During this period some of the alcohol is lost in elimination through the breath, sweat and urine, and through oxidation in the tissues.

It makes a difference whether the alcohol is taken all at one time or spread out over a long period. If a man weighing 150 pounds were to drink about two-thirds of an ounce of whisky or an eight-ounce glass of beer each hour in the twenty-four, his blood at the end of each hour might show practically no alcohol while resting. Even if (in the twenty-four hour period) he had drunk over a pint of whisky or a gallon and a half of beer, he could have burned up the alcohol imbibed. However, if he had drunk this much of either beverage *in one hour,* he would probably be in a reeling, incoherent condition.

Alcohol Can Kill You

It is possible for a person to drink so much alcohol within a restricted period of time that he will die from the experience. Dr. Sidney Kaye and Dr. Harvey Haag, of Richmond, Virigina, studied the blood alcohol levels of 94 persons who had died of acute alcoholism. These investigators found that when the blood concentration of alcohol reaches 500 milligrams per 100 milliliters of blood, death will occur unless prompt and vigorous medical treatment is obtained. Another investigator stated, after a study of about 2000 cases, that he had never seen a survival when the blood alcohol value was above this figure. Other investigators have accepted a blood concentration of 550 milligrams per 100 milliliters as the fatal level. It appears that from 0.50 to 0.55 per cent or more of alcohol in the blood will be fatal.

Tests for Drunkenness

A concentration percentage up to 0.05 to 0.1 per cent of alcohol in the blood stream might cause no perceptible signs of drunkenness. A percentage as high as 0.3 or 0.4, however, would usually mean severe intoxication.

IN THE UNITED STATES
"More than one million persons, 60 per cent of those arrested for all causes (are arrested) annually . . . on charges associated with heavy drinking . . ."
U.S. News and World Report, 1957

Traffic accidents today cause injuries and deaths equal to those of whole wars in previous generations. To drive a car while you are under the influence of alcohol is to endanger not only your own life, but also the lives of others. It is very important if you have been drinking to delay driving until the concentration of alcohol in the blood has fallen to safe levels.

When a motorist is given a sobriety test, a concentration of less than 0.05 per cent of alcohol in the blood stream is usually accepted as proof that he is not intoxicated. Studies indicate that it is probably not safe to drive an automobile for at least one hour after a couple of highballs or three bottles of beer, since the blood level of alcohol will likely remain above 0.05 per cent for this length of time. After four cocktails, studies suggest it is unsafe to drive for five to six hours or longer if the alcohol is consumed within a short period of time on an empty stomach.

Alcohol and Alertness

Alcohol spoils muscular coordination and hinders skillful movement. Tests show that even the little alcohol that a person would get out of half a glass of mild beer is enough to spoil driving precision. What is worse, some people, though actually driving far worse than usual, think that they are driving better than ordinarily. Experiments have shown that alcohol dulls the attention, so that a driver is less aware of traffic lights and signals from other motorists. The responses of eyes, hands and feet are slower; and the results of this lowered awareness and lowered ability to respond when driving at high speed should be obvious. A delayed reaction time too often results in failure to bring a car to a stop, to swerve around an obstruction, or to perform any act which must be done swiftly and accurately in order to prevent damage and injury.

The Alcoholic Hangover

Too much drink usually results in a hangover, and a hangover is a far from pleasant experience. Physically and psychologically it is punishing.

The hangover begins when the alcohol has been almost or entirely oxidized by the body and the sedative effect has worn off. Then the drinker is aware of aches and pains. The hangover lasts until the sufferer returns to the condition that is "normal" for him, or again starts drinking to blot out his physical and mental torment.

Remorse is characteristic of the hangover period. Loss of self-esteem is profound. Fear and acute anxiety are present, and inability to sleep is a frequent and disturbing symptom.

Physically, thirst is one of the tortures of the hangover period; headache is another. Another symptom is stomach ache, which develops from indigestion and is due to the delay in emptying of the stomach because of alcohol, and because large amounts of alcohol in concentrations above 20 per cent cause a direct irritation of the stomach mucosa. Sweating occurs; a runaway pounding of the heart may develop. Extreme fatigue, the result of much emotional tension and expenditure of energy, is another symptom.

Alcohol and Nutrition

People who drink too much are likely not to eat enough. Their diet consists of too much alcohol and too little food. Alcohol, as a food, is a contradictory one; it is rich in calories, but completely deficient in minerals and vitamins. In a sense, you can get fat on alcohol while you starve to death.

An essential problem in nutrition for people who drink excessively is that of maintaining a proper balance of vitamin intake. The basis of most of our so-called alcoholic disease today is a deficiency of the B complex vitamins.

The person who drinks alcoholic beverages to excess may consume several thousand calories daily from alcohol alone, in addition to those in his food. These extra calories cut down the ratio between the vitamins and calories in his diet, so that the margin of safety, already slim, is substantially reduced. It may be still further reduced by another effect of alcohol: by irritating the stomach lining, alcohol may cause gastritis. The resulting distress and indigestion may turn the sufferer away from food.

Alcoholic beverages, used in moderation, do not disturb nutrition any more than would an amount of sugar cane having the same caloric value. However, the person who uses alcohol to excess is usually liable to neglect other food, and by failing to eat properly, he fails to supply his system with the vitamins, minerals and proteins necessary to maintain good health. Alcohol does not contain these vital food elements. Their absence in the human body brings on various nutritional deficiency diseases. Practically all chronic alcoholics suffer from a deficiency of diet.

Such deficiencies, for half or more of all chronic alcoholics, have already become so severe that such persons have passed from vague ill health into recognizable disease. In general, the condition is due to lack of several of the vitamins; typically, however, the chief lack is of the B vitamins.

Put Vitamins in Alcohol?

It has been suggested, since chronic alcoholics drink too much and eat too little, that alcoholic beverages be fortified with the necessary vitamin B complex. Government regulations make this illegal. However, it has been tried as a laboratory experiment. Results showed that riboflavin is unstable in whisky, in either paper-wrapped or amber bottles; in six months a 50 per cent loss of riboflavin occurred. On the other hand, niacin (nicotinic acid) and thiamine did prove stable in whisky. Even so, it is not recommended that alcoholic drinks be fortified with vitamins. Physio-

logic considerations make such formulas undesirable. The real solution to the problem lies in a well rounded diet and the cessation of excessive consumption of alcohol.

Alcohol: Stimulant or Sedative?

Many people regard alcohol as a stimulant. Often when a person faints, a bystander may put a bottle to the victim's lips in an attempt to let the whisky gurgle into his mouth. Of course the unconscious person cannot swallow. Neither is alcohol a stimulant; it is a sedative and acts as a depressant on the nervous system.

Just how intense a depressant it proves, and to what extent it affects various activities of mind and body, differs with different people, and with the individual at different times, depending upon fatigue, sugar metabolism, emotional state and other conditions.

POSSIBLY FATAL

"Barbiturates and alcohol both act in the same direction as sedative drugs and together may produce exaggerated anesthesia, even leading to death."

Target, May 1956

By the word "depressant" is meant that the alcohol works to reduce the activity of the brain center. This results in a reduction of attention, a blunting of keen judgment, and easing of critical attitude, a lessening of discretion and control. And herein lies the danger of using alcohol for anyone doing something that requires a maximum of alertness, such as driving a car in traffic, or evaluating subtle clues in a diagnosis, or making the fine distinctions of motion and color and space necessary to piloting a plane.

The effect of alcohol on the human organism has been tested in a variety of ways. In the Hollingworth test, men were asked to name the opposites of given words. After drinking the amount of alcohol equivalent to one glass of whisky, the subjects' ability to perform *decreased* by 29 per cent. After taking several more drinks, efficiency was *cut by 52 per cent.*

In tests made by the British Medical Council to appraise judgment of lapse of time, motorists were directed to drive over a given course. Afterward they were given 1½ glasses of whisky and sent over the course again. They drove faster—*but thought that they had taken a longer time.*

Alcohol and Reaction Time

Reaction time is the interval between getting a signal and acting upon it: i.e., the time it takes you to see a sudden flash of light and press a button in answer to it; the time it takes you to put on the brake when you see a car skid to a stop in front of you; or to reach up and catch a ball coming at you in a line drive; or to press a trigger when an enemy plane zooms into your sights.

A normal person ordinarily requires about 1/5 second to respond to a signal to perform a simple motion, like pressing a button. This simple performance has been tested many times by psychologists. After the consumption of as much as 3½ glasses of whisky, reaction time one hour later has been found to be on the average about 34 per cent slower. This slowing of reaction time is one reason why alcohol is not advisable for athletes.

A difference of 34 per cent in reaction time can be crucial under some circumstances. For instance, if you're driving a car at 50 miles an hour, this difference means that you will travel about 17 more feet before stopping. That distance can be the difference between stopping safely or going through a railroad barrier or hitting a small child or smashing into the rear of a truck.

Alcohol and Resistance to Disease

Alcohol lowers body resistance to disease. As far back as 1884 Robert Koch observed that in cholera epidemics more patients died who were excessive drinkers of alcohol than those who were nondrinkers. He concluded that alcoholic intoxication lowers the body's natural resistance to the *Cholera vibrio.* It is believed that this holds true of other microbes as well.

This belief was tested in laboratory experiments by C. C. Lushbaugh at the University of Chicago. Immunity against pneumococci was built up in rabbits by injections of vaccine. A control group was given no vaccine. Pneumococci were administered. The immunized rabbits all lived; the nonimmunized rabbits all died.

Then alcohol was given orally. to the rabbits, by means of a stomach tube, in an amount sufficient to produce stupor. Two hours after intoxication was begun, each rabbit was given the routine test dose of pneumococci. Of 27 nonintoxicated immune rabbits, only *one* died—a death rate of 3.7 per cent. Of 49 intoxicated and immune rabbits, 32 died—a death rate of 65 per cent. Two hours of intoxication had almost completely destroyed the immunity built up in the rabbits by previous vaccination.

Among humans, physicians have long noted that the death rate of alcoholics from pneumonia has been greater than that of nonalcoholics. The use of modern drugs such as sulfonamides and the antibiotics in the treatment of pneumonia has changed this picture somewhat in terms of lives saved, but not in terms of basic principles.

Many people believe that moderate and heavy drinkers are far more apt to be victims of tuberculosis than are nondrinkers. However, it may not be the alcohol itself that is to blame, but the nutritional and social effects of heavy drinking.

Some enlightenment on this possible relationship may be found in a study conducted at the Olive View Sanatorium. At this institution the records of 2000 patients were studied for significant findings. Of the entire group of 2000, approximately 1 in 4 drank; and of those who drank, 1 in 6 drank excessively. Those patients who had a history of drinking were much more likely to have a *far-advanced* case of tuberculosis.

The records on these patients, five years after discharge from the sanatorium, revealed that, on the whole, nondrinkers were in slightly better health than drinkers. For the *immoderate* drinkers, after discharge, the death rate was more than 50 per cent higher than that of the moderate or nondrinkers who had also had severe tuberculosis.

Alcohol and Liver Disease

In time past, cirrhosis, or hardening of the liver, was considered to be the most characteristic "alcohol disease," the specific and inevitable consequence of overindulgence. Today, however, it is generally known that cirrhosis occurs not only among people who drink heavily, but among abstainers as well. It is still true, though, that cirrhosis occurs most frequently among those who drink alcohol excessively.

In cirrhosis of the liver a condition develops in which there is an increase in the supporting, connective or fibrous tissue at the expense of the liver cells. The disease has variations. In general, the liver shrinks in size and hardens. Sometimes the reverse occurs—the liver enlarges.

Formerly, it was supposed that the liver and other organs of the chronic alcoholic functioned practically in a bath of alcohol. And, since alcohol burns the throat when drunk, it was assumed that alcohol was so corrosive that it destroyed the delicate internal tissues, acting on the liver somewhat like a bath of sheep dip or battery acid, scarring and eroding it. It is known now, of course, that alcohol is so diluted

in the stomach and intestines and in the blood that by the time it reaches the liver it is too low in concentration to harm by direct contact.

The theory that alcohol was the direct and positive cause of cirrhosis began to be shaken when it was observed that people who drank no alcohol whatsoever sometimes suffered from cirrhosis. Even children occasionally are afflicted with it. In fact, it occurs among inhabitants of countries where religion forbids drinking alcoholic beverages. Obviously, alcohol was not the specific and predictable cause of cirrhosis.

Now it is known that cirrhosis of the liver in the alcoholic person is only indirectly caused by alcohol. This form of liver disease is directly caused by a dietary deficiency, especially of certain of the vitamin B complex group. It has been noted already that in the heavy drinker there is apt to be a serious deficiency in the consumption of vitamins as well as of other food essentials. It is this nutritional deficiency that produces the harmful effects upon the liver. From a practical viewpoint, however, alcohol must still be blamed when it has resulted in a neglect of the diet with subsequent cirrhosis of the liver.

Alcohol and Delirium Tremens

Delirium tremens is a mental disorder, lasting a few days to a week, which afflicts about 4 per cent of very heavy drinkers. Far more men than women are stricken by it.

It seems to come on suddenly. Actually, certain signs may betray its onset several days, or even a week or two, in advance. The sufferer may be revolted by food, may be unable to keep any nourishment down; he may be jittery and restless, and be prey to a brooding anxiety that seems without cause. His sleep is broken and tormented by nightmares. His eyes and ears become abnormally acute; a bright light or sudden sound may cause him a violent start, and leave an aftermath of intense irritation. His head aches, and his breathing is difficult; he sweats profusely. These symptoms seem to occur mostly at night; in fact, delirium tremens usually begins at night.

In the course of delirium tremens, a patient suffers an onset of ceaseless, sometimes violent, activity. He trembles. His whole body shakes. Tongue, face, fingers, legs, all shiver and quiver in a helpless, exhausting vibration. Also characteristic of delirium tremens are hallucinations, both oral and visual. The patient sees images of animals that do not exist and hears voices of people who aren't there.

Anxiety, vague but oppressive, felt in the period before delirium, becomes very acute during the actual delirium. Often this anxiety is dramatized: the patient believes that he is straining like mad to do what can never be finished. Here, too, some logic still holds: he slaves away at something related to his actual job. A fireman may imagine that he is helplessly spraying extinguisher upon a conflagration that is growing every minute bigger and hotter. A barber may imagine that he's clipping an endless head of hair. A Congressman may believe that he is orating in a filibuster that never terminates. Such hallucinations result in an unceasing intensity of emotion that wears the patient out.

Besides hallucinations, patients may suffer disorientation for space, time and persons. Such patients may look at objects and mistake them for something else; at people, and mistake them for the wrong individuals. The hospital, similarly, may seem to be a resort, a theatre, a gymnasium. Such patients may "recognize" hospital personnel, whom they've never encountered before, as old college roommates, or relatives, or lodge brothers, or famous personalities in the news.

Very marked among the physical symptoms which are characteristic of delirium tremens is a severe and ceaseless trembling. Patients also suffer nausea and constipation. And they perspire very heavily. This excessive sweating leads to dehydration of the body through the loss of water and of salt, which in turn upsets the system's normal functioning. This loss, unless the patient receives treatment, can cause him serious harm. Changes in the pulse rate and blood pressure also occur, heightening as the delirium rises to its peak on the third or fourth day. The liver, also, seems to do its work badly.

The brain of a patient who has died in delirium tremens proves, in seemingly every case, to have undergone a change: a watery swelling. This is so usual that sometimes delirium tremens is referred to as "wet brain."

Fever also occurs in most cases of delirium tremens. In some instances the patient is affected with another disease besides the delirium tremens, such as pneumonia, disease of the nervous system, or severe head injury. It is difficult, therefore, to tell whether the fever is the result of the delirium tremens or the accompanying disease.

Delirium tremens usually lasts four or five days. When the patient's excitement eases and he falls asleep, recovery is beginning. From the terminal sleep the sufferer usually awakes much improved. By the seventh day, ordinarily, he is well.

Wood Alcohol—Poison!

A group of men on a South Sea island, during the war, found some cases of alcohol. The men were members of a construction battalion who had been working hard on this lonely, rugged island for months. They wanted a drink. So they mixed some of the alcohol with water and fruit juices to make highballs, and drank it.

The alcohol was methyl alcohol (better known as wood alcohol) intended for use in testing for leaks of Freon gas in refrigerators. All the eighteen men reported to the hospital in bad condition. Six died—one in three.

In another area forty-two patients, enlisted personnel and natives, came to the hospital suffering from acute methyl alcohol poisoning. Of the forty-two patients, thirteen died. Again, a mortality of about one in three.

The patients reported to the hospital from one to three days after drinking the wood alcohol. Investigation revealed that the men had been mildly drunk a few hours after the drinks. Gradually they had become drowsy, felt headache and nausea. Their vision began to blur, and they could not stand strong light. Their breathing became labored, and they started vomiting. When they arrived at the hospital, the odor of methyl alcohol was on their breath. They were drowsy and confused, their faces flushed; they had low-grade fever, and their pulse was rapid, and breathing difficult.

Their vision was impaired. At first they had lost ability to detect green color; then, successively, they could not see red, yellow and blue. Impairment of vision, for some of the patients, was so severe that all color sense was lost, and vision was limited to hand movements at a distance of about a foot. Some of the patients, furthermore, had numbness of all toes about six days after drinking poison.

Of the severe cases who died most were brought to the hospital in profound coma, their faces a deeply purplish livid hue, eye pupils dilated and unresponsive to light, their breathing very slow and difficult. Autopsies of the dead men revealed damage to the lungs, liver, stomach, kidneys and brain.

According to the doctors in charge of treatment, most of the symptoms of the poisoning, and probably even the deaths, were caused by acute acidosis.

The acidosis, in turn, was likely caused by the accumulation of formic acid in the tissues and body fluids, derived from the methyl alcohol. Formic acid is a poisonous corrosive.

The story of poisoning, blindness and death from methyl or wood alcohol is an old one. This is a different kind of alcohol which cannot be consumed safely, regardless of the circumstances. To drink wood alcohol is a sure and certain way for anyone to court death or chronic impairment of health. This is one brand of alcohol that must be left alone.

Another epidemic of wood alcohol poisoning which gives additional evidence of the fatal or injurious effects of this substance occurred at Atlanta, Georgia. In this outbreak 323 persons consumed bootleg whisky that resulted in the death of forty-one of the persons affected. Visual disturbances, abdominal and back pains, headache, vomiting, dizziness, difficult breathing, diarrhea and death occurred in various patients.

Great differences in susceptibility to wood alcohol were found among the various patients. The smallest amount that produced death was three teaspoonsful, whereas the largest amount taken by a survivor was one pint. This, definitely, is one kind of alcohol that must be left alone.

RESPONSIBILITIES OF A HOST

1. Never give a party for the main or sole purpose of drinking.

2. Always serve food with alcoholic drinks.

3. Always serve the meal without prolonged delay if alcoholic drinks precede it.

4. If alcoholic drinks are served, serve always with them, and as attractively, nonalcoholic drinks.

5. Never violate courtesy by allowing pressure to be put on guests to drink if they do not wish to do so.

6. Never delegate to cocktails the host's responsibility to create an atmosphere, and to encourage relationships, conducive to wholesome recreation.

7. Avoid drawing attention to a guest who is known to have the illness of alcoholism.

Joint Commission on Alcoholism of the Protestant Episcopal Church, 1958

Questions

1. Why is it that alcoholics of long standing can sometimes give up alcohol without evidence of having
   sustained any serious effects upon the body?
2. If alcohol does not damage the brain, why is there
   a disproportionate share of alcoholics in mental
   institutions?
3. Why is the nutritional status of the alcoholic apt to
   be poor?
4. Why do some doctors prescribe moderate drinking
   of alcohol for some forms of heart disease?
5. Is alcohol a stimulant or a depressant?
6. Should a person who commits a crime while intoxicated be partially exonerated of blame?
7. What kind of personal program can a college student evolve on the matter of drinking that will
   give most hope of reasonable control?

For Further Reading

1. Adams, Leon D.: *The Commonsense Book of Drinking.* New York, David McKay Company, 1960.
2. King, Albion Roy: *Basic Information on Alcohol.*
   Mount Vernon, Iowa, Cornell College Press,
   1960.
3. McCarthy, Raymond G.: *Drinking and Intoxication
   —Selected Readings in Social Attitudes and
   Controls.* Glencoe, Ill., Free Press, 1959.
4. Roueché, Berton: *Neutral Spirit: A Portrait of Alcohol.* Boston, Little, Brown and Company, 1960.

Recommended Film

To Your Health. Boston, 16 mm. sound, color, 10 minutes, New York, Columbia University Press, 1956.

15

ALCOHOLISM

IT IS THOUGHT that there are about five million alcoholics in the United States. Not more than about seven per cent of these live on Skid Rows in the cities of America. Only about six per cent of this group can be identified as a member of any group seeking help. Some investigators have concluded that the remainder of the group might well be called the "hidden alcoholics." These alcoholics have occupational stability and many of them have stable marriages although problems centered around excessive drinking undoubtedly exist.

These hidden alcoholics often conceal their drinking habits from employers, friends and family physicians. In fact, some physicians are treating alcoholics without realizing that they are such. The hidden alcoholic does not report to his physician the full extent of his drinking or

> **SHRINKING CIRCLES**
>
> "In the beginning, the alcoholic belongs to the big circle . . . of family, friends, work, recreation . . . then, inch by inch, his drinking pattern changes. He gets drunk more often than his friends do . . . he finds excuses to keep drinking . . . people start to criticize . . . the circle is closing in. Relationships with the outside world deteriorate by slow but steady steps . . . the circle will become a narrow enclosure and he will live inside it all alone, trapped and helpless."
>
> *C. S. Clifton, 1956*

the effects that alcohol may be having upon his health.

There is no sharp definition of an alcoholic. He or she is simply a person who drinks too much and whose life has been adversely affected by alcohol. The alcoholic is a person who can no longer control his drinking: "one drink is too much, and a thousand drinks are not enough."

Alcohol has been accepted in virtually all societies and civilizations for thousands of years. It is unrealistic to believe that efforts directed at stopping the manufacture of alcohol will be able to overcome the traditions and desires of a large segment of our population.

In this day and age alcohol has assumed tremendous significance in industrial processes. It is completely unrealistic to believe that we can stop the manufacture of alcohol completely. To do so would have serious consequences, even upon our health. Alcohol, for example, is used in the manufacture of DDT, which, in turn, is used in worldwide control of malaria and many other insect-borne diseases.

If we are to prevent alcoholism, we must find ways of doing so even though alcohol is still available. We must continue to search for more effective ways of treating alcoholism, for as long as we have alcohol we shall have alcoholics.

Certainly the alcoholic who no longer drinks must be considered a wholesome force in the community for the direction of young people and others away from the multiple problems that excessive drinking creates.

In the past, alcohol education in the schools was largely centered upon teaching about the physiologic effects of alcohol in the body. Modern research and medical evidence now suggest that these effects are not as harmful as was once believed. Education would probably be more effective if a shift were made toward teaching about the *social* effects of the excessive drinking of alcohol. Such instruction should probably also be done in direct association with everyday problems of the high school and college students, for it is at this age that the great majority of persons begin the drinking of alcohol.

The churches must assume responsibility for leading people to the discovery that spiritual resources may give sufficient strength so that flight from the difficulties of life need not be attempted through the means of alcohol. Though many other community organizations also have responsibilities for character development, it must be emphasized that the major obligation lies with parents and family members in this respect.

Perhaps most important in the prevention of alcoholism is the acceptance of responsibility by the individual himself in regard to this problem. No matter what others say or do, the decision about starting to drink eventually rests with the individual and with no one else. A sensible examination of the facts about excessive drinking will be a wise prelude to any decision on the matter.

Each person should have a sufficient philosophy in life so that he or she is able to recognize and work for values that the unthinking person may never see. To drink excessively is to create problems rather than to resolve them. Such problems should be discussed openly and candidly by young people. Agreements and decisions should be reached by them, both individually and in groups. Social influences in regard to drinking are very powerful among young people, so that often an individual decision may recede in the face of group pressures toward social drinking. When there is basic agreement within the group itself, however, based upon a sensible discussion, there is less apt to be this conflict between the individual and those with whom he or she wishes to associate. The final decision about drinking, however, rests with you and with no one else in the world.

Who Can Become an Alcoholic?

One reason why medical or psychiatric treatment will not stop addiction to alcohol in all cases is the fact that there are various types of chronic alcoholism. What helps one person to rehabilitate himself may not help another. Drugs, moreover, cannot get at the emotional factors which often are the cause of overindulgence in liquor.

According to some authorities in the field of alcoholism, out of every 100 excessive drinkers, some 40 are neurotic inebriates, 10 are psychotic (mentally deranged), and another 10 are of low mentality. Among alcoholics, thus, some investigators believe that 60 per cent have succumbed to alcoholism because of some physical or psychic ailment or deficiency. To give a patient among this 60 per cent a "cure" that is aimed at a symptom (the drinking) will not heal the disease that is causing the symptom.

The remaining alcoholics, who are neither emotionally ill, nor mentally deranged, nor feeble-minded, to begin with, are considered to be "normal" excessive drinkers. However, too much drinking over a long time has made them as helpless in the grip of their craving for alcohol as the other types of addicts. And, like all the others, these "normal" excessive drinkers have finally become chronic alcoholics, just as ill and discouraged and desperate as the other types.

Contrary to the foregoing study, there are others that indicate that there is no clearcut personality characteristic of the chronic alcoholic. In one study, thirty-seven different investigations of organized research on the personalities of chronic alcoholics were made. There was conflicting evidence from these investigations, but the primary conclusion was that *there is no alcoholic personality prior to alcoholism.* In other words, *anyone can become a chronic alcoholic under certain circumstances.*

Undoubtedly, this last type of drinker, the person who is relatively stable or "normal," but who has become an alcoholic through excessive social drinking and a particular set of circumstances, offers the best chance for successful treatment, *provided he wants to be cured.*

Oddly enough, experience has shown that no matter how extreme alcoholism may be, there is always a possibility that the patient may be successfully rehabilitated. In other words, every alcoholic should be regarded as one who can be brought back to a more normal way of living, provided the key to his particular personality can be found in relation to his drinking. Fundamental to any attempt at rehabilitation is the patient's desire to be cured. Some authorities now believe, however, that even compulsory treatment is worth while and that good results may be obtained.

Rehabilitation of the Alcoholic

There is some promise that alcoholics can be rehabilitated and that their abilities to make good social and physical adjustments can be restored. In California a follow-up study by the State Department of Public Health of 1,256 alcoholic patients who were treated at a public health clinic showed that over 600 of these drinkers had been rehabilitated.

After these alcoholics had received treatment, only 15 per cent were arrested for drunkenness as compared with 48 per cent before treatment. Only 12 per cent were hospitalized for drinking after they had received treatment, whereas 46 per cent had received this care before treatment. It was found that approximately 50 per cent of the group were making good or excellent social adjustments after treatment. Approximately 70 per cent of those capable of working were found to be currently employed after treatment and only 18 per cent were actually unemployed as compared to 60 per cent who were unemployed before treatment.

Alcoholism is recognized as a national problem in Switzerland and treatment is required by law for this disease. Those alcoholics who do not respond to treatment are put in institutions such as psychiatric hospitals, work houses, or "closed" establishments. Those alcoholics who are judged to be capable of responding to treatment are required by law to appear before responsible health authorities. They receive an invitation for such an appearance and the first session is an educational one in which they are told why the authorities think they are alcoholics and why they ought to seek professional care. They are also told that compulsory legal measures may be taken if they fail to seek voluntary help.

Often hospital treatment is provided for alcoholic detoxication; thus, treatment is not restricted to psychotherapy and case work.

How Doctors Treat Alcoholics

Doctors, in general, have done good work on the medical aspects of treatment for alcoholism, but have been inadequate in treating the social and psychologic aspects of the patients' problem.

A study made by Dr. Riley and Dr. Marden, of Rutgers University, of the ways in which 455 physicians treated alcoholic patients in forty-two New Jersey communities showed that:

(1) 25 per cent of the physicians handled acute cases of alcoholism by giving only sobering-up treatment;

(2) 25 per cent referred the alcoholic patient elsewhere;

(3) 50 per cent of the physicians treated other illnesses of an alcoholic, but made no effort to help the patient with his problem of excessive drinking.

Those physicians who did make some superficial effort to treat patients for acute alcoholism during the sobering-up period used the following methods:

(1) 43 per cent gave sedatives;

(2) 42 per cent administered vitamins;

(3) 16 per cent prescribed a diet for the patients; and

(4) 13 per cent used psychotherapy.

It is obvious that most of the doctors gave their patients only temporary relief, and not basic treatment for chronic alcoholism. The fact is that physicians in general practice lack time, facilities, and cooperation from the patient for the long, difficult process of rehabilitating alcoholics.

Most of the doctors were reluctant to accept alcoholics as patients, because such patients, having imbibed, were hazy about following instructions, were unreliable, would call a doctor at any hour of the day or night, and in general were a nuisance to handle. Furthermore, hardly a third of the doctors thought that alcoholism could be cured at all.

The point made by this study is that most doctors give only temporary relief to alcoholics, not basic treatment, for the reasons that the medical men have neither time nor facilities to do otherwise. The conclusion is, of course, that the rehabilitation of alcoholics is a job for special personnel and special facilities.

Hospital Treatment

Most people who are picked up on the streets in a state of drunkenness spend their time in jails rather than in hospitals during the sobering-up process. In fact, most hospitals still do not admit a patient for treatment during a period of acute drunkenness. Since the hospital is generally filled with patients suffering from serious illnesses, it is not good to have them disturbed by the noisy, boisterous conduct of a drunk. Unless the inebriated person is in a stuporous condition, he is apt to be undependable, often obnoxious, and sometimes actually vicious.

In addition to the fact that the alcoholic may be disturbing patients who are sick, hospital treatment for the drunken person does not offer any permanent cure in the great majority of cases. What service is to be rendered is usually associated with the sobering-up process or the treatment of some complication that has occurred along with the intoxication.

Nevertheless some hospitals have made an attempt to be of service to alcoholics. The Knickerbocker Hospital is reputed to have been the first hospital in New York City to provide both sobering-up treatment and a more extended approach to the problem of alcoholism. At the Chicago State Hospital separate facilities have been provided for the exclusive treatment of inebriates. The treatment given at this institution is offered in conjunction with individual and group psychotherapy by competent psychiatrists, the organization of Alcoholics Anonymous clubs, and the provision of the conditioned-reflex treatment for alcoholism.

In some hospitals admission of a drunken patient is obtained through approval by some member of the Alcoholics Anonymous organization who agrees to act as sponsor for the intoxicated person. Medical treatment, proper diet, good nursing care, and psychotherapy are started at once with each alcoholic patient. No visitors are permitted, and no repeat visit is possible. Release from the hospital is generally permitted no earlier than five days after admittance. When the patient is dismissed from the hospital, he is taken over by Alcoholics Anonymous. Early hospitalization and medical treatment appears to be an important step in the treatment of alcoholism, for a large percentage of the patients treated in this manner have remained total abstainers.

Sobering-Up Treatment

One of the medical problems in the treatment of alcoholism is to shorten the period of great distress and intense illness that often follows a drunken spree.

Many individual drugs have been used by physicians for helping patients sober up. Great progress in this direction has been made in recent years. Alcoholic intoxication can now be cleared up rapidly and distressing hang-overs prevented by the use of ACTH or adrenocortical hormones. Other drugs have also been used with somewhat comparable results.

One of the newer drugs that has been used for about five years is hydroxyzine hydrochloride. This drug appears to be outstandingly safe without major damaging side effects. No liver damage has been reported in almost a billion doses. The drug helps to control hallucinations, irregularities of heart beat and certain types of circulatory disorder and to foster in general a more rapid recovery from acute drunkenness.

Treatment of any patient with drugs, of course, is a medical problem. Because drugs must be given in proper dosage and under restricted conditions to selected patients only, it is unwise for any person to use drugs of any sort on his own initiative for sobering up. When prescribed by a physician, however, various drugs can shorten substantially the intense discomfort of the after-effects of drunkenness. This type of treatment, however, makes no fundamental contribution to the cure of alcoholism. It is not to be looked upon as anything more than temporary relief of symptoms.

The Conditioned-Reflex Treatment

The conditioned-reflex treatment consists in giving the patient alcoholic beverages and some drug that will induce nausea and vomiting simultaneously. The patient is "conditioned" to react to the mere thought, sight, smell or taste of liquor with nausea and retching. His craving for liquor is transformed into revulsion against it. As a cure, it's fine while it lasts. But it does not usually last more than a few months. It has to be backed up with efforts that are more basic, by attempts to get the patient into a way of life which satisfies his deepest needs so that he will not turn to liquor for escape and comfort when the temporary effects of the conditioned-reflex treatment wear off. Nevertheless, in some cases this form of help to the alcoholic patient does bring good results, as shown at a number of institutions that specialize in the treatment of alcoholism.

The conditioned-reflex treatment of alcoholic patients has been used at the Washingtonian Hospital in Boston with some success. Various drugs are prescribed, although emetine is used most frequently at this institution. The patient is first treated with the drug and is then exposed to the sight, smell and taste of alcohol immediately before the expected vomiting begins. Drinks are offered to the patient in various mixtures, including both straight and highball forms.

The treatments last from twenty to thirty minutes and are repeated daily for five or six days. Later, six or seven such treatments are given at intervals of four to twelve weeks and are called reinforcements. Sometimes patients need these reinforcements extending into the second year.

In addition to the conditioned-reflex treatment, the staff of this hospital works with relatives and enters into group therapy work with former patients. Some of these come back for part-time hospitalization. Sometimes this type of treatment provides a balance in favor of abstention which the psychiatrist or other therapist can use to good advantage in dealing more effectively with the patient by other means.

Treatment with Drugs

Many drugs have been used on alcoholics in recent years. Sedatives, tranquilizers, steroids with tranquilizing action (Cetadiol), antihistamines, antidipsotrophics (Antabus), central nervous stimulants (Ritalin) and cerebral circulatory tonics (Niacin) have been used both in experimental studies and practical trials for the reduction of alcoholism. None of the drugs have been effective as a cure for alcoholism although some have improved the mood of the drinker. On the other hand, placebos (such as sugar pills) have also improved the mood of the drinker as much as 25 to 40 per cent of the time. A drug is not considered to be effective in improving the outlook of the alcoholic unless it can do better than placebos.

In recent years a considerable amount of publicity has been given to the use of Antabus in the treatment of alcoholism. This drug was first used abroad (especially in Denmark, Iceland and Finland), on thousands of patients.

To be effective in the control of drinking, Antabus must be taken about twelve hours before alcohol is consumed. Under these circumstances the drinking of alcohol brings on a number of distressing symptoms that prompt the person to forego his liquor.

The drinker is apt to experience first a feeling of heat in the face followed by an intense flushing of the face and neck. The whole area becomes purple-red. The eyelids often become puffy and swollen. Some patients become nauseated in thirty to sixty minutes after the drinking of alcohol. In these patients the severe flushing of the face disappears and is replaced by pallor and a drop in blood pressure. More alcohol is apt to result in dizziness and unconsciousness.

The discomfort experienced by the patient is so distressing that the great majority will not consume alcohol while under the influence of Antabus. This sensitivity begins to develop about three to four hours after Antabus has been taken, but does not develop to its fullest extent until about twenty-four hours.

Some patients have suffered mental illness during the first weeks of treatment with this drug. On hospitalization and discontinuance of Antabus, however, the psychiatric symptoms disappeared within a few days. Some deaths have been reported from the use of this drug, and it has been shown that persons with heart or liver disease should not be treated with Antabus.

The general medical conclusion in the United States is that Antabus is not a safe drug to be used in the treatment of alcoholism, except under careful medical supervision and on carefully selected patients. Since Antabus does not resolve the emotional problems that many alcoholics have, and does not alter the basic personality of the drinker, no long-term cure can be expected from its use. It must therefore be used in conjunction with other methods of treatment for best results. In short, the drug is dangerous and does not produce a permanent or long-lasting cure of the drinking habit. In this country Antabus has been used largely on an experimental basis in an effort to appraise its value. Most physicians do not prescribe the drug.

Recently citrated calcium carbamide has been used to render the effect of alcohol unpleasant to the drinker. As with Antabus, the discomfort of the drinker is such that he is not disposed to drink. The severity of the reaction depends upon how much of the drug the drinker has previously consumed and how much alcohol he takes. The drinker's face and neck (and often the entire body) flush, his heart pounds, his pulse races, and he breathes rapidly. The drinker may become nauseated, he may vomit, and his blood pressure may fall in dramatic fashion.

Although the effects of Antabus may persist for a week or more, those of carbamide last for only one or two days. Sensitization to the drug develops much more rapidly in the case of the citrated calcium carbamide. Usually one dose of the medicine is sufficient, in contrast to one or two weeks of treatment often necessary with Antabus.

It is likely that citrated calcium carbamide will have the same basic limitations and hazards that are characteristic of Antabus. Neither drug gets at the fundamental deficiency of the alcoholic, nor can results be expected on a lasting basis. Medical supervision of the drinker is essential with both drugs, and at best the drugs must be considered of temporary value while more productive measures are taken for rehabilitation of the drinker over a longer period of time.

Psychotherapy and Alcoholism

Many alcoholics drink because of fundamental insecurities, tensions, conflicts and other emotional disturbances. For these persons alcohol gives a temporary escape from emotional problems, even though the patient may not be aware of why he seeks alcohol. Other persons with more serious forms of mental illness may also become alcoholics. Frequently, then, the problem of alcoholism is a problem of mental health.

Psychotherapy for this type of alcoholic may produce substantially favorable results. The first step in psychiatric treatment is one of establishing favorable rapport between the psychiatrist and the patient. It also entails finding out things about the drinker, in order that the psychiatrist may proceed with more effective treatment. The appraisal of the drinker's personality may be extensive and may involve the use of many psychologic tests.

Numerous interviews with the psychiatrist will probably be needed. Even when the patient has been helped a good deal, it is frequently necessary for him to continue at least occasional interviews with the psychiatrist, and a continuous follow-up may be advisable.

All this adds up to the fact that although psychotherapy can be very effective in individual cases of alcoholism, the process of rehabilitating the patient by this means is apt to be long, expensive and often incomplete in results.

The great shortage of psychiatrists in the United States, the number of interviews needed before assistance to the patient begins to be substantial, and the lack of sufficient funds on the part of the average patient make it almost certain that the resources of the psychiatrist will not be used extensively by alcoholics in the United States.

This does not mean that psychotherapy will be absent from treatment of the alcoholic. In fact, it is very likely that one of the most effective aspects of the Alcoholics Anonymous approach to the problem of alcoholism is that of group psychotherapy. Even though members of this organization probably never think of themselves as being psychiatrists, it is likely that the crude form of psychotherapy which is involved in the Alcoholics Anonymous meetings is of real value to the patient.

Psychotherapy will undoubtedly play a large part in the rehabilitation of many alcoholics, but many practical problems associated with this form of treatment indicate that it is unlikely that the total national problem will be resolved by psychotherapy.

Alcoholics Anonymous

Alcoholics Anonymous is a loosely knit fellowship of alcoholics. The organization has several hundred thousand members and has been remarkably successful in getting alcoholics to stop drinking. Membership in Alcoholics Anonymous is open to anyone who is an alcoholic regardless of sex, religion, color or economic status. The only provision for membership is that the drinker wants to be cured.

Actually, the purpose of the organization is to get the alcoholic to stop drinking rather than to cure him. A fundamental tenet of the organization is that no true alcoholic ever actually becomes cured. The concept appears to be that the only difference between a "cured" alcoholic and an uncured one is a single glass of whisky. If the drinker who goes off alcohol ever takes another drink, he will find that he is still an alcoholic. The purpose of the organization, then, is to get alcoholics to stop drinking alcohol.

From 75 to 80 per cent of the alcoholics who join this organization of their own free will and with a real desire to stop drinking will be able to achieve this purpose. This is the highest rate of achievement in the promotion of sobriety that has been obtained from any method of treatment of the alcoholic.

> **ALCOHOLICS ANONYMOUS**
> "The fact remains, and the proof is in the final results, that the simple program of Alcoholics Anonymous is the answer to the problems of a greater number of alcoholics than from combined efforts of all others interested in contributing to the rehabilitation of alcoholics."
> *Robert J. Conner, Sr., 1957*

The attitude of Alcoholics Anonymous toward the drinker is the same as that of the medical profession, namely, that the alcoholic is a sick person who needs help. When the alcoholic accepts this viewpoint that he is ill and needs help, he is relieved of a sense of guilt or moral responsibility for his past drinking behavior. This is definitely of psychiatric value in the treatment of the illness in a person who has a genuine desire to stop drinking.

At the informal group meetings the new member finds himself in company with other alcoholics who understand his problem completely for the simple reason that they have been through the same experiences he has suffered. He is put in a social situation in which he has status and prestige. This, too, has great psychotherapeutic value, for the alcoholic, because of his extended misconduct over a number of years, has probably been shunned by others for some time.

The working principle of Alcoholics Anonymous is that of achieving sobriety for a period of twenty-four hours at a time. This practical approach is embedded in the acceptance of a basic philosophy that there is a power greater than the individual drinker and that help from this source can be obtained if the alcoholic desires it.

Proof of the value of Alcoholics Anonymous lies in their accomplishments. About 50 per cent of those who join this organization in real hope of help never take another drink for the rest of their lives. It is stated that about 25 per cent will have several relapses, but ultimately are able to overcome the habit of drinking. In the remaining approximately 25 per cent, the organization will fail to achieve results. Often this is because some members join under compulsion from others and have no genuine desire to be helped or have no fundamental faith in what the organization can give them.

Chapters of this organization are now established in virtually all the major cities of the United States and in many smaller communities also. Often the organization advertises in the "Personal" columns of the local newspapers. Sometimes a telephone number is listed in the telephone directory. A person in need of help who wishes to communicate with some member of the organization can search these two sources for directions that should permit him to get in touch with the nearest Alcoholics Anonymous group. If no local address can be found, the organization can be reached through the Alcoholic Foundation, Inc., 141 E. 44th St., New York 17, New York.

Questions

1. What should be done with the many alcoholics of the Skid Row areas in large cities?
2. What is the main cause of failure in most treatments of alcoholics?
3. Why is it that some nationalities have more alcoholics than others?
4. Why is it that most drugs used in the treatment of alcoholism achieve only a temporary success?
5. Is there any justification for putting intoxicated persons in jail rather than in hospitals?
6. Should a college student take the car key of a friend who is intoxicated and insists on driving?
7. Who is the "wet blanket" at a party: the drunken person or the sober person?
8. What can college students do to reduce social drinking on campus?

For Further Reading

1. *Alcoholics Anonymous.* New York, Works Publishing Company, 1955.
2. Habas, Ralph A.: *How to Live without Liquor.* New York, New American Library, 1955.
3. Kruse, H. D.: *Alcoholism as a Medical Problem.* New York, Paul B. Hoeber, Inc., 1956.
4. McCarthy, Raymond G.: *Drinking and Intoxication—Selective Readings in Social Attitudes and Controls.* Glencoe, Illinois, Free Press, 1959.
5. Pittman, David J.: *Alcoholism, An Interdisciplinary Approach.* Springfield, Ill., Charles C Thomas, 1959.
6. Rea, Frederick B.: *Alcoholism, Its Psychology and Cure.* New York, Philosophical Library, 1956.
7. Williams, Roger J.: *Alcoholism.* Austin, Texas, University of Texas Press, 1960.

For Advanced Reading

Himwich, Harold E.: *Alcoholism.* Washington, D.C., American Association for the Advancement of Science, 1957.

16

TOBACCO AND HEALTH

THERE ARE new facts about tobacco that you should know.

Studies of the past few years have shown that the smoking of tobacco is associated with shorter length of life, more lung cancer, more heart and circulatory disease and many other aspects of human health.

The studies have also shown that it is not easy to change the smoking habits of a person who has used tobacco for years. Success in getting people to do less smoking of tobacco is greater if the facts are presented to young people.

As a college student you are more intelligent than the average person. You can use this intelligence to get the facts about smoking. Can you use this same intelligence in reaching a rational decision about whether or not *you* should smoke? Whether or not a person decides to smoke tobacco is largely a matter of individual decision. Before a decision is reached, however, it makes good sense to know the facts about tobacco.

Even if tobacco is injurious to health, it may be that some persons will want to smoke purely because of the pleasure and satisfaction they get from the habit. The point is that people should know the facts before a decision is reached, not after the habit has been established.

Most people know, in a vague way, that nicotine occurs in tobacco, and that nicotine is a poison. Few people are aware, however, how extremely powerful and deadly it is. Fortunately, a smoker absorbs only a relatively small portion of this toxic substance from any single cigarette.

Sixty milligrams of nicotine constitute a lethal dose if placed directly into a human being's blood stream. Considering that a milligram is 1/1000 of a gram, and that a gram is only 1/28 of an ounce, a killing amount of nicotine is a small amount indeed. In pure form, just one drop of it placed on the tongue of a guinea pig or on the shaven skin of a rabbit will cause the animal to die. And if the amount of nicotine which is contained in just one cigar were divided in half, and each half injected into the veins of two different men, both would die.

Tobacco smoke, in addition to nicotine, may contain carbon monoxide, carbon dioxide, hydrogen sulfide, hydrocyanic acid, quinoline, ammonia, furfural, phenols, pyridine, irritant aldehydes, and other substances.

Excessive smokers may also run the risk of some lead and arsenic intake, because

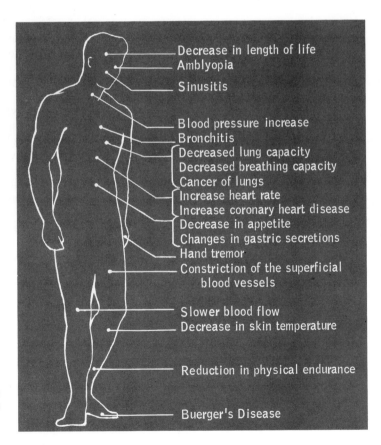

Figure 21. Some of the effects of tobacco on the human body.

Decrease in length of life
Amblyopia
Sinusitis

Blood pressure increase
Bronchitis
Decreased lung capacity
Decreased breathing capacity
Cancer of lungs
Increase heart rate
Increase coronary heart disease
Decrease in appetite
Changes in gastric secretions
Hand tremor
Constriction of the superficial blood vessels

Slower blood flow
Decrease in skin temperature

Reduction in physical endurance

Buerger's Disease

tobacco plants, while growing, are sometimes protected from insect damage by sprays of lead arsenate. The result is that tobacco, whether used in cigars, cigarettes or pipe mixtures, sometimes contains substantial amounts of both lead and arsenic.

The arsenic content of fifteen brands of cigarettes was investigated in one instance and found to vary among brands from zero to 106 micrograms of arsenic trioxide per gram of tobacco.

Obviously the question to be answered is whether any or all of these substances in tobacco are damaging to health and life, and if so, to what extent. It makes better sense to reach a decision about smoking before one begins rather than to drift into the habit carelessly and without thought.

Absorption of Harmful Substances

Nicotine is probably the chief poison in tobacco, and the one which requires most concern unless subsequent research reveals a more harmful ingredient.

Fortunately, part of the poison volatilized by smoking escapes while the cigarette or cigar is not in the user's mouth; and, even more luckily, part of the poison is exhaled when the smoke is blown out. The amount actually retained by the smoker is small.

In rapid smoking, more of the smoke may be breathed into the mouth than escapes into the outside air. The result may be that nearly half of the nicotine content of the cigarette is drawn into the mouth. Inhaling makes a difference; when the smoke is breathed into the lungs, it passes over a much greater area of absorbing surface than if it touches only the mouth and nasal passages.

It makes a difference how completely a cigarette is smoked, for the cigarette itself acts as a filter to some degree. As the smoke is drawn through a cigarette

from the burning end, some of the nicotine adheres to the tobacco through which it is being pulled. The result is that the "butt" contains a higher concentration of nicotine than does the front end of the cigarette. Therefore people who never smoke more than half a cigarette are apt to absorb *less than half* of its nicotine content.

Slow, intermittent smoking allows more of the nicotine to escape into the air than does rapid, continuous smoking. The fast chainsmoker, therefore, draws more nicotine into his system than does the leisurely smoker.

The amount of nicotine absorbed by a smoker will also vary with the nicotine content of the tobacco he smokes: some brands have a high content, others a low content. The use of a filter can reduce the amount of nicotine absorbed by about 25 to 75 per cent.

Obviously, a person's health will be affected the least by smoking if he absorbs a minimum of nicotine and tobacco tars. Whether you take in a lot of nicotine or only a little depends on your smoking habits.

The smoker who inhales deeply and frequently, who smokes a cigarette down to the last half-inch, who keeps the smoke in his lungs and who lights one cigarette upon the fading butt of its predecessor in a long chain, will absorb a maximum of nicotine and tobacco resins.

It can thus be seen that the amount of nicotine or other ingredient of tobacco that the smoker takes into his body will depend upon a variety of factors. Some smokers absorb very little, while others absorb a considerably larger amount of nicotine.

The question may well be asked: If nicotine is such a deadly poison, why don't heavy smokers drop dead? There are a number of reasons; among them:

About 25 per cent of the nicotine is destroyed in the zone of combustion.

About 30 per cent adheres to the tobacco in the butt.

About 30 per cent escapes into the air with the smoke.

About 15 per cent is drawn into the smoker's mouth, but only traces pass through the mucous membrane into the blood stream. If, however, the smoke is inhaled into the lungs, the amount absorbed by the body is greatly increased.

A lot of nicotine, of course, is exhaled as the user breathes out the smoke, and some of the absorbed nicotine is eliminated in the urine. Also, the human body, by exposure to small doses of nicotine over a period of time, is able to build up some degree of tolerance to it, as to other poisons.

The effects of smoking upon human health cannot be standardized easily. Tobacco affects people differently because people themselves vary in their resistance to the toxic substances encountered and differ greatly in their smoking habits.

Immediate Physiologic Effects

Nicotine causes a constriction of the superficial blood vessels. Because body temperature is maintained by the blood stream, the temperature of the fingers and toes is lowered when the supply of blood to the extremities is diminished by constriction of the blood vessels.

A number of experiments have established these facts. In one study, made at the University of Michigan, twenty-nine persons were selected as subjects. The purpose of the experiment was to measure the skin temperature, blood pressure and pulse rate in order to learn whether smoking caused any changes in them.

Heart rate and blood pressure were taken by the usual methods. To get the skin temperature, a sensitive electrical device called a thermocouple was used. Temperature readings were taken from the skin fold just behind the nail on fingers and toes.

Each of the subjects smoked two cigarettes.

Results revealed that in every case after smoking two cigarettes the skin temperature of the fingers dropped between 1° and 2° F., the blood pressure increased about 12 millimeters of mercury, and the pulse rate increased about 18 to 19 beats per minute.

In another study the drop in skin temperature of toes and fingers was even more marked, the average fall being 5.3°, with

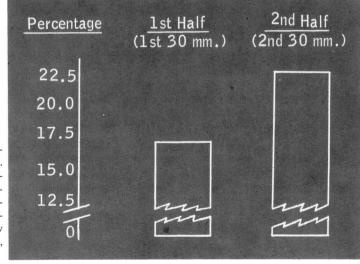

Figure 22. Smoke condensation from an 85-mm. nonfilter cigarette. (Wynder, Ernest L., and Hoffman, Dietrich: Some practical aspects of the smoking-cancer problem. New England J. Med., 262:542, March 17, 1960.)

a maximum drop in one case of 15.5°. Moreover, by observing under a microscope the blood capillaries of the fingernail fold, the investigators were able to see the flow of blood slow down or even stop very soon after the subjects began smoking.

These scientists ran a check on their experiment. On one occasion they gave their subjects "cigarettes" in which ashless filter paper had been substituted for tobacco. The result was no drop in skin temperature and no slowing of the blood flow.

Another check on the effect of nicotine on the circulatory system was made in which the investigators injected, directly into the blood stream, an amount of nicotine equivalent to that absorbed by smoking two cigarettes. The subjects revealed the same consequences that resulted from the previous experiments: a drop of skin temperature, and increases in blood pressure and pulse rate.

Although it has been well established that the primary immediate physiologic effects of tobacco smoking are to cause a constriction of the superficial blood vessels, to increase the heart rate, and to bring about an increase in blood pressure, there are great variations in the intensities of these effects. Most smokers will not have an increase in blood pressure of more than 6 or 8 millimeters of mercury or an increase in pulse rate of more than about 8 to 10 pulsations per minute. Probably most will experience a drop in skin temperature of less than one degree.

On the other hand, some extreme results have been noted. An increase of more than 100 beats per minute in the heart rate of one patient was reported by a physician. An increase in blood pressure of 30 to 40 millimeters of mercury is not at all rare; an opposite effect has been noted as well. In a minority of smokers there appears to be a vascular collapse and a *drop* in blood pressure after the smoking of tobacco.

It does appear to be definitely proved that the leading immediate effects of nico-

tine are on the circulatory system, except for those persons who are allergic to one or more ingredients of tobacco. In such cases the primary immediate effect may involve other tissues and organs, such as the respiratory system.

Smoking and Length of Life

The chances are that you'll live longer if you smoke only moderately or not at all. This is indicated by the results of several statistical surveys.

At the Seventh International Cancer Congress in London in 1957, Dr. Harold F. Dorn, Chief Statistician for the National Institutes of Health, reported a Public Health Service study of nearly 200,000 veterans that showed a significantly higher death rate among regular tobacco smokers than among non-smokers. Among all smokers in this group the death rate was 32 per cent higher for tobacco users than for persons who never smoked. For persons who smoked cigarettes only, rather than other forms of tobacco, the death rate was 58 per cent greater than for non-smokers.

In the study regular smokers had higher death rates from lung cancer, diseases of the heart, blood vessels, kidneys, stomach ulcers, liver disease and some respiratory disorders such as bronchitis, pleurisy, and emphysema.

The secretary of the class of 1868 of Dartmouth College kept a record, for fifty years after graduation, of the deaths of members of that class. His data showed that those members of the class who were habitual smokers in college died at an average age of 49 years and 9 months. Those members of the class who did not use tobacco died at an average age of 59 years and 4 months. The nonusers of tobacco, according to these data, lived on the average ten years longer than those who did use tobacco.

Statistics compiled by Raymond Pearl

of Johns Hopkins University in 1938 showed that:

Of 100,000 persons who were *non-smokers* aged thirty, a total of 66,565 reached the age of 60 years;

Of 100,000 persons who were *moderate smokers* aged thirty, 61,911 reached the age of 60 years;

Of 100,000 persons who were *heavy smokers* aged thirty, a total of 46,226 reached the age of 60 years.

Of this work Professor Pearl said: ". . . The net conclusion is clear. In this sizable material, the smoking of tobacco was statistically associated with an impairment of life duration, and the amount or degree of this impairment increased as the habitual amount of smoking increased."

Tobacco and Heart Disease

Until 1960 the American Heart Association had held that more evidence was needed before a definite conclusion could be reached as to whether the smoking of tobacco was a cause of heart and circulatory disease. By July of 1960, however, the medical leaders of this group had reviewed enough scientific studies to be convinced that there was an association between heavy smoking and death or illness from heart disease. In the many studies examined it was found that the death rates in middle-aged men from coronary heart disease were from 50 to 150 per cent higher than among those who do not smoke tobacco.

Such is the strength of the evidence that the American Heart Association now advocates that the association of heart disease and heavy smoking should be called to the attention of the medical profession, health leaders in general, health educators and the general public.

Other investigators at earlier dates had called attention to the apparent connection between the smoking of tobacco and heart and circulatory disorders.

Research men at the Mayo Clinic have studied the histories of thousands of smokers. *They did not find that smoking causes heart disease,* but they did find that heart disease occurs more often among tobacco smokers than among nonsmokers under fifty years of age. The researchers concluded that smoking contributes to the *earlier onset* of heart disease for persons who probably would have cardiac disturbances later in life, regardless of whether or not they smoked.

Some doctors report, however, that persons who have been heavy smokers for a long time may have a condition called "tobacco heart," or "tobacco angina." Such a person may suffer pains like those of angina pectoris during rest, and may even be awakened from sleep by them. The pains of true angina pectoris occur usually after exertion or after a meal. Other physicians doubt the existence of tobacco angina.

That there is often a cardiac irritability to nicotine has been demonstrated, even when there may be reasonable doubt that the reaction of the heart is in any way damaging. One study was made with the electrocardiograph to measure effects of smoking on the heart. Deviations in the normal electrocardiogram were found in nearly a third of the smokers studied, yet none of these aberrations indicated heart disease.

Many physicians advise their patients with heart disorders to reduce or eliminate the smoking of tobacco. Such advice is based upon consideration of the severity of the patient's cardiac condition and the satisfactions that he may derive from smoking. Often the use of tobacco is given medical approval solely because the physician judges that the patient is entitled to some of the satisfactions to which he has been accustomed, provided some moderation is achieved.

Tobacco usually makes the heart beat faster. In the heavy smoker, and especially in the chain smoker, this may in time be detrimental to health. Tobacco also tends to raise the blood pressure. In the heavy smoker this elevation of pressure may cause a sustained increase in the amount of work the heart has to do, which is not advantageous over a period of years. For a person with heart disease the increase in the rate and elevation of blood pressure may result in a real handicap. For the light or moderate smoker with a good heart it is doubtful whether any serious damage is done by smoking.

Tobacco and High Blood Pressure

For people with severe high blood pressure smoking can be a serious risk, because of the added elevation from the effects of nicotine. Dr. Hines and Dr. Roth, at the Mayo Clinic, made a study of the effect of nicotine on blood pressure. Identical tests were made on fifty-six people having high blood pressure and on thirty with normal blood pressure.

From this research the two physicians reached three conclusions:

1. People with high blood pressure as well as those with normal blood pressure have an increase in both systolic and diastolic blood pressure.
2. *Habitual smokers have a greater increase in blood pressure after smoking than do nonsmokers.*
3. The increases were due to actual smoking rather than to deeper breathing and mental associations.

Most people with normal blood pressure can easily stand the slight elevation that comes from light or moderate smoking. Most, in fact, can sustain good health even if their nicotine intake is heavy, so far as effects on blood pressure are concerned. People with borderline cases, between normal and elevated blood pressures, or those who have transient hypertension or permanently elevated pressure, can be adversely affected by smoking, primarily because of the added work for the heart.

There is another consideration. Since statistics on the length of life of tobacco smokers show a disadvantage on the part of both the moderate and heavy smokers as compared to the nonsmokers, it may be that the elevation of blood pressure from nicotine, however slight, can work to the disadvantage of the smoker over a period of years, in a slowly cumulative effect, especially in terms of the amount of work done by the heart. In other words, it is possible that moderate elevation of the blood pressure shortens length of life. If tobacco is consumed in sufficient quantity to raise the blood pressure, the day-to-day results may be negligible, but the lifetime results may be significant.

Buerger's Disease

Thromboangiitis obliterans is a very serious disease. This disorder is also known as Buerger's disease.

Buerger's disease is brought about by a constriction of the arterioles, or small arteries, inflammation, and slowing down of the blood flow to the affected parts. This occurs most often in the arms and legs. However, some cases have been found in which the arteries supplying the heart, brain and abdomen have been affected.

The result is often an occlusion of the small arteries by blood clots, which brings on pain and other symptoms and complications of the disease.

When an artery becomes plugged, movement of blood through it must, of course, cease. This results in a lack of blood moving to the tissues supplied by the damaged artery. Such tissues turn gangrenous and die unless they are adequately supplied by other undamaged blood vessels. To save the patient, if an arm or leg is affected, an amputation is sometimes necessary.

Dr. Leo Buerger and Dr. Samuel Silbert, of Mount Sinai Hospital in New York, studied and treated 1000 victims of this disease. *Among these thousand patients not one was a nonsmoker.*

Dr. Silbert reported that the disease was arrested, regularly, for patients who stopped smoking; whereas, for patients who continued to use tobacco, the disease grew worse. Many patients recovered after eliminating tobacco and receiving treatment. However, when patients who had recovered started smoking again, the disease returned. For very early cases, elimination of smoking without any other treatment was sufficient to cause all symptoms to disappear.

Another report on thromboangiitis obliterans has come from Dr. Bayard T. Horton of the Mayo Clinic. In his summary it is interesting to note that out of 948 patients, only twenty-one were women and that only sixty-eight of the total group were nonsmokers. Out of these 948 sufferers, 385 had an arm or a leg amputated. Dr. Horton advised all his patients having this disease to stop smoking. He found this part of his treatment hardest of all for patients to carry out.

Tobacco and Cancer

Many medical authorities now believe that it has been established with certainty that smoking is a direct cause of cancer, and many others are convinced that it is one of the contributing causes, if not the chief cause.

On March 22, 1957, a seven member "Study Group on Smoking and Health," which had been organized by the American Cancer Society and other groups, released a report that in their opinion cigarette smoking is a factor in the cause of human lung cancer.

Research conducted by the American Cancer Society and the United States Public Health Service on hundreds of thousands of persons has left no doubt in the minds of the health leaders of these organizations that there is an association between cancer of the lung and the smoking of tobacco. These studies showed that heavy cigarette smokers have at least twenty times more chance of developing lung cancer than do nonsmokers.

A large number of medical investigations are giving support to this conclusion. In California, for example, the State Department of Public Health studied the possible causes of lung cancer in terms of air pollution, occupational factors, and cigarette smoking, for a period of ten years. By 1960 the evidence had so convinced the health authorities of the state that the conclusion was reached that ". . . the weight of evidence with regard to cigarette smoking as a cause of lung cancer is now so great that the department must bring the matter to the attention of the public."

On the basis of current evidence it appears that 1 out of every 10 heavy smokers of cigarettes will die of lung cancer.

Even the courts have now given legal sanction to the fact that heavy smoking of tobacco may cause cancer of the lung. In Miami, Florida, the heirs of a man who had died of lung cancer after smoking two to three packs of cigarettes a day for about 30 years sued a large tobacco company as being responsible for the man's death.

The jury decided in 1960 that the death had been caused by the smoking of cigarettes, but that the tobacco company could not be held financially responsible because not enough had been known about the dangers of smoking before 1956 when the man's illness was diagnosed. The decision of the jury suggests that from now on cigarette manufacturers may be held legally liable for the death of a smoker from cancer of the lung because a sufficient link between smoking and cancer has been established scientifically. It remains to be seen whether substantial legal evidence can be produced in specific instances of death from lung cancer on such a basis as to incriminate a specific brand of cigarette or particular tobacco.

It is not yet known what specific ingredient of tobacco smoke is the cause of lung cancer. Tobacco smoke is a highly complex compound and additional ingredients are being identified by chemical research annually, but it will probably be many years before all of the chemical contents of a cigarette are known. At least one chemical, named benzpyrene, that has been proved to cause cancer has been recovered from tobacco. Possibly seven other substances in tobacco may cause cancer. Several investigators have produced cancer in mice and rabbits by repeatedly exposing their skin to material condensed from cigarette smoke.

Two substances especially have been suspected of causing cancer of the lung, tar and arsenic.

Dr. A. Roffo of Argentina estimates that the average smoker in ten years absorbs more than 8 quarts of tobacco tar into the tissues lining his breathing apparatus. Another authority, Dr. Edgar Mayer, New York University Medical School, has estimated that a smoker who uses more than one package of cigarettes a day absorbs into his system 1.7 pints of tar each year.

Dr. Wynder and Dr. Wright have tested many parts of the condensations of tobacco smoke on the skin of mice and have concluded that the cancer-producing element is contained in the tobacco tars, but the specific tar that causes cancer in humans has not yet been identified.

In the past twenty years arsenic has been widely used in the spraying of tobacco plants. During this time the arsenic content of individual cigarettes has increased about 300 per cent, according to one competent medical researcher. *Arsenic is the only part of tobacco smoke that is definitely known to be carcinogenic for man.* In other words, it *has been proved that arsenic can cause cancer in humans.* Although the evidence against tobacco tar is mounting, this product has not yet been *proven* to have caused cancer in humans through the smoking of tobacco.

Spokesmen for the American College of Chest Physicians point out that 98 per cent of all lung cancer victims are smokers. Furthermore, public health leaders stress the fact that the increase in lung cancer mortality shows what may be a meaningful parallel to the enormous increase in cigarette consumption in the past generation or two.

Official statistics released by the National Office of Vital Statistics indicate that about 32,000 persons now die each year from cancer of the respiratory system.

Lung cancer now affects 1 to 2 per cent of the male population over forty years of age. By the time the symptoms develop, only about seven cases out of a hundred can be saved by surgery; and even for these fortunate few, treatment means only a five-year prolongation of life at best.

The Medical Research Council of England and Wales carried out an investigation recently and concluded that "above the age of 45, the risk of developing the disease (lung cancer) increases in simple proportion with the amount smoked, and may be 50 times as great among those who smoked 25 or more cigarettes daily as among nonsmokers."

> "It is no longer an argument whether smoking affects the development of lung cancer, but rather a question of how the risk of the smoker can be avoided or reduced."
>
> *Dr. Ernest L. Wynder and*
> *Dietrich Hoffmann, PhD., March 17, 1960*

Smoking and Athletics

Athletes in training are usually requested by their coaches not to smoke, for the reason that tobacco is apt to hinder their performance. The question whether athletic ability is actually impaired has been answered in a number of tests.

In Dallas, Texas, a group of four scientists conducted research on 14 smokers and 14 nonsmokers that revealed extensive changes in the function of the lungs of the smokers. These scientists found that anyone who has smoked more than 20 cigarettes a day for a long period of time does not have normal lung function.

The volume of expiration, the total lung capacity, and the maximum breathing capacity of the two groups were measured scientifically. The functioning of the lungs was definitely not as good in the group of smokers when compared to the nonsmokers. The investigators found evidence that smoking damages lung tissue and depresses the functioning of the lungs.

In another study, H. Blackburn and his associates found, in a group of 221 persons, that lung volume had decreased in cigarette smokers, especially among heavy smokers.

The effects of smoking upon athletic participation has been measured in other ways.

An investigator at the army physical training center at Aldershot, England, kept records for seven years on the smoking habits of almost 2000 men who participated in an annual 3-mile cross-country run. These men were classified as "heavy smokers" (twenty or more cigarettes per day), "moderate smokers" (under twenty cigarettes per day), and "nonsmokers" (no cigarettes). Results showed that a nonsmoker had three times as much chance to be among the winners as did a heavy smoker.

Dr. T. K. Cureton at the University of Illinois tested 271 men swimmers for endurance. He found that swimmers who were nonsmokers were able, on the average, to hold their breaths 21 per cent longer than smokers. The nonsmokers, moreover, were 18 per cent faster in swimming the 100-yard distance.

Why should smoking affect physical endurance?

Tobacco appears to damage athletic performance by making the heart beat faster, which lessens its ability to pump at full capacity; and by diminishing the amount of oxygen which the cells in the blood are able to carry to muscle tissues.

The research of the preceding paragraphs also shows that athletic performance is impaired by the smoking of tobacco because the lungs themselves are damaged and the breathing capacity is reduced. The great importance of good "wind" in sports is universally recognized among coaches and athletes.

Tremor from Smoking

Many smokers believe that they are calmer, more relaxed, and steadier after smoking a cigarette. The scientific evidence suggests that this is not so.

One investigator subjected twenty men to a blindfolded smoking test. While their eyes were carefully bandaged, they were alternately given pipes full of tobacco to smoke, and dummy pipes rigged up with an electrically heated coil in the stem and a piece of water-soaked asbestos in the bowl. The result was that on some days each smoker drew real tobacco smoke into his mouth, and on other days he inhaled only hot, moist air. Not one of the subjects knew that some days he was drawing on a pipe that held no tobacco.

After smoking (whether real or dummy) each subject was given a metal stylus and told to hold it exactly in the center of a metal plate. Every time the metal rod wavered enough to touch the side of the hole, an electrical contact was made and the touch recorded.

After the habitual smokers had used real tobacco their hands wavered so much that they touched the side of the hole with the stylus 60 per cent more times than after a dummy smoke. Nonsmokers, on the contrary, touched the side of the hole only 41 per cent more times after smoking.

Both habitual smokers and nonsmokers, therefore, were less steady after smoking than before. An interesting sidelight on the test was that the habitual smoker proved to be more unsteady after smoking than the nonsmoker.

In another test, done at George Williams College, it was found that, for some persons, unsteadiness increased 100 per cent immediately after smoking two cigarettes. And in one case, after a person had smoked twelve cigarettes, a test showed that his unsteadiness had increased 230 per cent.

Such research is at variance with the claims made by many habitual smokers that tobacco brings them a reposing, stabilizing and tranquilizing effect. In some persons this stabilizing action has been demonstrated objectively by measurement of reactions to painful electrical stimulations. The excessive consumption of tobacco, however, even in these persons, tends to increase nervous excitability.

It is difficult to assess the exact nature of this tranquilizing factor in smoking. It may be that what appears to be a restful influence is actually the alleviation of nervousness that has developed because the person has gone a period of time without smoking. At least one pharmacologist has suggested that this nervousness from lack of tobacco may be analogous to the craving that develops in more serious drug habits when the addict goes without his narcotic.

If tobacco has a truly tranquilizing effect, it might be assumed that this would result in greater working efficiency, but studies are in fair agreement that nonsmokers are generally more efficient than smokers. Such studies do not prove, however, that relative inefficiency is due to tobacco, for it may be that a conscious or unconscious feeling of inferiority fosters the smoking habit, rather than the habit of smoking causing the inferior performance.

In general, it does appear that smoking, especially to excess, increases nervousness and tremor.

Tobacco and Gastrointestinal Functions

In experiments done at the University of Chicago and elsewhere it has been established that a strong stimulus, whether mental or physical, may remove feelings of hunger.

Smoking can provide such a stimulus and, by erasing the sensation of hunger, can suppress appetite and cause a reduction in eating. The habitual smoker may, therefore, actually so diminish his intake of food that he may lose body weight and even suffer undernourishment.

It is not wise to reduce by smoking, however, because of the variety of other effects that tobacco has upon the body.

Various forms of "nervous dyspepsia" have been found by physicians to be due to excessive smoking of tobacco. Signs and symptoms may include the loss or impairment of appetite, constipation or diarrhea, and loss of weight.

Whether the smoking of cigarettes causes an increased production of acid in the stomach has not been completely settled. Apparently, in a minority of persons the smoking of tobacco does cause an increase in stomach acidity, but this is apparently not true in the majority of smokers. Dr. Philip Cooper and Dr. James B. Knight of Providence, Rhode Island, studied the production of acid in the stomachs of 147 male patients who had a diagnosis of duodenal ulcer, but found no major differences in those who smoked for 30 minutes and those who refrained from smoking for the same length of time.

Since some physicians have found patients who have responded to the smoking of tobacco with a greater production of stomach acid it is not uncommon to hear of a person with an ulcer who has been advised by his doctor to give up cigarettes or at least to cut down on his smoking.

Experimental studies have shown that nicotine increases the motility of the intestines and that such accelerated movements begin within a few minutes after smoking is begun and persist for thirty minutes to an hour after smoking ceases. Depression of hunger contractions of the stomach appear to be brought about by reflex action following the smoking of tobacco. Because of these effects some people prefer to smoke after meals rather than before or in between.

The point to remember is that tobacco does significantly impair appetite. From the health viewpoint this is not generally advisable.

Tobacco Blindness

A very few heavy smokers suffer from an impairment of vision characterized by dimness or partial blindness, dilation of the pupils, and inflammation of the optic nerve, which is called tobacco amblyopia.

Nicotine causes blood vessels to constrict, and some people are specially susceptible to this effect from nicotine. This effect is considered to be the cause of tobacco blindness among certain heavy smokers. When the blood vessels of the retina constrict in this way, the supply of blood is diminished in the retina and vision is impaired. Such a patient's eyes usually recover when he stops smoking. It must be emphasized that only a few smokers are affected in this manner by tobacco, so this complication must be considered a relative rarity, although it is sufficiently common to cause repeated comment by physicians in medical literature on the problem.

Tobacco blindness usually comes on suddenly, although it has been known to develop gradually. The loss of visual acuity appears to be greater for colored objects.

If smoking is reduced or discontinued, recovery of vision can be expected, but symptoms return when persons affected by this disorder begin smoking again. From the visual and medical standpoints it should be obvious that people who are affected in this manner by nicotine ought not to smoke.

Tobacco Allergy

Many people are probably mildly allergic to tobacco smoke; a few are extremely allergic to it, and suffer keenly, as the following description of one man's sensitivity reveals: Only a small concentration of tobacco smoke in the air was enough to give him a persistent sensation of tightness in the chest. Unless he was able to get away immediately from the smoke, he would start getting pains in the chest, and these pains would radiate into both shoulders and would move up into the neck and jaw and along the inner side of the left arm. His pulse rate would increase and his blood pressure rise.

If he walked into a room in which people had been smoking hours before, so that the smoke had caught in the drapes or curtains, he would suffer; if he lay down in bed in a room in which clothes and bedding had picked up smoke, he would have an allergic attack.

For persons with a mild allergy to tobacco smoke the result is mere discomfort, but for persons with severe allergy the problem is more serious. For this reason, anyone who smokes tobacco among other people is truly considerate if he takes the trouble to find out whether his smoking may cause actual distress to his neighbors.

Some smokers suffer severe throat irritations because of allergic reactions to various ingredients of tobacco smoke.

Not all irritation of the respiratory tract

is due to an allergic reaction, but when allergy is present in addition to other irritating effects of nicotine on the mucous membranes of the nose, throat, bronchial tubes, and lungs, inflammation is apt to be severe.

Bronchial and lung complications after surgery have been observed to be more numerous in smokers than in nonsmokers. Some physicians and surgeons believe this is because of the greater production of mucous in the air passageways due to inflammatory effects of tobacco smoke. Failure to keep the airways clear fosters infection in the lungs and bronchial tubes. Whether tobacco allergy is involved in such cases has not been sufficiently established.

Breast Nursing and Tobacco

Dr. W. B. Thompson of Los Angeles, among others, has investigated the effect of smoking upon the breast milk of nursing mothers. In one experiment, milk from a nursing mother who was a heavy smoker was found to contain enough nicotine to cause very marked effects of poisoning when injected into a frog. Though this amount of nicotine is still small, it is enough to upset the digestive processes of a delicate baby. Thompson also found that all but two of his patients who smoked more than eight cigarettes a day could not nurse their babies because they did not have enough milk. Of course, this lack may have been due to nervousness or some other factor.

It was found that the breast milk of women who worked in the Royal Tobacco Factory of old Austria smelled of nicotine. Babies absorbed this nicotine and suffered from chronic nicotine poisoning. One out of every five of those children showed evidence of this poisoning.

From these and other studies it appears that for the welfare of the baby the nursing mother should either greatly restrict her smoking or should not smoke at all.

The Smoking Habit

It is difficult to get smokers to stop smoking. Public health authorities in the city of Edinburgh, Scotland, found this out when they attempted to inform the community about the relationship between smoking and cancer of the lung.

City authorities provided $12,000 for an intensive campaign to get smokers to quit their smoking because of the hazard of lung cancer. The facts about smoking were brought to the attention of the public through advertisements, verbal comment, news broadcasts, sports columns, posters, billboards, leaflets, letters to every household, public meetings, rallies, distribution of 30,000 copies of a British Medical Association pamphlet on the subject and the release of 150,000 leaflets specially prepared for the campaign.

Nearly 600 smokers who were interviewed before the campaign were interviewed again six months afterward. There was no significant change in their smoking habits, although two-fifths of the group indicated that they would *like* to stop smoking. The lesson of this experience seems quite clear: adult confirmed smokers do not easily change their smoking habits, even if their lives will be affected adversely.

The research is more encouraging for younger people.

Studies by the American Cancer Society have shown that when parents smoke tobacco in a family their children are more apt to smoke, and that poor students and inactive or non-participating students are more apt to smoke than those with good academic records or athletic and other extracurricular abilities.

When the new research on the smoking of tobacco is presented to young people and when an appeal is made to their intelligence in a fair and unbiased manner a more thoughtful approach to the whole problem of smoking is achieved. When the young person is encouraged to think about smoking before he starts the habit there is a better chance that he will not smoke at all.

It is possible, even for heavy smokers, to stop the use of tobacco, but success along these lines is apt to be an individual phenomenon.

Some time ago the staff of The Psychological Corporation made a study of 1000 men who were or had been heavy smokers. Only 145 had succeeded in stopping smoking, although nearly one half of the remaining 855 had given up smoking for brief periods of time in an attempt to quit. The percentage of success in this group was low.

It seems much simpler not to start smoking in the first place, if your judgment tells you the habit is harmful.

Questions

1. If tobacco is harmful to health, why do some doctors smoke?
2. Why should a person who desires to smoke among strangers first make a courteous inquiry as to whether or not there are objections?
3. Should women give up smoking during periods of pregnancy and nursing?
4. If nicotine is a deadly poison, why don't smokers obviously suffer impairment of health?
5. Why is it so difficult to stop smoking?

For Further Reading

1. Koskowski, W.: *Habit of Tobacco Smoking.* New York, John de Graff, 1956.
2. Ochsner, Alton: *Smoking and Health.* New York, Julian Messner, Inc., 1959.
3. Weller, Carl V.: *Causal Factors in Cancer of the Lung.* Springfield, Ill., Charles C Thomas, 1955.
4. Wynder, Ernest L.: *The Biologic Effects of Tobacco.* Boston, Little, Brown and Company, 1955.

17

NARCOTICS

NEARLY 80 per cent of the narcotic addicts in the United States are men. Nearly 60 per cent of all addicts in this country are Negroes and the largest concentration of those who are addicted to narcotic drugs reside in New York State. In that state during the year 1958, 60 per cent of all addicts were under 20 years of age. Nine out of ten *registered* addicts in this country use heroin.

Addiction to narcotics is a health and social problem in the United States, not because of the number of persons who are addicts, but because of the possibility of an increase in their numbers and because of the profoundly degenerating effects upon any individual and society in which addiction becomes established.

Contrary to popular belief, the number of drug addicts has been substantially diminished in the United States over the past two generations. When the Harrison Narcotic Act was passed in 1914, there were approximately 200,000 narcotic addicts in the United States. By 1960 this number had diminished to less than 50,000.

AN OLD PERSIAN TALE

"Three men arrived at Ispahan at night. The gates of the town were closed. One of the men was an alcoholic, another an opium-addict, and the third took hashish.

The alcoholic said: 'Let us break down the gate,' the opium smoker suggested: 'Let us lie down and sleep until tomorrow,' but the hashish addict said: 'Let us pass through the keyhole.'"

Dr. Tigani El Mahi, 1960

The problem of narcotics gained prominence in the mind of the American public within the last few years because of two primary reasons. First, the lawless element moved into the illicit market for drugs and began to make large supplies of heroin and other habit-forming substances available in numerous communities. Second, there has been a sharp rise in the number of juvenile and adolescent addicts.

Currently the government is moving vigorously against the drug market, and there is every reason to believe that the problem will be brought under control, although it is imperative that the American public be educated to the dangerous possibilities of addiction to drugs.

International Aspects

The narcotic problem is international in scope. It is quite unlikely that the black market in drugs can be controlled in the United States until there is greater international cooperation in the restriction of production, transportation and sale of narcotics.

Smugglers from China take huge amounts of opium to Thailand and other oriental countries, and from these areas opium is smuggled to cities in the United States and other countries throughout the world. Narcotics officials in the United States report that there is no evidence that Communist China is going to cooperate in keeping huge stocks of narcotics out of illegal channels.

GEOGRAPHY AND NARCOTICS

"Today your narcotics problem is in New York City, Philadelphia, Pittsburgh, Washington, D.C., Detroit, Chicago, all through Texas and all through California. You don't see addiction in New England. A little in Boston, but not very much.... Sixty-five per cent of the illicit opium came out of Red China last year. Most of it came across the Burma border ... there were 10,000 arrests of Red smugglers in Hong Kong ... this underground trade flows right across the world ... to the sidewalks of New York."

H. J. Anslinger,
Commissioner of Narcotics, New York City

Many countries, however, are now making sincere efforts to cooperate in the control of the illicit narcotic trade. Authorities in Hong Kong and Singapore have made thousands of arrests for opium law violations. Seizures of 500 to 600 pounds of opium have been common in Thailand, Malaya and Singapore. The authorities in Thailand seized about 15,000 pounds of raw opium in one raid. Indian authorities annually seize more than 2,000 pounds of opium at ports and borders, but the narcotic traffic continues to flourish across the borders of India, Pakistan, Afghanistan and Iran, although the latter country has vigorously enforced the ban on production and export of opium, and Afghanistan has prohibited the cultivation of the opium poppy.

Mexico has cooperated vigorously with the United States in an effort to suppress the illicit traffic in opium and marijuana. During 1958 Mexican authorities seized about 36 tons of marijuana and destroyed more than 27,000 square meters of mari-juana plants under cultivation.

There is need for constant vigilance for the control of the sale of narcotics on the black market and for much greater co-operation among nations in respect to the control over drug production. Until unity is achieved on an international scale, it is unlikely that the problem of drug addic-tion in any one country will be solved.

What Is Drug Addiction?

In the United States drug addiction is thought of mostly in terms of heroin and marijuana. This is because these two drugs constitute the great narcotics problem at present in this country. Habituation is a better term to use in respect to marijuana, since true addiction to this drug probably does not occur. Actually, a person may become addicted to a variety of drugs.

Drug addiction is a state or condition in which a person has lost the power of self-control with reference to the particu-lar drug. There may be both physical and emotional dependence upon it. The basic feature of addiction is that the person cannot get along in comfort or well-being without the drug he has come to crave.

Addiction to narcotics is actually a symptom of immaturity, for psychiatric studies have shown that practically all drug addicts are unstable. Addiction can happen by accident, however, as when a normal person has been given some drug for medical reasons over such a period of time that addiction has developed.

In general, it can be said that drug ad-diction is a symptom of emotional malad-justment to life. Addiction represents an attempt to escape the tensions and un-happiness that an unstable person has encountered in his family and community.

Addiction to narcotic drugs involves three different phenomena: tolerance, physical dependence and habituation.

Tolerance is characterized by a dimin-ished effect on the addict of the same dose of the drug over a period of time. In other words, to get the same results from the drug the addict must continu-ally increase the dosage.

Physical dependence is illustrated by what happens to the addict when he does not get his drug. He experiences the in-tense discomfort of withdrawal symptoms which are described in another section of this chapter. These withdrawal symptoms are so disagreeable that the addict is apt to become frantic for his next dose of the drug. When he gets his next dose he gets relief from the physical signs and symp-toms of discomfort. In other words, he has come to have an actual physical de-pendence on the drug.

Habituation refers to the emotional or psychologic dependence of the addict on the narcotic drug. In other words, he seeks the drug to escape from emotional prob-lems that would be better approached in other ways. The drug gives temporary re-lief from the psychologic problems that plague the addict.

Addiction in Special Groups

It is to be expected that narcotic ad-diction may be highest among those groups who have access to morphine and other drugs.

Dr. J. DeWitt Fox has reported a study of narcotic addiction among physicians. This investigator found that addiction to drugs is approximately 100 times more common among physicians than among the general population. Dr. Fox con-cluded from his study that a combination of accessibility to drugs and the profes-sional pressures involved in the practice of medicine makes the physician more susceptible to the use of narcotics. Dr. Harris Isbell, Director of the Public Health Service Hospital in Lexington, Kentucky, has reported that physician addicts fall into three common patterns: (1) alcoholic

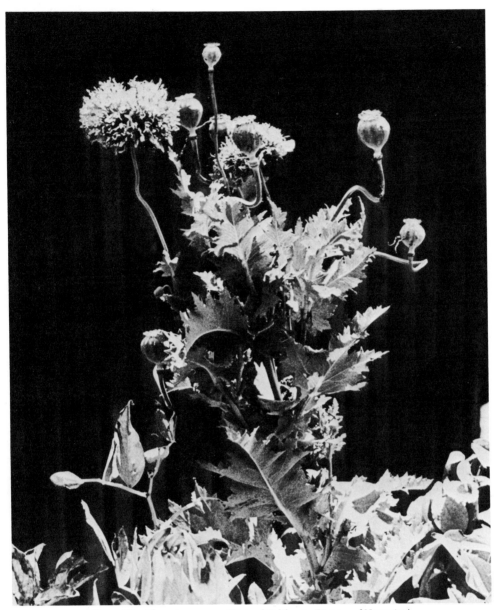

Figure 23.   The opium poppy. (State of California, Division of Narcotics.)

physicians who relieve hangovers with opiates, (2) tired doctors who habitually blot out fatigue with a narcotic and (3) doctors suffering pain from disease who overdose themselves with opiates.

Many physicians succumb to the use of narcotics because of fatigue and urgent demands for their services. A physician may lose sleep on successive nights and may be nearly disabled by fatigue when he receives another request for his medical services. Under these circumstances

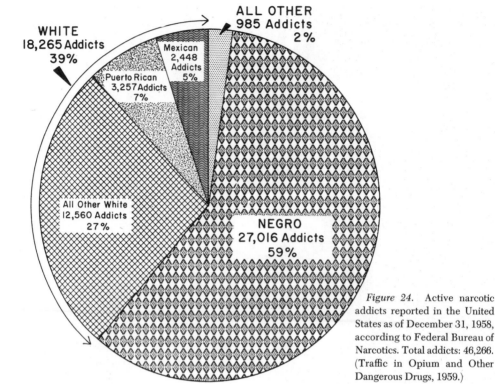

Figure 24. Active narcotic addicts reported in the United States as of December 31, 1958, according to Federal Bureau of Narcotics. Total addicts: 46,266. (Traffic in Opium and Other Dangerous Drugs, 1959.)

some physicians may resort to the use of a drug to relieve the fatigue so that the medical call can be made. The relief obtained may cause the physician to use the drug over and over again and soon he is a narcotic addict.

A study of drug addiction in Great Britain showed that the number of known addicts in the United Kingdom is remarkably small. In 1956 only 333 addicts were known in the entire country. Of this number, 77 were doctors, 20 were nurses, and two were dentists. All of these professional persons have access to narcotic drugs.

In this English study only one other occupational group appeared to be associated with a high rate of addiction. It was found that an appreciable number of dance band musicians were known narcotic addicts.

From the foregoing investigations it would appear that physicians, nurses, dentists and musicians are in occupations in which there is a greater hazard of narcotic addiction.

Signs and Symptoms of Narcotic Addiction

It is not easy to recognize a person who is addicted to drugs. Even a physician may find it most difficult. This is because there are no clear-cut obvious symptoms of addiction to narcotics as long as the addict is able to get his drug.

In general, morphine, opium and related drugs decrease the susceptibility to fatigue, hunger, discomfort, pain and other disagreeable sensations. Obviously, these symptoms are not such as can be readily recognized. The drugs also tend to depress attention, but many people are easily distracted, so that this is not a definite clue to addiction either. Somewhat larger doses may create a "mental fog," but such abstraction can occur from other causes or may go undetected. Some people, on the other hand, are more excited than depressed by narcotics. The drugs cause a depression of respiration, but since most people are not in the habit of counting the number of breaths per minute, this, too, is no important clue to narcotic addiction. There may be constriction of the pupils, but many people differ in the size of their pupils, and the degree of constriction depends on the amount of drug consumed. Other symptoms and signs include dryness of the mouth, thirst, constipation, reduced body temperature and decreased urinary output. None of these are likely to be observed by other people. In short, it can be said that the signs and symptoms of narcotic addiction are such as to be easily overlooked.

If the physician examines a suspected addict, he may find evidence of repeated injections of heroin or other drugs in the form of needle marks and fibrous changes in certain blood vessels that have been used for injections. This is circumstantial evidence, however, since needle marks could conceivably come from other factors.

Narcotic Poisoning

One of the great dangers of addiction to narcotics is the possibility that an overdose may be taken by the addict. Since the peddlers of narcotics have a general practice of diluting such drugs as heroin in order to make a greater profit, it sometimes happens that an addict may receive a stronger drug if he changes peddlers or gets a different supply of the drug. Numerous deaths have been traced to exactly these circumstances.

An overdose of morphine or opium and their derivatives is liable to cause a gradual development of coma and unconsciousness. Symmetrical, pinpoint pupils are characteristic, although the pupils dilate as death approaches. There is general relaxation of the muscles, especially of the jaw, so that the mouth drops open. There is slow, irregular respiration, and paralysis of this system is the cause of death. In other words, respiration stops before the heart ceases to function. With an overdose of heroin, the patient is apt to go into convulsions before death. The overdose is liable to have a fatal result within two to twelve hours.

The recent discovery of narcotic antagonists such as Nalline and Lorfan have made it possible to counteract the results of drug overdosage much more effectively than in the past. These antagonist drugs are described in more detail in the next section.

Narcotic Antagonists

The two most useful narcotic antagonists currently in use are called Nalline and Lorfan—trade names for nalorphine and levallorphan.

The value of Nalline lies in its ability to neutralize or counteract the effects of morphine and its synthetic derivatives. The most valuable feature of the antagonist is that it overcomes the respiratory depression that may result from the use of morphine. It may therefore save the life of a person suffering from an overdose of this narcotic.

Nalline has proved to be a useful substance for the diagnosis of addiction. If a person is a well-established drug addict using morphine or one of its derivatives, definite withdrawal symptoms will be noted within 20 minutes after he has been given an injection of Nalline. A second and third injection of Nalline may be given in suspected cases of narcotic ad-

diction where the patient does not respond to a first test. The pupils in the eyes
of the narcotics addict will dilate or expand, whereas they will constrict under
the influence of Nalline if the person is
not a narcotic addict. The patient's consent for the test is necessary and it is recommended that at least two physicians be
present. A number of police departments
now use this test for drug addiction.

Lorfan is a synthetic substance that is
not a narcotic. Its effects are the same as
those of Nalline, but the drug is ten times
more potent than the latter. Neither of
these substances is effective against respiratory depression due to non-narcotic
drugs or other conditions.

Signs and Symptoms of Withdrawal

Although addiction to narcotics does
not give rise to signs and symptoms that
are easily recognized so long as the addict
can get his drug, this is not the case when
he is unable to secure his next dose on
time.

At first, when the addict cannot get his
drug, he is likely to demonstrate irritability, bad temper and restlessness. He
then begins to yawn, sneeze, to have
watery eyes and hoarseness of the voice.
Muscular weakness also develops. The addict experiences hot flashes, chills, vomiting and diarrhea. His muscles begin to
twitch, and painful muscle cramps develop. He will have violent pain in the
legs, arms or abdomen as well as severe
headache. He then has severe tremors or
tremblings, inability to sleep, and other
symptoms. He may go into hysteria, delirium or mania, depending upon his basic
personality structure.

Sometimes there is a sudden circulatory collapse with heart failure that results in death. Whereas narcotic poisoning is liable to cause death through
paralysis of respiration, withdrawal from

the drug may cause death because of
heart failure.

It can be seen that these distressing
withdrawal signs and symptoms are one
explanation of why the addict craves his
drug. He needs to restore his sense of
well-being.

When a person is suspected of being a
narcotic addict, diagnosis becomes easy
if the patient can be isolated from any
possibility of getting his drug. Medical
observation of the addict with the appearance of the signs and symptoms just
described makes recognition a simple matter. Also, if all the signs and symptoms
disappear when the drug is given to the
patient, then a diagnosis of addiction is
further verified.

Marijuana (Hashish)

Marijuana is a drug obtained from the
hemp plant. Marijuana is not strictly a
narcotic, since true addiction does not
generally occur. From a practical standpoint, however, the drug is associated
with the problem of narcotics, and its control is an important function of local, state
and federal narcotic bureaus. In the
United States the drug is usually sold illegally in the form of cigarettes.

> **HASHISH**
> "...A drug consumed by some 200 million
> people all over the world...is being used in-
> creasingly since World War II, in spite of the
> drastic measures taken to check its trade and
> prohibit its use...it may even be one of the
> most widespread narcotics...Owing to its wide
> use among the youth of some countries, to its
> influence on criminality and to the active trade
> to which it gives rise, it is considered a major
> social hazard."
> *World Health Organization Committee
> on Addiction-Producing Drugs, 1960*

The use of marijuana is injurious to
health for several different reasons. First,

the drug is apt to accentuate the instabilities of the disorganized personality. Marijuana is usually smoked by a person who is not emotionally stable to begin with. The drug relaxes inhibitions and sometimes precipitates a dangerous disregard for others. A person who is already emotionally unstable will be made more so by the drug. Many persons under the influence of marijuana become violent, abusive and antisocial. Second, when marijuana is used over a long time, the mind appears to be damaged by it. Studies conducted in India, South Africa and other areas where the drug has been known to medical and public health authorities for some time indicate that mental illness is one of the common effects when the drug is used for an extended time. Third, the smoking of marijuana

tends to lead a person toward the use of heroin. The tendency is for the user of this drug to look for a more powerful narcotic. Heroin is almost always the choice.

Marijuana is known as hashish in many parts of the world where centuries-old experience with this drug has shown that even the most inoffensive person may become violently irritated and commit acts of destruction. When the drug is taken by a habitual hashish smoker in large amounts, delirium and raving madness often occur. Sometimes these states are followed by exhaustion and even death. The destruction of a sense of moral values while under the influence of marijuana or hashish is implied in the origin of the word assassin which is derived from "hashashin" which means a hashish-eater.

People can be taken off marijuana suc-

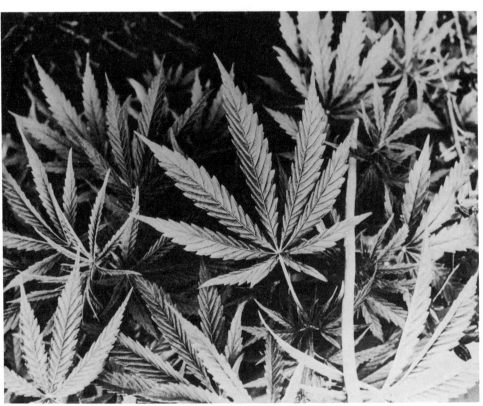

Figure 25.   Marijuana shrubbery. (State of California, Division of Narcotics.)

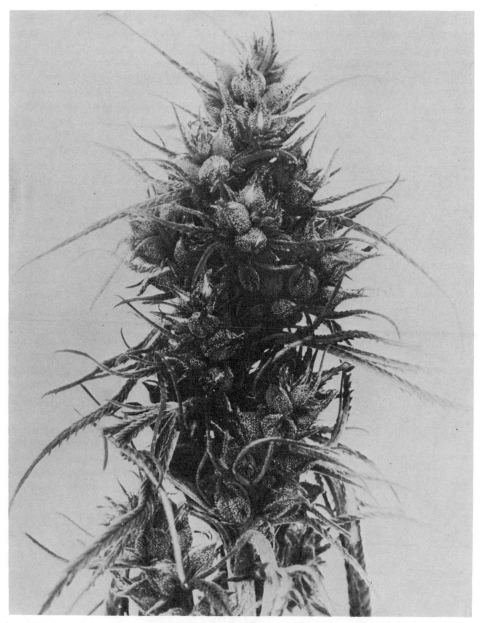

Figure 26.   Flowering top of the female marijuana plant. (State of California, Division of Narcotics.)

cessfully in a much greater percentage of cases than with heroin, morphine or the opium derivatives in general. Getting the user off marijuana, however, is not the sole solution to the problem. His malad-justed personality is still where it was, if not worse than before he started using marijuana. The use of marijuana is often associated with crime such as robbery and violence, and removal from the drug does not rehabilitate the patient so far as his antisocial behavior is concerned. Rejection of the drug, of course, would be one step in the total rehabilitation.

Marijuana cigarettes are often supplied free of charge or at low cost to young people by peddlers of narcotics in an effort to build up their trade. Once the use of marijuana has been established, it is a simpler process for the peddler to lead the victim on to the use of heroin, the sale of which is a much more profitable procedure for the peddler.

There is no standard picture of reaction to marijuana, and it is this very fact that makes the drug dangerous. Its strong association with the later use of more powerful drugs and with crime and prostitution makes marijuana a public health problem of some significance in the United States.

Heroin

Heroin is a derivative of morphine. It is prepared artificially from morphine and is a stronger drug than the latter. According to a report by H. J. Anslinger, United States Commissioner of Narcotics, about 90 per cent of the known registered narcotic addicts in this country use heroin.

The drug is usually taken by injection into the larger blood vessels that can be reached with the needle. Addiction to the drug usually requires more than two weeks, but often occurs within a few days and in some unstable persons after only a few doses of the drug. Some authorities in the field of narcotics believe that a person will be "hooked" by heroin after as few as two or three doses. The speed of addiction appears to be related to the basic personality maladjustment of the individual.

The use of heroin by pregnant women can have disastrous effects upon newborn babies. In a study of eighteen babies born to women using this drug, Dr. Samuel A.

Krause of New York City found that the average infant was underweight at birth and that nearly all would develop withdrawal symptoms within one to 56 hours after birth. In this small group of babies the physician also found that two were born with congenital defects. Nearly 25 per cent of the babies died at birth, or shortly after.

Heroin is a very expensive drug. The buyer usually pays from five to ten dollars per capsule or even more. As tolerance builds up in the addict, he needs stronger and stronger doses. This means that the price of his habit goes up. It is common for addicts to pay as much as twenty to sixty dollars a day in order to get the drug to which they have become enslaved.

Average people do not have this much money; so the inevitable result is that the addict turns to crime to get enough money to buy his drug. He may need a thousand dollars a month in order to keep himself supplied with the drug. Male addicts turn to robbery, safe cracking, pandering and other illegal procedures. Women resort to petty thievery, shoplifting and other crimes, but mostly they turn to prostitution as a means of raising money for the drug. Crimes associated with the use of narcotics in Chicago during 1955 are indicated in the table on page 219.

The length of time a patient can go between injections of his drug depends partly upon his level of tolerance and partly on the size of the dose of the drug he receives. An injection of morphine may be needed about every two hours. An injection of heroin may be needed every four hours, more or less. Withdrawal symptoms usually begin within four to twelve hours after the last dose of the drug. In other words, the addict usually needs another injection within four hours following his previous shot. If he does not get this injection, he begins to experience distressing and painful symptoms, which are described in another section of this chapter.

It is inevitable that the use of heroin will be associated with violence, crime and prostitution in the great majority of cases.

The Barbiturates

The principal medical uses of the sedative-hypnotic drugs such as the barbiturates are for sudden stressful situations such as insomnia and hypertension in which sedation of the patient is needed until a more relaxed state of mind and body can be achieved. These drugs are also used for the control of convulsions, to assist in the suppression of epileptic seizures, in childbirth and to prepare the patient in advance of surgery. There are many other medical uses of the barbiturates.

The abuse of the barbiturates seems to center around insomnia and a stressful situation. When a person is in a state of tension and stress over an extended period of time the use of barbiturates to relieve the situation may result in addiction. The use of the drug for overcoming insomnia may also lead a person to depend upon this product for regular sleep. If the barbiturates are taken only on medical prescription and are not abused, then they do have a constructive function in medicine.

SLEEPING PILLS
"It's all nonsense to say that sleeping pills are habit forming. I've taken one every night for years."
Anonymous

Many persons in the United States have developed the sleeping pill habit without realizing that they might become addicted to the use of barbiturates. Most states have now adopted legal restrictions governing the sale of these drugs. Despite this fact, addiction to barbiturates and overdosage of the drug have made a seri-

ous public health problem that centers around its use.

Several years ago a report from thirteen hospitals showed that they had received 643 persons suffering from acute barbiturate poisoning over a period of ten years. Of this number approximately 7 per cent died.

Studies conducted by members of the Harvard Medical School and the Massachusetts General Hospital staff, as well as by medical personnel in other institutions, have shown that the brain center that regulates breathing loses its sensitivity to carbon dioxide when the barbiturates have been taken by a patient. This results in a dangerous accumulation of carbon dioxide in the blood. This interference with the normal respiratory mechanism may be the explanation of some sudden deaths in persons who have taken barbiturates.

The main action of the barbiturates is that of depressing the central nervous system. Taken in proper dosage, such drugs produce calmness, relieve anxiety, and tend to promote sleep. The drugs have other medical uses as well.

A great danger of the barbiturates is that a person may become accidentally poisoned or may attempt suicide with one of this group of drugs.

"The suicide death rate from barbiturates has increased 400 per cent since 1935 . . . The annual consumption . . . now is over 350 tons . . ."
Dr. Dale G. Friend and Dr. George A. McLemore, Jr.

An excessive or toxic dose of a barbiturate usually results in drowsiness, weakness, headache, mental confusion and unconsciousness. The heart and respiration are depressed, and the lungs are apt to become filled with fluid. The blood pressure falls to shock levels. Body temperature also drops, but later may rise to fever levels. The heart is not usually damaged early in the poisoning.

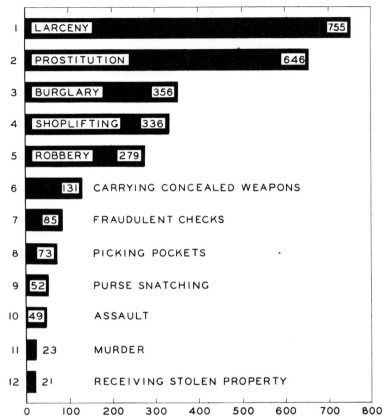

Figure 27. Leading crimes associated with narcotic addiction in Chicago during 1955.

Treatment

Addiction to drugs should be looked upon as evidence of a basic personality maladjustment. Treatment directed solely at getting the person to stop taking narcotics will ordinarily make little or no contribution to the solution of the addict's real problem. One authority in the field of narcotics, for example, studied the personalities of 1000 addicts and concluded that 97 per cent were suffering from anxieties, obsessions, compulsions, aggressions, hostilities, tensions, borderline mental illnesses and sometimes actual mental disease.

From the medical viewpoint there are two standard methods of taking the addict off his drug. These two approaches are known as the gradual and abrupt withdrawal treatments.

In the *gradual withdrawal* treatment the patient is permitted to continue his narcotic addiction, but under control and direction of a physician or psychiatrist. His dosage of drugs is gradually reduced over a period of weeks or months. Even after the patient has been completely taken off the drug he continues to receive doses of innocuous materials which he believes to be the drug he has been craving. Eventually he is informed that he has been off the drug for a period of time. There is obviously some psychologic value in telling the addict that he has been able to get along without his drug. However, this gradual withdrawal method has not been an effective means of curing patients, and the time involved, as well as the cost of extended supervision, has caused its replacement with the abrupt withdrawal type of treatment in most institutions.

> WITHDRAWAL SYMPTOMS IN
> BARBITURATE ADDICTION
>
> "It was long thought that barbiturates were not addicting . . . it is now known that if barbiturates are withdrawn (from an addict) . . . weakness, tremor, anxiety occur in all cases; 75 per cent . . . will have one or more convulsions and 60 per cent will develop a toxic psychosis closely resembling delirium tremens. Even death has been reported during abstinence from barbiturates in a strongly addicted patient . . ."
>
> *Dr. Harris Isbell, 1956*

In the *abrupt withdrawal* type of treatment the patient is simply taken off his drug. For this treatment to be successful even in the preliminary stages, the patient must be in an institution or in some other situation where he cannot possibly gain access to the drug he craves.

Within about twelve to fourteen hours the patient will begin to experience withdrawal symptoms which increase in intensity and complexity within the first twenty-four hours. The acute distress of the patient reaches a peak about forty-eight hours after the last dose of his drug has been taken. Then it gradually subsides, and within five to ten days the symptoms disappear. Usually by about the eighth day the patient is free of his withdrawal symptoms and can be said to have been taken off the drug.

Unfortunately, no method known to medical science has been found that will keep a patient off the drug. In other words, the patient is apt to go back to the use of drugs again when he gets the opportunity. Usually the patient returns to the same environment in which he originally acquired the drug habit. His basic personality structure has not been changed; therefore, he finds himself in the same emotional status and the same community environment which precipitated

his addiction to drugs in the first place. Studies indicate that from 95 to 100 per cent of such patients relapse.

Under the Harrison Narcotic Act, federal prisoners, federal probationers and voluntary patients may be treated at the Lexington and Fort Worth hospitals, which are maintained for the treatment of narcotic addicts. Applicants for voluntary treatment must make their requests for this service to the Surgeon General of the United States Public Health Service in Washington, D.C.

Public health authorities recommend that a person undergoing treatment for narcotic addiction should remain in an institution for at least four to six months so that there will be sufficient time to relieve him of any physical illnesses as well as to have a better chance for rehabilitation in general. Addicts need to develop new ways of living and working as well as new types of recreation. Psychiatric treatment is also basic, since this begins to get at the addict's fundamental emotional problems.

The present status of treatment for narcotic addiction appears to be rather discouraging. No simple, economical and effective treatment has been discovered. The real solution to the problem of narcotic addiction does not appear to lie in the field of treatment, but in the area of prevention.

There is some variation in treatment for addiction, depending upon the drug involved. Addiction to barbiturates is best treated by the gradual withdrawal method, since, if the patient is taken off barbiturates abruptly, convulsions may develop in three to four days and severe psychotic reactions may be expected in some cases within a week to ten days. The gradual reduction of the daily dose of barbiturates over a period of three weeks can avoid these complications and still get the patient off the drug.

Addiction to bromides can be treated successfully by the abrupt withdrawal method, since there appears to be little if any physical dependence upon this drug.

Free Narcotics for Addicts?

Some physicians have favored the legalizing of the distribution of free narcotics to addicts in order to reduce the incentive for these persons to resort to crime and violence to secure money for the purchase of drugs on the illicit market.

A principal advocate of the controlled distribution of free drugs to narcotic addicts has been Dr. Herbert Berger of Staten Island, New York. Dr. Berger has advocated the establishment of narcotics clinics in cities under the direction of the United States Public Health Service. He has also suggested that each narcotic addict be registered and fingerprinted and that they be given narcotics at a cost of 15 to 30 cents while an effort is being made to bring about a cure with hospitalization if the patient cooperates.

ILLNESS OR CRIME?

"For more than 40 years our lawmakers . . . have been trying to cure an illness by treating it as a crime. That illness . . . is addiction to narcotic drugs . . . We have created a new criminal class. We have a flourishing narcotics racket. We have ever more drug addicts . . . Since society shuns and abhors him (the drug addict) he must turn to the underworld . . ."

Dr. Herbert Berger, 1956

In Great Britain, physicians are permitted to prescribe narcotics for addicts as a part of their medical treatment. The British program has often been cited by persons advocating the establishment of narcotic clinics for the provision of free drugs in the United States.

Two New York physicians who made an on-the-scene study of the British narcotics control system reported in 1960 that under the British plan, morphine or heroin may be given to addicts only when they are under treatment by the gradual withdrawal method; when prolonged attempts at curing the addict have demonstrated that the use of the drug cannot be discontinued completely because of severe withdrawal symptoms; or when it has been demonstrated that the addict is incapable of leading a useful life when the drug is discontinued completely. These two physicians found that dangerous drugs could not be used for any other purpose than that of administering to the strictly medical or dental needs of the patients and that the continued supply of dangerous drugs to a patient solely for gratification of addiction is not regarded as medical need in England. No formal registry of addicts in England was found nor were any "narcotics clinics" to which addicts may report for drugs.

Dr. E. Vincent Askey, president-elect of the American Medical Association, indicated in 1959 that a version of the British plan under which a physician is allowed to prescribe narcotics to an addict was tried in Los Angeles, California. In this trial experience it was found that addicts frequently disagreed with physicians as to the amount of drugs they needed and often committed crimes to get money for extra allowances. Some investigators have found that addicts may request higher dosages in order to secure an extra supply which they then sell on the illicit market for large sums of money. Other narcotic addicts refuse to register at clinics because they do not wish to be identified.

Whether or not the provision of narcotic clinics for the provision of low cost drugs to addicts would reduce crime and other social problems in this country remains to be seen.

The Prevention of Addiction to Narcotics

Studies show that those who are most apt to become drug addicts are the ones who suffer from insecurity, poor home conditions, emotional instability, economic pressures and mental illness.

Most likely the family influence is a large factor in the long-run determination of who is to become a narcotic addict. A child who has affection and security in a

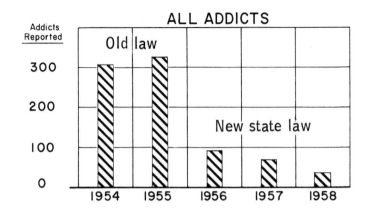

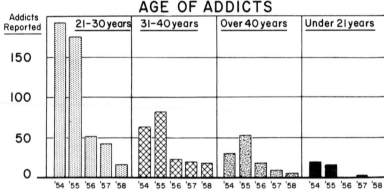

Figure 28. Results of effective legislation on drug addiction in Ohio, calendar years 1954–1958 (state law became effective September, 1955). According to Federal Bureau of Narcotics. (Traffic in Opium and Other Dangerous Drugs, 1959.)

well ordered home and experiences a gradual development of independence coupled with a growth in responsibility is most unlikely to suffer from those psychologic problems and deficiencies that may cause others less fortunate to seek ultimately an escape with narcotics.

Intelligent home supervision and early guidance in the creation of wholesome friendships are also strong forces making for the well adjusted personality. When children grow up to become narcotic addicts, parents cannot escape a heavy share of psychologic and moral responsibility.

The prevention of drug addiction through the improvement of family life is a social problem of the greatest significance. Although this is an indirect approach to the control of the narcotics problem in the United States, it is nevertheless a most basic one. Only through a long-range program of education, social betterment and moral enlightenment can we hope to raise the spiritual and psychologic level of family life in this country to the point at which that segment of our population to which narcotics has an appeal has been reduced to a minimum.

More immediate results can be expected from a direct attack on the narcotics problem by local, state and national law enforcement agencies and other community groups.

Vigorous suppression of the criminal element that keeps the narcotic trade alive is perhaps the most important immediate community measure in the prevention of addiction to narcotics. If the drug is not available, the individual cannot become addicted to it.

The local police department should be well supported by community members in its efforts to stamp out the illegal drug trade. Full cooperation with state and federal narcotics officials is also necessary, but an alert and interested police department must carry the main responsibility for keeping crime out of the local area.

The Boggs Act, which was approved as Public Law 255 on November 2, 1952, substantially increased penalities for violation of narcotic laws in the United States.

An important aspect of this law was that no probation or suspension of sentence is legally possible for a second or subsequent conviction. The law specified that for the first offense of importing, receiving, concealing, buying, selling or transporting narcotic drugs illegally in this country the penalty shall consist of a fine of not more than $2000 and imprisonment of not less than two or more than four years.

For the second offense the fine remains the same, but the guilty person must be imprisoned for not less than five years and not more than ten years. For the third and subsequent offenses the guilty party must spend at least ten years in prison, but no more than twenty years.

The Boggs Act was followed in 1956 by the Narcotics Control Act which made the death penalty applicable to persons convicted of selling heroin to minors and increased jail sentences to a maximum of 40 years in other cases.

The prevention of addiction to narcotics is not solely a matter of police and community action, however. Studies show that there is a certain pattern of behavior that the adolescent follows before he becomes a drug addict. As a rule, the chain of events that leads to narcotic addiction begins with the drinking of alcohol in association with others of similar age, then progresses to the use of marijuana on the suggestion or dare of others in the group,

and finally ends up with the use of heroin.

The responsibility of the normal individual should be quite clear. If he hears about the use of narcotics in his own community, he should report such information to the police so that trained narcotics agents may track down the source and arrest the peddler. The normal person should not under any circumstances submit to the use of any drug except on prescription for illness and under the supervision of a physician.

Questions

1. Does knowledge of the effects of narcotics create an abnormal interest in the subject and stimulate the desire to try a drug, or does it afford better control over the problem?

2. Why does the narcotic addict almost invariably become a criminal of one kind or another?

3. What kind of person is most apt to become a narcotic addict?

4. Is the control of narcotics likely to succeed on an international scale? Why or why not?

5. Why do some authorities believe that the roots of the narcotic addiction problem lie in the realm of parent-child relationships?

6. What advantages, if any, would be gained by society if narcotics were given free to addicts? What hazards would there be in this practice?

For Further Reading

1. Bureau of Narcotics, U.S. Government: *Traffic in Opium and Other Dangerous Drugs.* Washington, D.C., Government Printing Office, Annual Report.

2. Deutsch, Albert: *What We Can Do about the Drug Menace.* New York, Public Affairs Committee, 1952.

3. Hock, Paul H., and Zubin, Joseph: *Problems of Addiction and Habituation.* New York, Grune and Stratton, 1958.

4. Murtagh, John M., and Harris, Sara: *Who Live in Shadow.* New York, McGraw-Hill Book Company, 1959.

5. Nyswander, Marie: *The Drug Addict as a Patient.* New York, Grune and Stratton, 1956.

6. Reynolds, A. K., and Randall, Lowell O.: *Morphine and Allied Drugs.* London, England, Oxford University Press, 1957.

7. Spillard, William J.: *Needle in a Haystack: The Exciting Adventures of a Federal Narcotic Agent.* New York, McGraw-Hill Book Company, Inc., 1946.

8. Street, Leroy: *I Was a Drug Addict.* New York, Random House, 1953.

9. Weston, Paul B., editor: *Narcotics in U.S.A.* New York, Greenberg, 1952.

Recommended Film

Ivy, Andrew C. *Drug Addiction,* Sound, 20 minutes. Encyclopedia Britannica Films, 1958.

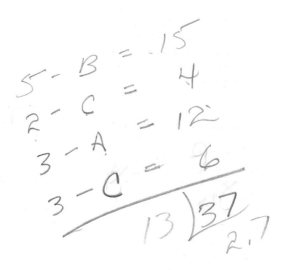

18

LEADING COMMUNICABLE DISEASES

ANTIBIOTICS have changed the importance of communicable diseases in human affairs. Many infections have come under almost complete control. Others have declined in importance although they still exist as potential threats to human health.

Some communicable diseases resist all antibiotics and remain as serious, unconquered problems. Some microorganisms have developed effective resistance to antibiotics and have taught physicians and research specialists that there is a continuing need for further research and control efforts.

The virus diseases are notable for their freedom from the effects of the antibiotics, although a few have yielded. The fungus diseases, too, are generally resistant and the staphylococci have proven to be tough and resistant enemies.

There are about 25 or 30 highly effective antibiotics that have changed the course of destiny in the field of communicable diseases.

> "... The influence of the antibiotics is so great that this may be called the age of the antibiotics as well as the age of the atom ..."
> *Selman A. Waksman, Ph.D., 1958*

Some diseases are widespread, but do not result in a great number of deaths. The industrial and financial losses from the common cold, for example, run into millions of dollars annually because of the absences from work for which they are responsible. Other infections take their heaviest toll during the early years of childhood. In a sense, these diseases may be considered more important than others which take a greater toll of life at a much later age. Some diseases, too, are debilitating rather than killing.

Generally, the greatest problems are those that take human lives. Pneumonia now leads all other causes of death among the communicable diseases. During 1958 there were 52,997 people who died from this disease. An additional 4,442 persons died from influenza which is often linked with pneumonia for statistical purposes in studies of deaths from infectious diseases.

Tuberculosis ranked second as a cause of death from communicable diseases, with 12,361 fatalities in 1958. Pneumonia and tuberculosis combined accounted for approximately 15 times more deaths than the third ranking, influenza, as well as the fourth and fifth ranking infections which were bronchitis with 3,973 deaths and syphilis with 3,469 fatalities.

From the standpoint of deaths alone, pneumonia and tuberculosis stand out head and shoulders as the leading communicable diseases in the United States. As is indicated in the chapter on tuberculosis, the latter disease is rapidly declining as a cause of death in the United States.

Sickness statistics generally resemble those of previous years. Although there is

Rank°	Deaths per 100,000 Population		
	1949	1954	1958
1. Influenza and pneumonia	30.0	25.4	33.2
2. Tuberculosis	26.3	10.2	6.6
3. Syphilis	5.8	3.0	2.0
4. Poliomyelitis	1.8	0.8	0.2
5. Rheumatic fever	1.6	0.8	0.5
6. Meningococcal infections	2.0	0.6	0.4
7. Dysentery	1.0	0.4	0.1
8. Measles	0.6	0.3	0.3
9. Whooping cough	0.5	0.2	0.1
10. Scarlet fever	0.0	0.2	0.0

° Among the communicable diseases, not among the total causes of death.

inevitably some variation from year to year, the communicable disease picture in the United States remains substantially the same. The total pattern changes slowly.

Tuberculosis and the venereal diseases are discussed in separate chapters, because of their worldwide significance as well as their importance in the United States. The major remaining communicable diseases in this country are evaluated briefly in the following pages.

Influenza and Pneumonia

As a team, influenza and pneumonia constitute the greatest communicable disease problem in the United States so far as deaths are concerned. In 1918 approximately 15,000,000 people throughout the world died of influenza. In the United States during this same worldwide epidemic there were about 20,000,000 cases and about 500,000 deaths in a period of six months.

Influenza can occur with dramatic suddenness. Within a period of two or three weeks as much as one third of a total population may be stricken by the disease.

Though it is possible that influenza itself may cause death, the greatest danger seems to come from the fact that influenza weakens resistance and makes possible secondary infections, such as pneumonia, which may be rapidly fatal.

Influenza is caused by a virus, various types of which have been identified. The latest additions to our knowledge of the types of viruses that cause influenza are represented by the so-called Asian strains. Pneumonia also may be caused by a number of different organisms including the viruses.

Because we now have immunizing substances that protect against certain viruses, it is important to identify the specific virus involved in a particular influenza outbreak. Unless mixed vaccines are used, immunization against one type of virus that causes influenza does not give protection against other types; however, a multiple type vaccine is now available for immunization against influenza including the Asian strains.

Protection by immunization is relatively short in duration, lasting no more than six months to one year at best. It is therefore advisable to be immunized annually against influenza.

Pneumonia can be treated effectively with sulfa drugs, penicillin and other antibiotics in many cases. However, *influenza cannot be cured with these drugs, nor can all cases of pneumonia be cured with these substances.* We are currently, therefore, in a state of partial control over influenza and pneumonia, with the possibility that if either of the two diseases should become more virulent, even existing measures of control might be highly inadequate.

Deaths from influenza and pneumonia may be as much as 65 per cent greater among men than among women. This may be because many men will attempt to work while suffering from one or both of these diseases. The failure to go to bed and secure proper medical treatment may prove fatal in such cases. Whether or not there is true sexual difference in respect to immunity to these diseases has not been proved.

It is interesting to note that in an epidemic of Asian influenza in Kansas City approximately one-third of the total population was affected and that 253 deaths were due to a combination of influenza and pneumonia. In this epidemic it was found that 73 per cent of the deaths occurred in persons *with a pre-existing chronic disease,* mostly of the heart, respiratory, and circulatory systems. Influenza thus appears to *collaborate with pneumonia in destroying people who already have a serious, chronic health problem.* As a life-saving device, it would appear to be especially important for people with chronic illness to be immunized against influenza.

Influenza is being intensively studied in this country. The National Institute of Health maintains eight regional laboratories throughout the country which gather scientific information on the disease and transmit these data to the Influenza Information Center. The World Health Organization also maintains an influenza center which studies reports from all over the world. Prompt information on the hazard of pneumonia is sent to all member nations when this is advisable.

Rheumatic Fever

Rheumatic fever is a disease in which three factors appear to be important. The disease develops only in certain persons who have suffered from a throat or respiratory infection caused by a certain type of streptococcus organism. Not all people who have this infection get rheumatic fever, however. Only those patients who have an allergic and inflammatory reaction to the infection get rheumatic fever. This particular type of reaction to the kind of streptococcus involved or to specific products produced by the organism appears to occur only in those who have inherited a particular type of constitution predisposed to allergies. Thus heredity, allergy and a particular kind of streptococcus infection appear to be necessary for the development of rheumatic fever.

The disease is characterized by fatigue, loss of appetite, fever, pain in the joints, nosebleed and rapid pulse. Other symptoms and signs may be present. Many cases of rheumatic fever, however, do not exhibit these signs, and diagnosis may be difficult. Rheumatic fever is particularly important because it may result in rheumatic heart disease.

The death rate for both rheumatic fever and the heart disease that may be caused by this disorder has been declining for many years. In 1960 the National Office of Vital Statistics reported from the latest data only 806 deaths from rheumatic fever in a year, although nearly 18,000 persons had died during the same time from chronic rheumatic heart disease. Better recognition of the disease in the early stages with subsequent treatment by sulfa drugs and antibiotics and the effective eradication of many infections (including those of the streptococcal group) before there has been time for an allergic reaction to develop, has undoubtedly prevented considerable rheumatic fever. It is likely that such prompt treatment of streptococcal infections has been a main cause of reduced illness from rheumatic fever. It must be remembered that the streptococcal infection *precedes* the onset of rheumatic fever and that the two are different phenomena.

Complete bed rest, often for an extended time, is the basic treatment for rheumatic fever. Penicillin and other antibiotics are of no value *once this disease has developed*, except for controlling recurrent episodes and secondary infections. *The most effective method of preventing rheumatic fever would appear to be prompt treatment for sore throats and respiratory illnesses.* Although the majority of these will not be due to the streptococcus germ that causes rheumatic fever, it would appear to be a wise precaution to seek medical care promptly, especially by members of families in which there is a history of rheumatic fever.

Poliomyelitis

Poliomyelitis is a generalized disease of the body caused by a virus. Although inflammation of various parts of the nervous system occurs when a person suffers from this disease, the large motor cells in the spinal cord seem to be especially susceptible to damage. When this part of the nervous system is injured, there is paralysis of the voluntary muscles which receive their nervous impulses through this part of the spinal cord.

It used to be thought that poliomyelitis was a disease of infancy and childhood exclusively. For this reason the disorder was called infantile paralysis, and it is still known by this name to many people. However, medical and public health experience has shown that the disease may occur at any age. For this reason the disorder is no longer known by its former name, but is called poliomyelitis by physicians and public health workers.

We do not have accurate statistics as to how prevalent poliomyelitis may be. Probably a majority of the population has suffered from this disease at one time or another. Poliomyelitis begins with symptoms that are very similar to those of many other communicable diseases. Digestive disturbance, headache, a feeling of general indisposition, fever, and occasionally nose and throat irritations are characteristic. In many cases even these symptoms may be so mild as to cause only a slight illness.

It should be understood that in the great majority of cases of poliomyelitis there is no paralysis. Some authorities estimate that as many as 75 per cent of our adult population has had this disease at one time or another during their lifetime, without even knowing it. The number of cases of poliomyelitis diagnosed by physicians and reported to public health authorities will vary from year to year, depending on whether or not epidemic conditions exist.

How Poliomyelitis Is Spread

Modern evidence indicates that poliomyelitis is spread primarily through intestinal discharges. This means that ordinarily the disease will not spread unless a person touches something or someone that has been contaminated with feces containing the virus of poliomyelitis. The direct spread of the disease from person to person is likely to occur only within family groups or groups in which there is close association of individuals with a maximum of uncleanliness.

As in other feces-borne diseases, poliomyelitis is likely to be spread also through contaminated food or drink and by flies or other insects that may contaminate food or drink.

Although it was formerly thought that poliomyelitis might be spread through nose and throat discharges, this concept is gradually being abandoned. If the disease were spread primarily in this manner, large gatherings of people during the time of epidemics would be a special hazard. The evidence indicates, however, that attendance in school, at theaters, dances and other group associations is not followed by more widespread dissemination of the disease.

On the other hand, it has been shown repeatedly that persons recovering from poliomyelitis do contain the virus of this disease in their intestinal discharges for days, weeks or even months after they

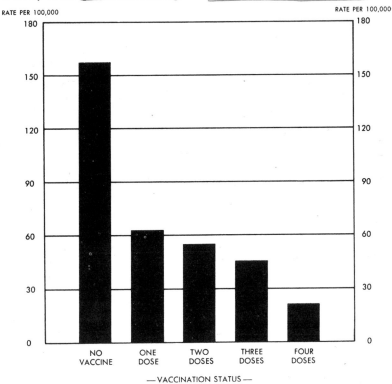

Figure 29. Paralytic attack rates in 3900 cases of poliomyelitis by vaccination status in Massachusetts in 1955. (Massachusetts Department of Public Health and the National Foundation for Infantile Paralysis.)

have apparently recovered from the disorder. In some cities the virus of poliomyelitis has been identified in sewage taken at random from the sewage disposal system. On occasions, flies trapped in the field have also been found to harbor poliomyelitis virus.

Most modern communities depend in part upon protection against the intestinal-borne diseases by chlorination of the water supplies, but recent research has shown that chlorination of water does not always kill the virus of poliomyelitis.

In some cases, outbreaks of poliomyelitis have been traced to contaminated food or drink. For example, the New York State Department of Health traced one epidemic of the disease to a dairy in which there were no toilet facilities, no soap or paper towels at the handwashing sink, and where it was found that cream was bottled by hand without proper sterilization of the milk bottles. Also, the only operator in the milk plant was the father of a child who had recently had poliomyelitis. The milk route of this dairy extended through the same area in which cases of poliomyelitis were occurring. Investigation of the individual cases of the disease showed that the great majority had consumed milk from this dairy. It was judged that the disease had definitely been spread through contaminated milk supplies.

Symptoms of Poliomyelitis

The signs and symptoms of poliomyelitis depend upon the severity of the disease. In a mild case a person suffering from this disease may have little more than a mild fever, headache, nausea, and perhaps a sore throat. Nausea and vomiting as well as headache are two of the earliest symptoms of the disease.

In the mild case of poliomyelitis the illness lasts only a short while, often being of no more than one to several days' duration. The vast majority of people who get poliomyelitis have the mild form of the disease. It is likely that the disorder will es-

cape diagnosis, and even the patient will not know that he has had the disease.

In the more severe, paralytic type of poliomyelitis the illness is of longer duration and the fever is sustained for a greater number of days. The earliest sign of involvement of the central nervous system is a relative inability to bend the head forward. This stiffness of the neck is an important sign. In its absence medical experience has shown that for at least twenty-four hours there will be no immediate danger of paralysis or death.

Headache may be very severe, and muscle soreness appears in various parts of the body. Muscle spasms are especially likely to occur in the back, neck and hamstring muscles.

Paralysis is likely to appear on the second to the fourth day and starts as a weakness of particular muscles. Within two to three days this paralysis reaches its maximum.

Although muscle spasm occurs commonly in early poliomyelitis of the paralytic type, the ultimate or residual paralysis is of the flaccid type with no spasms. In other words, the permanent paralysis is of a relaxed or flabby type, rather than the stiff or spastic type. The muscles are loose rather than in spasm. Death is relatively rare, but usually results from paralysis of the respiratory system when it does occur.

Life Expectancy after Poliomyelitis

Poliomyelitis is not the killing disease that many people think it is. In 1960, for example, the National Office of Vital Statistics released data showing that only 402 persons had died in a single year from acute poliomyelitis or as a result of this disease.

When it is recalled that the great majority of poliomyelitis cases are so mild that they are not even diagnosed as such, it can be seen that the disorder is not as dangerous as is frequently feared.

Even in the paralytic cases spontaneous

recovery can be expected in 35 to 60 per cent of the cases. With good medical care from 75 to 85 per cent of the patients who are paralyzed will show marked improvement or complete recovery. From 10 to 20 per cent will require the use of braces or some aid from reconstructive surgery, and about 2 per cent will remain completely disabled. However, *these percentages apply only to those patients paralyzed from the disease.* In the great majority no paralysis develops in the first place, and in those in whom this complication does ensue there is still an excellent chance for recovery. The person who survives poliomyelitis has as great a life expectancy as any other person.

The Salk Vaccine

In 1953 Dr. Jonas E. Salk of the University of Pittsburgh reported the preparation of a vaccine that has been found to be effective in the prevention of all three types of poliomyelitis. This immunizing substance is composed of viruses that have been killed by exposure to formaldehyde under certain controlled conditions. Dr. Salk was awarded a gold medal by the Congress of the United States on August 9, 1955, in recognition of his preparation of this vaccine.

An unfortunate error in its production was apparently to blame for the onset of 114 cases of poliomyelitis, with five deaths, during the same year when five and one-half million persons received their first injections. Although the attack rate was remarkably small, these few cases did temporarily shake the confidence of the American public in the vaccine. The error in production was discovered when the Public Health Service sent its experts to investigate. New government standards were established to make the vaccine 100 per cent safe, and the present vaccine is produced under rigid controls that have made it a completely safe yet effective product.

It is estimated that during 1955 the Salk vaccine prevented between 1250 and 1300 cases of paralytic poliomyelitis. The effect of the vaccine on nonparalytic poliomyelitis has not yet been determined.

Reports from all over the world have indicated that the product is now completely safe to use.

The Salk vaccine has no value in the treatment of poliomyelitis, but only in its prevention.

The development of a live vaccine against poliomyelitis has resulted in a challenge to the Salk vaccine. Both vaccines appear to give effective protection against the disease. The live vaccine is discussed more fully in the next chapter.

Colds

Colds are apparently caused by a number of different viruses. Symptoms of a cold, however, such as a watery discharge from the nose, coughing and sneezing, are also characteristic of many other infections in the early stages.

Overexposure and chilling often have some relationship to the onset of colds, but not as a direct cause. It is apparently the lowering of body resistance to the virus or viruses that promotes the onset of a cold when a person has been overexposed.

Colds appear to be spread in much the same manner as other virus diseases. In other words, coughing, sneezing, eating from the same utensils that a person with a cold has used, shaking hands, and any other method of transferring the virus from one person to another could be effective in spreading a cold.

It is likely that many colds are actually allergic reactions. The recent use of antihistamines for the treatment of colds is based upon this fact. When such drugs do give relief from the symptoms of a cold, it is likely that the allergic reaction is more important than the virus in that particular case.

Colds may be of such short duration in some cases that any type of treatment may apparently produce good results. Experimental studies have shown that some people will think they have been cured of a cold no matter how they are treated.

Recent research with volunteers from military service and other sources indicate that a group of viruses now known as the "adenoviruses" may be partially confused with colds. In this research evidence was secured that suggested the need for more careful exploration of the possible influence of nasal irritants, psychologic, allergic and other factors in the production of a cold. On the other hand, colds presumably due to viruses may be caused by infectious agents that do not produce lasting immunity. It is also possible that colds are caused by so many different viruses that immunity to one virus after a cold has little effect upon the onset of other colds due to other viruses. Some colds may be due to viruses, while others are due to totally different agents.

The most effective treatment for a cold is bed rest. This is important not only to establish greatest resistance to the cold itself, but also because the symptoms involved may actually be an early stage of a more serious respiratory illness.

Unless the symptoms of a cold are due primarily to allergic reaction, little specific treatment can be advised, The best procedure is to go to bed, get more rest, and, if a fever develops, call a physician.

The Adenovirus Diseases

The adenovirus group of infections consists of at least 23 distinct types, 18 of which are of human origin and 5 of which have been found in animals. During the first three years of life a great many children are infected with one or more of the adenoviruses. It is thought that the viruses may persist for years in tonsils, adenoids and other lymphoid tissues. Whether or not this is responsible for recurrent respir-

atory diseases has not been proven. Infections appear to be followed by lasting immunity especially when the adult has his first experience with the adenovirus.

Rabies

Rabies, often known as hydrophobia, is a disease caused by a virus that affects the brain and spinal cord. It is spread through the saliva of the biting infected animal. The incubation period, the time between infection with the virus and the appearance of symptoms may vary from days to months depending on how close the bite may be to the brain and the severity of the bite.

Human beings often develop rabies from dogs although many other animals may be infected with the disease such as cats, coyotes, skunks, squirrels, cows and bats. There is no successful medical treatment for rabies after the symptoms have begun. The person bitten by a rabid animal can be protected if he is immunized early enough before symptoms of the disease appear. It takes about 15 days for the human to develop enough antibodies to be protected against rabies. During this time he can be protected by the use of hyperimmune serum which should be given within 72 hours.

Animals other than dogs appear to be taking a more important role in the spread of rabies. In 1950 there were 4,979 dogs reported with rabies in the United States compared to 1,375 miscellaneous sources, including wild life. Ten years later in 1959 only 1,124 dogs were reported with rabies whereas those in the miscellaneous group had risen to 1,925 cases. The dog is still an important source of rabies but other animals now appear to have greater significance in the spread of this disease. In some states the fox and the skunk appear to be major hazards in wild animals.

Vaccination of dogs annually is now a

legal requirement in some states. This protects not only the dog from contacts with strays and wild animals but also protects the humans with whom the dogs associate.

The first case of rabies in a bat in the United States was reported in 1954, after a bat had attacked a boy near Tampa, Florida. Since that time rabies has been revealed in at least 15 different species of bats. In one instance a boy was bitten at school by a rabid bat that he had taken there as part of a nature study exhibit; in another instance a fisherman knocked a bat down with his fishing rod and the bat bit him; rabies in the mammal was confirmed. Rabies has occurred in livestock in the southwestern United States as a result of bat bites. Recent public health experience tends to confirm the old Pima Indian belief that "if a bat bites you, you will go crazy and die."

Measles

Measles, or rubeola, is a highly contagious disease caused by a virus. The disease is characterized by fever, inflammation of the respiratory mucous membranes, sensitivity of the eyes to light, loss of appetite, vomiting, and a rash or eruption of the skin.

Contrary to common belief, measles is not a disease that should be treated lightly, despite the fact that ordinarily less than 600 persons a year die from it. Not only is the child or adult who has this disease seriously ill in the majority of cases, but the possibility of complications is always present. Pneumonia, middle ear infections and inflammation of the brain are three of the complications most to be feared. In one group of children with measles at the Boston University School of Medicine, 25 per cent had pneumonia. In a Michigan outbreak of several years ago a relatively large number of cases resulted in inflammation of the brain, although this is a relatively

uncommon complication and probably occurs in no more than one in every 200 cases of the disease.

After a person has been exposed to measles it usually takes ten to twelve days before onset of the disorder.

One of the means of preventing measles is by injection of gamma globulin. This substance gives a passive immunity which lasts at most only about three weeks. If globulin is given within four days after exposure, the disease will be prevented, and if given six or seven days after exposure, the infection will be modified. It is not of value after the appearance of the rash.

For some children a *modifying* or partial dose of gamma globulin may be advised. The child then develops some active immunity against measles; whereas, he gets no *permanent* protection from the disease through a *full* dose of gamma globulin. On the other hand, infants under the age of six months will not need gamma globulin in most cases if the mothers have had measles. The baby will have acquired some passive immunity from the mother during the period of pregnancy. This immunity, however, wears off at about the age of six months. If the mother has not had measles, then the infant does not possess this passive immunity.

By 1960 a vaccine had been developed against measles. This vaccine, on experimental trial, appears to give more enduring protection against measles than gamma globulin provides.

Measles should not be confused with German measles (rubella), which is a much milder disease, except for its effects during pregnancy.

Scarlet Fever and "Strep" Throat

Scarlet fever is a serious disease characterized by fever, a bright red skin rash, sore throat, and frequent complications of the middle ear and kidneys. One attack of the disease usually gives sufficient immunity so that the rash is no longer repeated. Later infections may be recognized only as sore throat.

Scarlet fever is caused by a certain type of streptococcus germ. The disease usually develops within five to twelve days after a person has been exposed.

A study of nearly 8000 cases of scarlet fever in military personnel and their families showed that about 9 per cent had infections of the middle ear as a complication of the disease. Pneumonia occurred in about 2 per cent of the cases; rheumatic fever symptoms developed in 2 per cent also. Of five patients who died from the disease, three perished from pneumonia which complicated the disorder. Although scarlet fever spreads readily among children, only a small number of adults will get the disease. In one study of 250 cases of scarlet fever in which 550 adults were exposed, only 1 per cent got the disorder.

The Dick skin test has been widely used for the detection of persons susceptible to scarlet fever. It is possible to immunize against scarlet fever, but reactions are so severe in many cases that immunization is not widely practiced. It is unwise to immunize people against scarlet fever who have had a previous history of rheumatic fever, because an attack of the latter disease may be stimulated.

The disease can be successfully treated with sulfadiazine, sulfamerazine, penicillin, convalescent serum, antitoxin and gamma globulin. These substances are not equally good, and their use depends upon the particular case, since the severity of the disease may vary widely.

Under the modern treatment severe types of scarlet fever are not as commonplace as in former years, and complications are likely to be less severe also. When medical treatment is delayed, however, the disease is likely to be as severe as in previous years.

Whooping Cough

Whooping cough, or pertussis, is a highly contagious disease which attacks mostly children and infants. The microscopic organism that causes this disease is known as *Hemophilus pertussis*.

The disease usually starts much like a cold, but then gradually develops into a series of coughing attacks. After the coughing spell there is likely to be a loud whooping or crowing sound as the air rushes back into the lungs. It is this whooping sound that has given the disease its popular name. Among physicians the disease is known as pertussis. Frequently the attack is also followed by vomiting.

Since the disease is easily spread to others, the child suffering from this disorder should be isolated, or kept apart from others for a period of three to six weeks after the coughing has begun.

Since whooping cough is highly fatal to infants who receive no treatment, it is imperative that medical care be obtained when a child is suffering from this disease. The death rate is still about 95 per cent when a baby under the age of one year has not been immunized against whooping cough and gets the disease. Immunization, however, gives a very high level of protection. All babies should be immunized against this disease, starting at the age of two or three months.

Bacillary Dysentery

Bacillary dysentery is of worldwide distribution and is especially common in tropical and subtropical areas. It is spread by intestinal discharges, usually through food or drink which has been contaminated by flies, or by food handlers infected with the disease. The disease is caused by various strains of microscopic organisms known as *Shigella dysenteriae* or *S. paradysenteriae*. The disease develops within twenty-four hours to a few days after exposure and is characterized by bloody diarrhea with fever, weakness, and great loss of fluid. On the other hand, mild cases may occur in which there are only a few loose stools and slight fever.

In severe cases the onset of the disease is very abrupt, with fever, abdominal cramps, and loose stools that may soon become bloody.

Penicillin has no value in the treatment of this disease, although the sulfa drugs have been reported as being effective. Streptomycin, Aureomycin and Terramycin have all been reported as useful in the treatment of dysentery. Toxic side effects from the use of sulfa drugs may be severe unless the water loss of the body is replaced.

Protection against the disease is best achieved by protecting foods against flies, sanitary disposal of human excreta and other wastes, maintenance of proper sanitation in restaurants, removal of carriers of dysentery bacilli as food handlers, and prompt treatment for those who have the infection. Immunizations against the disease are available, but their exact value has not been determined. Overcrowding, poor sanitation and the presence of flies are all associated with diarrheal disorders. Finger contamination and direct person-to-person spread are often responsible for bacillary dysentery, especially in young children.

During World War II a large part of one Army division was incapacitated with bacillary dysentery when 1557 men came down with the disease. In this epidemic a marked deviation from the usual enforcement of well known military sanitary protective measures resulted in exposure of latrines to fly population. When the division was moved to an area free of flies, the epidemic stopped abruptly. When large numbers of the flies were trapped, it was found that 3 per cent were infected with the same dysentery organisms found in the intestinal discharges of the men suffering from this disease.

Infectious Hepatitis

Infectious hepatitis is a virus disease of the liver. The disease is characterized by loss of appetite, concentrated urine, nausea, fatigue, vomiting, abdominal pain, whitish stools, enlargement of the liver, itching and fever.

The disease is spread through intestinal discharges, usually by contamination of food or water. In some cases blood transfusions, in which blood from infected persons has been used, have resulted in spread of the disease.

Blood plasma and blood which is currently used for transfusions, however, are now treated to eradicate the virus of infectious hepatitis.

The most important single factor in the treatment of infectious hepatitis is bed rest. Physical activity is the one factor most likely to cause a relapse from infectious hepatitis after recovery is well under way. Exercise should therefore be restricted *for as much as one year* after a person has been sick with this disease.

The incubation period, or length of time needed for development of the disease after exposure, ranges between twenty and forty days. In experimental human cases the average incubation period has been about twenty-five days, but it may occasionally be as short as fifteen days or as prolonged as eighty-five days.

One attack of infectious hepatitis appears to give immunity against reinfection. Diet is also important in the treatment of the disease.

Meningitis

The term "meningitis" means an inflammation of the membranes surrounding the brain and spinal cord. Actually, there are many types of germs that can cause meningitis, but the most common organism affecting this part of the nervous system is the meningococcus.

Meningitis is a very serious disease which is characterized by severe headache, fever, nausea, often vomiting, delirium, coma and other signs of inflammation of the nervous system. A skin rash may also be present.

The disease is spread by discharges from the nose and throat of infected persons or of carriers of the disease. In some epidemics as many as 50 per cent of healthy people have been found to be carrying the microscopic organisms in their nose and throat without evidence of the disease.

Meningitis is always a serious disease, but variations in severity occur according to the kind of organism causing the disease. During 1923 and 1926, for example, 91 per cent of the people who had meningitis died. As late as 1935 approximately 50 per cent of the people with this disease died from it. Since that year, however, there has been a steady decline in the case fatality rate, or percentage of affected people dying from the disease.

Many complications can occur from a severe case of meningitis. Deafness, blindness, paralysis and other complications are sometimes found.

Great progress has been made in the treatment of this disease within recent years. The sulfa drugs, penicillin, Aureomycin and some of the other newer antibiotics are effective against the disease. As a consequence of newer treatment the death rate from meningitis has fallen substantially. Whereas the death rate used to be from 50 to 90 per cent or thereabouts, probably no more than 10 per cent of the cases today will be fatal.

Diphtheria

Diphtheria is a serious disease in which there is an oozing of semi-solid material in the throat which forms into a tough membrane. A severe general reaction to the disease is the body's response to a toxin or poisonous substance produced by the organisms causing the disease. This organism is known as the diphtheria bacillus, or *Corynebacterium diphtheriae.*

The disease usually develops within two to five days after exposure. Early symptoms may be slight, such as mild fever, sore throat and a general feeling of indisposition. Later, however, symptoms may be very severe. Numerous complications may arise. Among these is difficulty in breathing due to obstruction in the throat from the production of the membrane previously mentioned and general swelling and inflammation. In such a complication, surgery may be necessary in order to open a passage for breathing below the level of obstruction. If the heart is attacked by the diphtheria organisms, there may be a rapidly fatal heart block. Pneumonia is one of the most frequent complications of diphtheria, especially when the membrane extends downward. Paralysis may occur in about 10 per cent of the cases, especially those which are untreated or inadequately treated. Other complications may also occur.

Studies show that under normal conditions from 1 to 5 per cent of healthy persons are carriers of virulent diphtheria. In such people the diphtheria organisms can be found in the throat by bacteriologic study. The persons themselves, however, remain healthy, although they spread the disease to others. Fortunately these healthy carriers can now be cured with penicillin treatment.

Although most diphtheria occurs in children, the disease can also attack adults. In the United States about 80 per cent of the cases of this disease occur in children less than ten years of age. On the other hand, the disease can attack at any age.

In recent years diphtheria has spread on an international scale. In Europe diphtheria began to spread about 1930 from Germany to neighboring countries. By 1945 diphtheria had reached the point of being the most dangerous epidemic disease throughout most of Europe. By 1945 diphtheria was the leading cause of death except for war casualties in the Japanese army and navy, and the disease had become common throughout the entire country.

Immunization, which is described in the next chapter, can be remarkably effective in preventing this disease. In Michigan, for example, the State Department of Health reported that the diphtheria rate was the highest in the world in 1921 but that continued immunization had changed this picture so that by 1941 that state had one of the lowest diphtheria death rates in the world. In fact, diphtheria had been reduced 98 per cent. Diphtheria became so rare in Michigan that young mothers neglected to have their children immunized. As a result, the disease began to rise sharply by 1944. This experience and that of other states and countries has shown the great need for continuous education in the importance of immunization against diphtheria. Treatment for this disease is very effective if it is begun soon enough. Diphtheria antitoxin, when given within the first twelve to twenty-four hours of symptoms, completely neutralizes the toxin or poison produced in this disease and saves the patient from serious damage. If given after twenty-four hours, the largest dose may not save the patient from severe illness or death. Large doses of antitoxin can be given, as there is no harm from this. The antitoxin is given by injection, usually in a single dose. Although penicillin and other antibiotics may be helpful, the primary treatment resides in the prompt use of antitoxin.

Amebiasis

Amebiasis, or amebic dysentery, is a disease in which symptoms may vary greatly. In many cases there may be only slight abdominal discomfort, while in others there may be periodic attacks of diarrhea, and in still other cases the diarrhea may be very severe, with blood and mucus discharged in the stools.

The disease is spread by intestinal discharges from infected persons and is caused by the microscopic organism known as *Entamoeba histolytica*.

It is estimated that about 5 per cent of the population in the United States carry this germ in their bowel discharges in one form or another. Diagnosis of the disease is made by the symptoms and by finding of the cyst form of the ameba through microscopic examination of intestinal discharges.

This disease seldom occurs in epidemic form, although the 1933 Chicago hotel epidemic, which involved 1050 known cases and seventy dead, is one of the classic examples of an epidemic of amebiasis. In this epidemic it was proved that sewage drippings had contaminated a water cooler which supplied certain rooms of the hotel.

Since amebiasis is a disease spread by intestinal discharges, the disorder is best prevented by sanitary disposal of human feces, protection of the water supply against contamination by intestinal discharges, personal cleanliness such as washing the hands thoroughly before eating, eradication of flies and protection of foods against flies, safe plumbing, use of pasteurized milk, and medical care for all known cases of diarrhea.

One attack of amebic dysentery does not give protection against subsequent infections. Complications are relatively rare, although the liver is one of the particular sites for such complications. This usually takes the form of a liver abscess. The disease can be treated effectively with modern drugs.

Brucellosis

Brucellosis, or undulant fever, is a recurrent illness which may last for months or years. It is a disease characterized by fever, headache, weakness, sweating and general ache. The disease is caused by any one of three varieties of microscopic organisms known as *Brucella melitensis*, *Br. abortus* or *Br. suis.*

In the United States the principal source of the disease has been the consumption of raw milk from infected animals, especially cattle and goats. The disease may also be caught from hogs. The disease usually develops within six to thirty days after exposure.

Brucellosis can be prevented by the pasteurization of milk and by eradication of the disease in animals. Sustained efforts have been made to wipe out brucellosis in cattle in the United States. Formerly blood testing of all cattle in an area was done, and those found to be infected with the disease were marked for slaughter. The so-called cream-ring test is now used as a rapid and inexpensive method of locating infected herds. It is used in conjunction with the blood test. As milk is received at a dairy plant, a small sample of milk from each can is taken for testing with a test fluid. In milk from infected herds a deep blue cream line is formed. In negative milk the cream ring remains white. Blood tests are then made only in those herds from which milk shows a positive ring test. This saves much time and expense in locating cattle infected with brucellosis.

Cattle can be partially immunized against the disease. Heifers four to eight months of age usually develop fair resistance to brucellosis when they are immunized. The immunity, however, is not complete, and it decreases with time. Vaccination is used in conjunction with other measures for control of the disease among animals.

In human beings the disease can be treated with fair success with Aureomycin. Most drugs are not effective against this disease.

Trachoma

Trachoma is caused by a virus that invades the mucous membrane covering the surface of the eyeball and the lining of the lids. The disease is important because it may lead to scarring of the eye tissues and to blindness. This disorder is also known as granular lids or contagious granular conjunctivitis.

The disease may be spread by personal contact or through the handling of towels, handkerchiefs and other linen which has been handled by a person suffering from the disease.

Trachoma is one of the most widely distributed illnesses in the world. It is especially prevalent in the Orient, and it has been estimated that about 25 per cent of the people in China have the disease. The infection also exists in the United States on a larger scale than most people realize.

In former years the disease was likely to persist into a chronic and long-lasting stage, but with the discovery of the sulfa drugs it can now be cured rapidly.

Typhoid Fever

Typhoid fever is a disease caused by the microscopic organism known as *Salmonella typhosa*. The disorder is characterized by a continued fever, often with delirium, slow pulse, abdominal tenderness and a rose colored eruption or rash.

Typhoid fever occurs throughout the world; it is spread by intestinal discharges. Any person carrying the typhoid fever germs in his intestinal tract can spread the disease to others even though the person himself may not be suffering from the disorder. These persons are known as healthy carriers. In addition, every person who is ill with the disease is likely to spread the disorder to others. The principal means of spread is through contaminated water and food.

The disease was widespread in armies and wars of the past, and was epidemic in parts of Europe after World War II.

Special efforts to control this disease in the United States have been made in the field of water sanitation, food control and the location or detection of typhoid fever carriers. Some states maintain a typhoid fever registry in which the names and addresses of all known carriers of the disease in the state are listed and followed by public health authorities.

About 3 per cent of the people who have typhoid fever later become chronic carriers of the disease even though they may no longer be suffering from the illness. In recent years attempts to cure typhoid carriers have been made by surgical removal of the gallbladder, in which the germs appear to be concentrated, and by treatment with antibiotics. In Massachusetts, public health authorities reported that surgical removal of the gallbladder cured about 90 per cent of the carriers who submitted to this operation. The most effective drug treatment for typhoid fever appears to lie in the use of chloramphenicol. This drug is also known as Chloromycetin. It has been known to produce harmful side effects such as leukemia and should be used only under the guidance of a physician.

Pennsylvania passed a law in 1945 providing an income up to $600 per year for chronic typhoid fever carriers who suffer financial loss through unemployment or decrease in business because of public health restrictions on their activities.

The prevention of typhoid fever rests upon a good level of community sanitation, protection of the water supply, protection of food from contamination by flies, and by personal cleanliness such as washing hands before meals. Immunization against typhoid fever is described in the next chapter.

A great many complications can occur in typhoid fever. Intestinal hemorrhage, perforation of the intestines, inflammation of the gallbladder, formation of blood clots and other dangerous developments may ensue, particularly when the disease has not been adequately treated.

Diagnosis of typhoid fever is made primarily through laboratory detection of the germ which causes this disease in the intestinal discharges of the patient.

Paratyphoid Fever

Paratyphoid fever is a disease that resembles typhoid fever in many respects, but is caused by different microscopic organisms. The disease is also much milder than typhoid fever.

Three main types of germs are involved in this disease. These are *Salmonella paratyphi*, *S. schottmuelleri* and *S. hirschfeldii*. Symptoms of paratyphoid are similar to those of typhoid fever, and the complications resemble those of the latter disease also, although, in general, the infection is definitely milder. Practically all medical authorities agree that the two fevers cannot be distinguished except on laboratory grounds. In other words, the microscopic organisms must be identified, or blood tests must be used to distinguish between the two diseases.

Infectious Encephalitis

Encephalitis means inflammation of the brain. This inflammation can come from many different types of infections, such as measles, whooping cough and so on. A certain group of viruses appears to be specifically involved in certain cases of encephalitis.

Western equine encephalitis and St. Louis encephalitis are two of the most widely known types of brain inflammation spread by mosquitoes. The term Western equine encephalitis has originated because horses were found to be sources of the virus. When it was proven that the virus was spread by a certain type of mosquito such as *Culex tarsalis* it became possible for public health authorities to test them for evidences of viruses. Research in California, however, suggests that other factors besides mosquito density are related to epidemics of encephalitis despite the fact that it is well proven that the mosquito is involved in the spread of the disease. It is known that the virus that causes encephalitis is kept alive by wild birds, chickens, bats and other such fowl. Horses appear to be a minor source of encephalitis compared to the great fowl reservoir. The antibiotics are not effective against encephalitis so that treatment has not been truly effective.

Several types of mosquitoes are capable of spreading infectious encephalitis.

The disease often begins with a mild fever with later development of symptoms suggesting inflammation of the brain or other nervous tissues. Restlessness, twitching, paralysis and other disturbances involving the brain or central nervous system, including psychologic symptoms, may arise.

Blood tests are of value in diagnosis of the disease. In an autopsy on animals, fowls or humans the virus may be isolated from nervous tissues.

The principal method of control of this disease lies in the eradication of mosquitoes in a community and in effective home screening. Horses and mules may be immunized against the disorder and thus reduce the source of the infection in some cases. Primary emphasis in the control of this inflammation of the brain type of disease must be placed on prevention, since there is no effective drug treatment for the disorder at this time. Immunization is possible for horses and will probably be available for human use before long. A vaccine for both Western equine encephalitis and St. Louis encephalitis would be desirable.

Tetanus

Tetanus occurs all over the world and is most likely to develop after penetrating wounds or injuries. The disease is caused by the tetanus bacillus. It is the toxin or poisonous substance produced by this bacillus that causes the symptoms of the disease.

Another name for the disease is lockjaw. The organisms are found especially in soil which has been contaminated with animal or human intestinal discharges. The disease usually develops within five to ten days after contamination of a wound with *Clostridium tetani*. The poison produced by this germ is probably one of the most potent known to man.

Muscle stiffness, especially of the jaw, may be the only early symptom of the disease, although irritability, stiffness of the neck and difficulty in swallowing may also indicate onset of the disease. Stiffness and muscle spasm develop over other parts of the body, and headache, fever, chills and convulsions may then follow. The disease is almost always fatal unless treatment is prompt and effective.

The treatment of tetanus is basically a matter of giving sedatives to control convulsions, administering antitoxin as promptly as possible to counteract the effects of the poison generated by the tetanus organisms, and giving antibiotics to control secondary infections. The newer drugs, however, are not markedly effective against tetanus itself.

Best control of this disease is achieved by active immunization. This is described in the next chaper.

Trichinosis

Trichinosis is a disease caused by intestinal parasites. *Trichinella spiralis* is the specific organism which causes this disease.

Trichinosis is a disease which has persisted in the United States because in some cities we have allowed hogs to be fed uncooked garbage which contains meat scraps with live *Trichinella* parasites, and for that reason some authorities have stated that trichinosis is a disease of "garbage worms."

The symptoms of trichinosis include swelling of the eyelids, muscle pains, fever, diarrhea, headache, abdominal cramps, nausea, vomiting, and sometimes restricted hemorrhage.

The disease is occasionally fatal, although not usually, and is confined almost entirely to people who have eaten raw pork, or pork products which have not been sufficiently cooked. Since pork is sometimes used in hamburgers, it is essential that this type of meat product be thoroughly cooked. Trichinosis has also been spread through undercooked bear meat.

The disease develops usually within six or seven days after the infected meat has been consumed. In heavy infections, however, symptoms may begin within twenty-four hours. No immunity is known to the disease.

The disease has been kept alive in the United States by the practice of feeding pork scraps back to hogs, usually through the feeding of garbage to these animals. By this means the disease has been kept alive in hogs and thus transmitted to human beings. A number of cities now have regulations requiring the cooking of pork scraps or garbage before this refuse can be fed to hogs. Such local legislation should be very helpful in the control of trichinosis.

On a personal basis, the disease can be prevented by insisting on a thorough cooking of all pork products.

Typhus Fever

There are two types of typhus fever, one known as the epidemic form and the other as the endemic form. The latter, or murine type, is the one in existence in the United States today. Epidemic typhus fever is spread by body lice from person to person, but has not been a problem in the United States.

Endemic or murine typhus is spread by fleas from infected rats. The disorder is most likely to occur in those who live or work in close proximity to rats.

The disease develops within fourteen to sixteen days after the bite of the flea and usually starts with fever, chills, headache and generalized muscular aching. Respiratory inflammation and coughing may be present. When the central nervous system is involved, as is sometimes the case, delirium may be present as well as other signs of nervous involvement. Vomiting and diarrhea are common, as are other intestinal upsets. A characteristic rash or skin disorder usually appears on about the fourth or fifth day. About 5 per cent of the people who get murine typhus will die from the disease.

The disease can be effectively prevented by programs of rat eradication or by the use of DDT for the destruction of fleas on the rats. In the latter case the dusting of rat runways or burrows has been found to destroy as many as 99 per cent of the fleas harbored by the rats. This suggests that if rats cannot be wiped out, control may be sustained through the use of DDT powder.

Rocky Mountain Spotted Fever

Rocky Mountain spotted fever is one of the typhus group of diseases. It is known by many different names in various parts of the world. The disorder is spread by the bite of a tick containing rickettsial organisms which cause the disease.

The disease is usually not definitely diagnosed until the appearance of a characteristic rash. Aureomycin, Chloromycetin and para-aminobenzoic acid (PABA) are all effective in the treatment of this disease.

The most serious complication, and the one most likely to result in death of the patient, is pneumonia. Penicillin, which is not effective against Rocky Mountain spotted fever itself, can be used effectively to control the pneumonia if this complication develops. Circulatory and heart failure may also result as a complication. An effective vaccine has been prepared against Rocky Mountain fever. This is described in the next chapter.

Questions

1. Why do some persons think that it would be unwise to wipe out a communicable disease entirely so that it would no longer be present in a particular population?

2. Why do public health statistics fail to reveal the actual incidence of many communicable diseases?

3. Should any child ever be deliberately exposed to any of the so-called "children's diseases" in an effort to "get it over with"?

4. Is there a moral obligation on the part of a person suffering from a communicable disease to protect others from the infection?

5. How important are insects in the spread of infections?

6. What protections do we have against the communicable diseases that would be most apt to be used against us in case of bacteriologic warfare?

7. Which is the most fatal communicable disease under current conditions and what can be done about it?

For Further Reading

1. American Public Health Association: *Control of Communicable Diseases in Man.* New York, American Public Health Association, 1960.

2. Hare, Ronald: *Pomp and Pestilence: Infectious Disease: Its Origins and Conquest.* New York, Philosophical Library, 1955.

3. Williams, Greer: *Virus Hunters.* New York, Alfred A. Knopf, 1959.

4. Winslow, C. E. A., Smillie, Wilson G., Doull, James A., and Gordon, John E.: *The History of American Epidemiology.* St. Louis, C. V. Mosby Company, 1952.

For Advanced Reading

1. Baron, A. L.: *Man Against Germs.* New York, E. P. Dutton and Company, 1957.

2. Simon, Harold J.: *Attenuated Infection—The Germ Theory in Contemporary Perspective.* Philadelphia, J. B. Lippincott Company, 1960.

3. Top, Franklin H.: *Communicable and Infectious Diseases.* St. Louis, C. V. Mosby Company, 1960.

Recommended Films

1. Agress, Harry and William A. Hagan: *Rabies: Its Cause, Its Effect, Its Control.* 16 mm., black and white, sound, showing time 13 minutes, 1957. American Medical Association Motion Picture Library, 535 North Dearborn St., Chicago 10, Ill.

2. *The Infectious Diarrheas.* 16 mm., color, sound, showing time 15 minutes, 1960. United World Films, Inc., 1445 Park Avenue, New York 29, New York. For purchase. Communicable Disease Center, Attention, Audio Visual, Atlanta 22, Georgia. For loan.

3. *Management of the Leprosy Patient.* 16 mm. color, sound, showing time 19 minutes, 1960. United World Films, Inc., 1445 Park Avenue, New York 29, New York. For purchase. Communicable Disease Center, Attention, Audio Visual, Atlanta 22, Georgia. For loan.

4. *Stop Rheumatic Fever.* 16 mm., black and white, sound, showing time 13 minutes, 1955. Communicable Disease Center, Attention, Audio Visual, Atlanta 22, Georgia.

19

TWENTY IMMUNIZATIONS

SOME college health service departments report more student calls for immunizations than for any other single service. At the Stanford University Student Health Service for the first seven months of 1960, there were 4,340 calls by students for immunization purposes.

A knowledge of immunizations is important to the college student from several viewpoints. First, he should understand what protection he can personally achieve from the use of immunization services; second, he should learn what protection is advisable for the children of his future family; third, in case of epidemics of any particular disease the student should know whether or not immunization can be used as a protection; and fourth, there should be a thorough understanding of the immunization requirements for international travel.

243

Despite great progress in sanitation and the treatment of diseases with the so-called miracle drugs, vaccination still remains as a strong weapon against many diseases. In some cases immunization constitutes the only effective method of controlling a disease.

PREVENTION

"To cure is the voice of the past, to prevent is the divine whisper of today."

Kate Douglas Wiggin

In accordance with the international sanitary regulations adopted on October 1, 1952, under the auspices of the World Health Organization, certificates of vaccination are now required for only three diseases, namely, smallpox, yellow fever and cholera.

The international control of disease, however, is vastly different from the saving of lives on a community basis. Immunization against poliomyelitis, diphtheria, whooping cough, tetanus and smallpox has become routine pediatric procedure in the United States. This practice has undoubtedly saved hundreds of thousands of lives.

Other vaccinations are advisable and used on special occasions and during epidemics rather than on a routine basis. Decisions on such matters must rest with the physician and public health officer if the individual is to be sensibly guided.

Not all the vaccines or immunizing substances for the diseases discussed in this chapter are available in the office of the average physician. It must not be assumed that the physician is unaware of available vaccines merely because he does not have them immediately at hand. Some of the vaccines are prepared on a very small scale because they are used only during epidemics or for international travel. Yellow fever, for example, is not present in the United States; hence there is no reason to maintain a constant supply of yellow fever vaccine in every community. On the other hand, the supply of this vaccine is kept at certain central depots where it will be available when needed.

Some immunizing substances are still in the experimental stage. The reluctance of a physician to use a certain vaccine for a given disease may be based upon the fact that its value has not been fully proved, or that possible complications may outweigh the value to be received, or the need in terms of possible exposure is remote. In other words, the guidance of the physician should be sought as to when and against what diseases immunizations should be attempted.

The status and value of immunizations for twenty different diseases are described in this chapter. Only those diseases for which known vaccines or other immunizing agents are available are discussed in this part of the book.

NEW NEIGHBORS

"In this age of jet air travel our public health is really no better than that of our neighbors, and our neighbors include the whole world."

Dr. Verne Jackson

Adenovirus Vaccines

Adenovirus infections, some of which resemble colds, have recently been identified as causing disease characterized by eye irritation and discharge, nasal discharge and obstruction, sore throat; and occasionally cough, fever and headache.

A number of different types of adenoviruses have been identified by laboratory techniques, and heat-and-formaldehyde-inactivated virus vaccines have been prepared for protection against this group of virus diseases. Type 3 adenovirus vaccine was found to give evidence of immunization in 78 per cent of a group of adult volunteers inoculated with the virus. These vaccinated persons were protected when efforts were made to infect them with the disorder.

It appears likely that the adenovirus

vaccines will be developed soon to a point at which they may be used on a widespread scale for the prevention of the type of nose and throat disease described in the foregoing paragraphs. Whether or not the vaccines will prove to be of value in the prevention of the typical cold remains to be seen.

The adenoviruses are also known as the APC viruses because they were secured from the adenoidal, pharyngeal and conjunctival tissue of the nose and throat.

Cholera

Cholera vaccine is made from dead organisms prepared according to government specifications. The organism that causes cholera may be killed by heat and injected under the skin with very little inconvenience to the patient. The cholera vaccine used most widely consists of a suspension of approximately eight billion dead organisms per milliliter. The first vaccination is likely to consist of two injections seven to ten days apart. The resulting immunity lasts about four to six months. Subsequent immunizations are therefore made after this period of time as needed.

It is very important to realize that immunization alone against cholera will not protect fully against the disease. The level of immunity is likely to be incomplete and of relatively short duration. Since cholera is usually transmitted by food or drink contaminated with intestinal discharges, it is possible to secure adequate protection against cholera by thorough heating or cooking of food and drink. Nevertheless, immunization gives an added protection which is advisable when a person is traveling in regions where cholera is present or during an epidemic of the disorder.

It should be noted, however, that no case of cholera has existed in the United States for the past fifty years. Immunization against this disease in the continental United States is therefore not advisable and is not necessary. Only when a person leaves the United States for certain other areas is it advisable to be immunized.

Diphtheria

Contrary to popular belief, persons of all ages are susceptible to diphtheria. In other words, diphtheria should not be regarded solely as a problem of infancy and childhood.

When children are immunized against diphtheria, the immunity does not last for a lifetime. Studies show that approximately 20 per cent will have lost their immunity by the time of high school.

In most parts of the United States it is now customary to immunize against diphtheria in conjunction with poliomyelitis, tetanus and whooping cough. This multiple vaccine is intended for the simultaneous immunization of children against these four diseases.

The four-way vaccine, also known as Quadrigen, may be given at about the age of three months, or as soon thereafter as possible. An initial series of three doses of the vaccine are given by injection into the muscles at intervals of four to six weeks. After these three injections one additional immunization is recommended after six to twelve months. The product is not recommended for immunization of persons over the age of six years because of a higher percentage of reactions, although the product can be given in smaller dosage or after testing for sensitivities.

A booster immunization is recommended about 15 to 18 months after the first immunization. If the first immunization against diphtheria and the other three diseases mentioned is given in infancy, a booster dose is recommended within one year followed by a second booster injection at three years of age, with still another dose about the fifth or sixth year or by the time of entry into school.

According to recent investigations only about 50 per cent of mothers are immune to diphtheria. Children born to mothers who are not immune are also susceptible to the disease. Some investigators have attempted to give the newborn baby protection against diphtheria by immunizing the mother during the late stages of pregnancy. This method has been shown to be effective in the immunization of the newly born baby. In one study 44 per cent of the babies retained their immunity over the first three months of life. By the age of six months, however, all indications of resistance to diphtheria from the prenatal immunization of the mothers had disappeared in the babies.

Immunization of the adult against diphtheria is often an uncomfortable experience for the patient. The adult may have a severe reaction sufficient to put him to bed for three or four days with a swollen arm. Such reactions are especially liable to occur in the person who has a negative reaction to the Schick test, which is used to measure the immunologic status of the individual. It is important to give the adult who is going to be immunized against diphtheria a Schick test to screen out those who may have violent reactions.

Smaller doses of toxoid may be well tolerated by the adult, however. The use of a purified toxoid has also helped to reduce reactions in adults. It is possible to maintain a good level of immunity in the adult by repeated small doses of the toxoid, and this is advisable in order to reduce severe reactions.

German Measles

Passive immunity to German measles can be achieved by the use of gamma globulin. Neither children nor adults, however, are generally immunized against this disease because of the mildness of the disorder. There are special occasions, however, when it is wise to protect an individual against German measles.

Because recent research has shown that, if a woman who is in the first three months of pregnancy gets German measles there is a high likelihood of damage to the unborn baby, it is advisable to protect the woman in this stage of pregnancy by vaccination if she has been exposed to the disease. Two injections of gamma globulin are given to such a patient at five- to seven-day intervals. This appears to be sufficient to give protection against the disease.

There will be occasions also when babies and small children should be immunized if they have been exposed to this disorder. Children weak from other illnesses, and premature infants, for example, may need temporary protection against German measles. The decision should rest with the medical adviser.

Infectious Hepatitis

It is possible to protect against this virus infection of the liver through the use of gamma globulin. A single injection of gamma globulin, in a quantity or amount adjusted to the body weight of the patient, can give protection for about five to nine months.

Since infectious hepatitis is spread through intestinal discharges, immunization should be attempted only when it is judged that there is a particular hazard to this disease. In other words, when there is likelihood of contamination of food or water with the virus of infectious hepatitis, it is then well to consider the advisability of achieving a temporary and passive immunization by means of gamma globulin.

Immunization is not recommended as a routine procedure for all children or adults. This is partly because the immunity is temporary and passive, but also because current supplies of gamma globulin should be preserved for more effective use against other diseases. Also, in a modern community with good sanitation, exposure to the disease should not be great.

Influenza

Vaccination is the only known effective method for the control of influenza epidemics. Research is currently being conducted in the preparation of a vaccine containing a multiple number of influenza strains. Experimentally it has been shown that from four to six strains may be contained in an influenza vaccine with good results. Most of the vaccines currently used for vaccination against influenza contain only types A and B, although the A type does include the Asian strain of influenza virus. Two injections of this vaccine are given at least two weeks apart.

Regular annual immunization against influenza in the autumn is recommended. Immunization is also recommended under certain special circumstances. For example, the California State Department of Public Health recommended that those people who planned to attend the Winter Olympics in Squaw Valley in February, 1960, should consider vaccination against influenza because of the crowding and close contact with so many people.

Some investigators have recommended that the influenza vaccines should be injected in emulsified mineral oil for the achievement of longer lasting immunity to the disease. Studies show that antibody levels may remain elevated for at least three years after vaccination with mineral oil containing the influenza vaccines. The use of this type of vaccine has not yet become general, however.

Although vaccination against influenza cannot be depended upon to protect a person completely, it appears that the vaccine can be relied upon to be from 50 to 75 per cent effective in the prevention of this disease. The influenza that may develop despite vaccination is also likely to be milder than in the unvaccinated person. In other words, the vaccine does appear to give some measure of protection and may prevent the disease entirely.

In about 50 per cent of those who are immunized against influenza there may be moderate reactions such as headache, fever and general aching.

There are a number of different strains of viruses that cause influenza. Vaccination against one strain may not protect against another. It is therefore important to know which type of virus is prevalent when an epidemic of influenza is in existence, although a vaccine of multiple strains is now available.

The immunity developed by vaccination against influenza is not of unlimited duration; it appears to last about one year or less. It is advisable to immunize against influenza about once a year.

The Russians consider active immunization with live influenza virus as the only practical method for the mass prevention of influenza. The Russians report that the efficiency of live vaccine is such that it will cause a reduction of two to three times the illness rate of unvaccinated people. Although the Russians advocate the use of live influenza vaccine directly into the respiratory tract, at least one American investigator who gave the vaccine by spraying it into the nasal passageways was able to find only a moderate improvement in antibody levels. This investigator found that inactivated vaccine given by injection was far more effective than the live vaccine in raising antibody levels.

Only about one person in 1000 will have a fever in reaction to influenza immunization. The Army has reported that of seven million men vaccinated against this disease, there were no reports of nerve or brain inflammation following the vaccination. This would seem to indicate that serious reactions to the immunizations are exceedingly rare. Previous vaccination against virus influenza appears to have no significant effect on reactions. The vaccine should not be given to persons who have an allergy to egg or chicken, however.

Measles

Considerable research is being conducted on the safety and value of an attenuated measles-virus vaccine. Although in the past it has not been possible to achieve a lasting method of immunization for this disease, the new vaccine appears to offer considerable promise. When the new measles vaccine was injected into 79 children, a modified form of measles occurred in 77 of them. The disease was of shorter duration, resulted in no complications, and did not disable those who developed the vaccine-induced illness. There also appeared to be no communication of the infection to others. Blood studies showed that the antibody response in these children was equal in quality and quantity to that of those children who had had the natural disease. Whether or not these children will be immune to measles, however, is not yet known.

It is likely that this modified live-virus vaccine may soon be available on more than an experimental scale. In the meantime, a temporary, passive immunity can be achieved against measles with gamma globulin. The immunity from this product will last about three weeks only.

Gamma globulin is one of the substances recovered from blood plasma. The antibodies produced by the human body are concentrated in the gamma globulin. This blood protein gives temporary immunity in a number of other diseases besides measles.

Because of the brief duration of the immunity obtained from the use of gamma globulin, it should be used only to immunize infants and very young children who have been exposed to measles, because the death rate from this disease is greatest in the very young. Most babies who are born to mothers who have had measles will have some immunity to the disease up to about the age of six months. If it is certain that the child has some level of resistance to measles, then a modified or smaller dose may be useful. Usually the gamma globulin is given, by intramuscular injection, between the fourth and eighth day after the child has been exposed to measles. Gamma globulin is quite safe, since reactions are rather rare.

Convalescent measles serum and placental globulin are two other substances which have been used for immunization against measles. Although convalescent measles serum gives a high level of protection, it is difficult to secure. Placental globulin, also known as immune human globulin, gives less protection and is often accompanied by fairly severe reactions.

Immunization for measles should be considered in the very young child or in the child whose health is already impaired so that it is not advisable that he be subjected to further illness. Since measles is a severe disease and complications such as bronchial pneumonia and inflammation of the eyes and even of the brain are fairly frequent, the very young or debilitated child should be protected, not only because of the severity of the disease, but also because of the danger of possible complications.

Since the immunity conferred by gamma globulin is of such short duration, it is used primarily for preventing onset of the disease after exposure has occurred. The mildness of the substance is shown by the fact that gamma globulin has been given to premature infants with no ill effects.

Mumps

A vaccine for mumps is now available. Some physicians still regard it as being in the experimental stage and it is not routinely used on infants or children. The vaccine is used on a limited scale for active immunization of adults when there is an epidemic of mumps in the community and the latter have not had the disease previously. Nonimmune parents whose children have been exposed to mumps, military personnel and others who have not had mumps should be immunized during an epidemic of the disease.

It is advisable for adults to be skin tested for susceptibility to mumps before immunization. Material for this purpose is also available now.

The active immunity produced by the mumps vaccine is thought to last about six to twelve months. The mumps vaccine consists of a killed virus, and is effective within four to five weeks. Routine immunization of children is not advisable.

Hyperimmune mumps serum has also been used for passive immunization of certain patients who have been exposed to mumps. This serum must be used in large doses, and it does not give an extended immunity.

Attenuated live-virus vaccines have been used extensively in the Soviet Union for the prevention of mumps. This vaccine is injected into the skin in a single dose. Immunity appears to develop within 14 to 21 days and to persist at a high level for three years or more; at least, in a group of 35,000 pre-school children the vaccine appeared to give at least 90 per cent protection for a period of three years. Cases which occurred in the remaining 10 per cent of the children were very mild and apparently not contagious. The Russians are now producing this attenuated mumps virus on a large scale in a massive program to control this disease among children.

Plague

Under international agreements adopted in 1952, anti-plague vaccination can no longer be required for admission to any country. This is not because vaccination against plague is inefficient or ineffective, but because better methods of controlling the disease have been found.

Since plague is a disease spread by fleas from infected rats to human beings, and since the disease is spread on an international scale mostly through infected rats on ships, the control measures have shifted away from vaccination of the individual to the rat-proofing of ships and the destruction of rats and insects.

Under international agreements, for example, it is compulsory that every ship be examined every six months to see whether rats are aboard. A large majority of modern ships are now rat-proofed.

The World Health Organization has expressed the opinion that vaccination against plague is of value for the individual, but has no place in international quarantine practice.

Within recent years very few cases of plague have occurred in the United States. In fact, from the years 1900 to 1945, inclusive, only 504 cases of this disease were reported to public health authorities. Of this number, however, 318 cases resulted in the death of the patient. In 1958 there was not a single death from plague in the United States. Nevertheless, sporadic cases of plague may be expected to develop in this country since there is a constant reservoir of the disease among certain wild animals. These cases may be expected to be so rare, however, that immunization against this disease is not advisable as a routine procedure.

The vaccine used for immunization against plague consists of a suspension of two billion dead plague organisms per milliliter. The vaccination is given in two injections under the skin with an interval of about seven to ten days between the two shots. The International Quarantine Measures now recommend plague inoculations only during an epidemic of the disease.

Poliomyelitis

Poliomyelitis vaccine has now been proved to be both safe and effective. Despite the unfortunate and tragic experience with the Salk vaccine in the spring of 1955, technical improvements in production have now made the product safe. As of 1960 many millions of children throughout the world had been safely vaccinated against poliomyelitis with the Salk vaccine.

The recommended procedure now calls for a multiple vaccine to be given infants about the age of three months for protection against poliomyelitis, diphtheria, tetanus and whooping cough simultaneously. Three injections are given about four to six weeks apart, followed by later booster immunization of the multiple vaccine.

It is not yet known how long a person will be protected against poliomyelitis after a series of three doses of the vaccine. Only time can decide this question, although there is some possibility that a lifetime immunity may be conferred.

The poliomyelitis vaccine is a "killed virus," containing no living material. It consists of each of the three known types of virus which have been killed with formalin and heat. Every bit of poliomyelitis vaccine released for use by the public has the approval of the U.S. Public Health Service as safe, pure and potent.

Live poliomyelitis vaccine has been developed and used on a broad scale by three different medical leaders. Dr. Albert B. Sabin, Dr. Hilary Koprowski, and Dr. Herald R. Cox, Sc.D., have used a live polio virus vaccine in Europe, Mexico, Singapore, Latin America and the Belgian Congo, apparently with good results. The Russians have also used a live poliomyelitis vaccine. In field trials on nearly two million children under the age of 15 years it was found that no poliomyelitis occurred due to the vaccine. Later experience with 12 million children resulted in the conclusion that a live polio virus vaccine can be used safely. The Russians found the live polio virus vaccine to be about 20 times more effective than non-vaccination so far as illness from poliomyelitis is concerned.

The World Health Organization Expert Committee on poliomyelitis reported in 1960 that both the killed-virus of the Salk vaccine and the attenuated live-virus vaccine play a major role in the control of this disease. This committee also reported that more than 60 million children had then been vaccinated in the Soviet Union with live polio virus without any reported ill effects.

A statement by the Surgeon General of the United States indicates that the live polio virus vaccines have not produced harm to individuals, but that there is already at hand a potent weapon against poliomyelitis in the Salk vaccine whose value and effectiveness have been proved.

For people who have not previously been immunized against poliomyelitis it is possible to reach a protective level of antibodies through a single injection of poliomyelitis vaccine. This single injection may be at ten times the strength of the regular injections. A group of five physicians at the National Institute of Health have reported that a single injection of ten cc. of poliomyelitis vaccine resulted in rapid immunization. These investigators recommend that a single large dose is desirable before and during epidemics of poliomyelitis for people who have not completed the usual three-dose schedule of immunization.

Rabies

Immunization against rabies should not be attempted unless there has been exposure to the infection. Only after rabies has been diagnosed in animals that have bitten the patients should the latter be immunized. This is because some persons may have a reaction to the vaccine, although newer and safer vaccines are being prepared. On the other hand, it should be remembered that if a person has been bitten by a rabid dog or other animal, the death rate is virtually 100 per cent unless treatment and immunization are used. Immunization can be safely delayed for as long as ten to fourteen days after the patient has been bitten by a rabid dog.

Antirabic vaccine is prepared from brain tissue. The possibilities of severe reaction are increased in persons who have been previously immunized, even though the second treatment comes many years later. There may be redness and swelling at the site of the injections, or there may be fever, rashes, swelling of the joints and inflammation of the brain. If headache, nausea and vomiting develop, treatments need to be discontinued, since these symptoms often precede paralysis. The vaccine is given daily for fourteen to twenty-one days.

Recent research has indicated that a rabies vaccine prepared from a duck embryo culture is much safer than the older vaccine which has been traditionally prepared from a suspension of rabbit brain which has been infected with the rabies virus. The Semple vaccine which has been widely used in the United States consists of dead rabies virus. Death of the virus has been achieved by the addition of phenol or by exposure to ultraviolet light. The duck embryo rabies vaccine has been found to stimulate an earlier production of antibodies than the Semple vaccine. It has also been found that the duck embryo vaccine apparently does not result in the inflammation of the brain that sometimes occurs with the older rabies vaccine. It is likely that a modified vaccine of this type will ultimately supplant the previously widely used product.

Complications are sufficiently infrequent so that anyone who has been bitten by a mad dog should be immunized with one or the other of the foregoing vaccines. The risk in ignoring treatment of this type is too great, and once the disease has developed it is invariably fatal. The danger of treatment paralysis is sufficiently great with the older vaccine, however, that at no time should a person be routinely immunized against rabies *when there has been no exposure to the disease*.

It has been reported that the Pasteur Institute of Southern India gave treatment to immunize 40,421 persons who had been bitten or scratched by mad animals. Of these patients, 402 died of rabies, a death rate of approximately 1 per cent. A death rate of well under 1 per cent was observed in a still larger group immunized against rabies after exposure to the disease.

In the United States it was reported in 1949 that approximately 30,000 persons each year were being immunized against rabies because of exposure to rabid or rabid-suspected dogs. By 1956 about 60,000 persons were receiving vaccine or serum treatment for prevention of the disease each year. By 1958 only 5 persons died of rabies in the United States, signifying the very great value of immunization when people are bitten by rabid dogs. Since the death rate from untreated rabies is generally accepted as being 100 per cent, the great value of rabies immunization should be obvious.

The mass immunization of dogs against rabies has proved to be a very effective means of controlling this disease. Many communities throughout the United States have now used this method of control. Obviously if the dogs themselves are protected against rabies, there is less chance of exposure so far as human beings are concerned.

It appears that dogs must be vaccinated against rabies each year if they are to be protected against the disease with the older type of vaccine. Recently, however, a new, so-called avianized rabies vaccine has been developed for the active immunization of dogs. The active, life-long type of immunization that this vaccine confers may make it unnecessary to vaccinate dogs each year. In Detroit only one unfavorable reaction was observed in over 7000 inoculations, so the vaccine appears safe. A policy of immunizing all stray dogs that are apprehended is one aspect of a broader rabies control program which is based upon widespread vaccination of all dogs.

Another illustration of the value of vaccination of dogs against rabies may be found in the experience of Memphis and Shelby County, Tennessee, where an alarming epidemic of this disease occurred some years ago. During a six-day period 23,000 dogs were inoculated at seventy emergency clinics set up for that purpose. The results were phenomenal, both the city and county remaining entirely free of rabies in dogs for more than one year.

It should be realized, of course, that most dog bites are not made by animals suffering from rabies. In the city of Los Angeles approximately 10,000 animal bites are reported each year. It has been estimated on the basis of the Los Angeles experience that the chance of getting rabies from known animal bites is about one in 1400 or less.

Rocky Mountain Spotted Fever

A relative protection can be secured against Rocky Mountain spotted fever by means of immunization. Though the vaccine does not prevent the onset of the disease in all cases, especially in the more severe types of illness, it does reduce the severity of the disease, and this may be lifesaving. Milder forms of Rocky Mountain spotted fever may be prevented entirely by annual immunization.

The vaccine is injected under the skin or into the muscles in either two or three doses at intervals of five to seven days. Immunization should be completed, if possible, about one month before possible exposure in areas where the disease is always present. Since Rocky Mountain spotted fever is transmitted by the bites of the wood tick or the dog tick, it is wise to be immunized against this disease *any time when there is contemplated travel in an area where these ticks are prevalent.* The immunization should be accomplished in the late winter or early spring months if possible. The minimum length of time needed for immunity to develop to a satisfactory level is at least ten days.

Fishermen, hunters, trappers, campers and travelers in general are advised to be immunized against this disease in certain parts of the West where the disorder is more severe.

Scarlet Fever

Active immunization against scarlet fever can be obtained, but side reactions are so numerous and the modern treatment of this disease with penicillin and the sulfa drugs is so effective that immunization is not commonly done. When immunization against scarlet fever is attempted, it is done only on persons with a negative reaction to the Dick test.

Smallpox

The value of vaccination against smallpox has been demonstrated in various countries throughout the world as well as in the United States. Vaccination is achieved by means of the virus of cowpox. Smallpox is caused by a virus which closely resembles the virus that causes cowpox. When the smallpox virus is injected into cows, a change occurs in the nature of the virus so that it can no longer be used to cause typical smallpox. When the virus undergoes this change, it is known as vaccinia virus, the cause of cowpox.

When the virus of cowpox is used in vaccination, it does not revert to its previous status; hence it cannot produce typical smallpox in the human. The modern preparation of vaccinia virus is accomplished by means of growth in tissue cultures.

Smallpox vaccination is generally done today by the multiple pressure method. The skin on the arm or thigh is thoroughly cleansed with sterile cotton and acetone, ethyl alcohol or ether, and is then per-

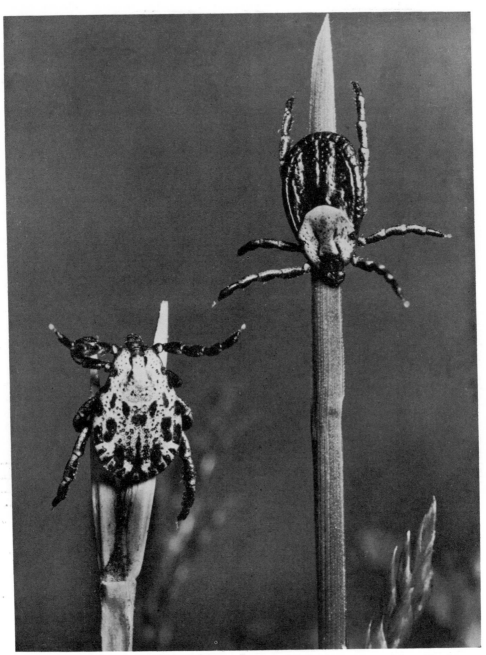

Figure 30. Ticks are a source of various diseases, including Rocky Mountain spotted fever. (Courtesy of N. J. Kramis for Photography and Scientific Monthly.)

mitted to dry thoroughly. When the skin is dry, a drop of the vaccine is placed on the surface of the skin and a needle or point is held at an angle of about 45 degrees with the skin surface and is then moved up and down rapidly in such a way that no blood is drawn, but a slight scraping or thinning of the skin occurs. After the vaccination has been completed the vaccine may be wiped off.

ANACHRONISM

"... The presence of smallpox in the world today is an anachronism, since vaccination against the disease has existed for more than 150 years and vaccine is now both effective and cheap. In spite of this fact, there were more than 200,000 cases of smallpox in Asia last year ... the disease was introduced into Europe, where several outbreaks occurred ..."

World Health Organization, 1959

Three general types of reactions to smallpox vaccination may occur. The first is the immune reaction, in which there is slight redness and swelling that develops within one or two days and then decreases fairly rapidly. This reaction may indicate a high level of immunity, but it could also mean that there is not a typical "take" even though immunity is not sufficiently high for adequate protection. A second type of reaction is known as the "vaccinoid," in which a vesicle or blister forms with considerable redness and swelling which develops in three to five days. This reaction may be accompanied by slight fever, a general feeling of indisposition, aching, tenderness and slight soreness of the area. In the third type of reaction, known as a primary or typical "take," the vesicle or blister does not appear until about the fifth day. There is then an increase in redness and size of the vesicle until about the ninth day, when the involved area is about the diameter of a half dollar or more.

A failure to react to smallpox vaccination in the foregoing ways does not indicate a well established immunity, but

usually is strong evidence of an inactive virus vaccine. In other words, the vaccinating material for one reason or another has lost its capacity to develop immunity.

It is sometimes claimed that smallpox vaccination is unsafe because inflammation of the brain may occur. On the other hand, the Pasteur Institute of Algeria accomplished more than fifty million smallpox vaccinations during the years 1910 to 1937 without a single case of inflammation of the brain being reported.

An epidemic of virulent smallpox that broke out in April, 1947, in New York City led to a tremendous public demand for vaccination. It was estimated that more than six million vaccinations were performed on New York citizens and people living in the surrounding area. In this epidemic it was judged that forty-two persons out of the six million who had been vaccinated had an inflammation of the brain. This was a rate of approximately one in every 150,000 vaccinations.

Generalized vaccinia occurred in thirty-six persons, but twenty-two of these were in children who had not themselves been vaccinated, but who acquired the disorder by contact with other members of the family. Two of these children died. It can thus be seen that complications do happen after smallpox vaccination, but these are very rare. In contrast to the number of lives saved by smallpox vaccination, there can be no doubt of its tremendous value.

In general, a person should be vaccinated every five to seven years, although it is advisable that this service be performed whenever an epidemic of smallpox occurs. No one has died of smallpox in the United States during the last few years.

It has been shown rather clearly that there is an association between the number of cases of smallpox that occur in a particular state or area and the presence or absence of vaccination laws.

Tetanus

It has become virtually routine in pediatric circles to immunize infants and children against tetanus in conjunction with poliomyelitis, diphtheria and whooping cough.

For routine immunization with the multiple preparation, three injections are given at intervals of about one month or more, with the first injection about the age of three months or slightly older.

Military experience has shown the value of immunization against tetanus. Early in 1941 immunization against tetanus was made routine for all military personnel on active duty. The fluid or plain tetanus toxoid was used and given in a series of three injections three weeks apart. One year later another injection was given, and a booster shot was required one month before the soldier departed for overseas duty.

Reactions to tetanus immunization have been mild in most cases. Headache, weakness, feeling of discomfort and local soreness of the arm with occasional chills and fever have been reported. More severe reactions consisted in flushing and itching of the skin and eruptions and swellings of the lips and eyelids. It was found that these reactions were due mostly to certain substances in the toxoid, which were eliminated. After this improvement of the toxoid, the reports of sensitivities became rare. The Army has reported that reactions are now less than one in 10,000 injections. The use of antihistamines, corticotropin (ACTH), cortisone and epinephrine has helped greatly to control sensitivity reactions when they do occur. Sometimes desensitization by small doses of serum gradually increased in magnitude is necessary.

When tetanus toxoid is used alone with children, the immunization can be delayed and the period between injections lengthened somewhat. Studies suggest that two injections of alum-precipitated tetanus toxoid can give immunity for about five years when the child is immunized between the ages of three and eight years. The two injections can be given three months apart. Under this plan of immunization against tetanus only about 10 per cent of the children will complain of soreness at the site of the injection, which is usually in the arm.

Temporary passive immunity can be established by the injection of tetanus antitoxin when a person has been exposed to tetanus. The patient should be tested for sensitivity to this substance, however, before it is given. The use of antitoxin is routine medical treatment for tetanus.

The value of tetanus immunization was clearly shown in World War II. During those years approximately one-half million soldiers were wounded, but only twelve cases of tetanus were known to have occurred. Of the twelve cases, six were in persons with no active immunization and two were in soldiers who had not been adequately treated even though they had been immunized.

In the Japanese army and navy, in which no routine immunization was done, about ten cases of tetanus occurred for every 100,000 men who were wounded. The incidence of tetanus for this group was much greater than that in the American army. The German army, too, had a high rate of tetanus in the nonimmunized ground forces in Normandy.

In the civilian population the greatest hazard from tetanus occurs in the age group up to fifteen years and in farmers, horsemen and others whose injuries are especially liable to be contaminated with tetanus spores. For these people and for children, routine immunization against tetanus is especially advised by public health authorities.

> "Tetanus remains a highly fatal disease with about 60 deaths occurring for every 100 cases reported in the United States..."
>
> *Norman W. Axnick, M.S., and E. Russell Alexander*

It must be remembered that tetanus is highly fatal if there has been no previous immunization. Dr. Harold Bedell and Dr. Samuel S. Paley, of New York City, reported on seventeen patients who had acquired tetanus through various minor wounds. Out of this group thirteen patients died despite the most vigorous medical treatment.

One patient became infected with tetanus through a cut on the leg, another from puncturing her foot with a splinter and a third from cutting his finger on a can. Still another patient got the disease after cutting and treating a corn himself. One patient got tetanus through injuries sustained when he fell down an elevator shaft. Another got the disease after burns to his right elbow, and six had it from the injection of drugs with unsterilized needles. All these drug addicts died from tetanus.

There is no known method of controlling tetanus after the exotoxin (the poison produced by the tetanus organisms) has become fixed to nerve tissue. The only satisfactory protection is obtained by immunization against the disease. Vaccination with tetanus toxoid is desirable for the entire population, according to some medical authorities. During 1958 there were 303 persons in the United States who died of tetanus.

Tuberculosis

Vaccination against tuberculosis is not widespread in the United States, although a great deal of interest has been created recently in the use of BCG (bacille Calmette Guérin) vaccine for the prevention of this disease.

It appears to be well established that when BCG vaccination is done properly, it is safe. This is in keeping with the European experience, in which millions of people have been vaccinated against tu-

berculosis, especially in Norway, Sweden and Denmark.

Although there is reported to be considerable opposition to vaccination against smallpox in Norway, there is practically no resistance to vaccination against tuberculosis. In fact, during 1947 a law was passed in that country providing for the compulsory tuberculin testing and vaccination against tuberculosis of certain groups in the community.

The foreign experience with BCG vaccine seems to indicate that vaccination against tuberculosis does give considerable protection against the disease. No one has been able to judge accurately, however, the value of immunization alone, since in all countries where vaccination against tuberculosis is practiced, there are also many other measures in operation for the control of the disease. Controversy on the value of BCG has raged for about 40 years and has limited its use in the United States.

One of the possible hazards in widespread vaccination against tuberculosis is that older, more established methods of fighting this disease may be abandoned in the false hope that tuberculosis can be controlled by vaccination alone. Public health and medical experts have cautioned that BCG vaccination should be used to supplement rather than replace other measures of control.

> **BCG OR DRUGS?**
> "Apparently we are in the dawn of the day of treating tuberculosis successfully with drugs. And . . . the possibility looms of destroying all tubercle bacilli . . . this opportunity . . . is nullified if BCG has previously been administered."
> **Dr. J. A. Myers, 1958**

Foreign experience with BCG vaccination has led to the conclusion that only tuberculin-negative reactors should be immunized with this substance. When persons who have a positive reaction to the tuberculin test are vaccinated with

BCG, the disease is sometimes activated. By this is meant that the disease becomes more active in the person.

The BCG vaccine is injected into the skin rather than under it. A small nodule or lump usually appears at the site of the injection in about four or five weeks. This increases in size slowly, and in about a month and a half after the vaccination the nodule erupts and discharges one or two drops of pus. This small ulceration may persist from a few weeks to several months and then heal. Only a small scar is left. About 97 per cent of those who are vaccinated with BCG give a positive tuberculin reaction in about six to nine weeks after the vaccination.

At the current time it is felt that those who are especially exposed to tuberculosis, such as nurses, medical students, hospital employees and resident physicians, should be immunized against tuberculosis if they are nonreactors to tuberculin.

Typhoid Fever

Typhoid vaccine gives a high level of protection, but may not prevent entirely the onset of typhoid fever. There have been repeated reports in medical literature of people recently immunized against typhoid fever who got the disease when sufficiently exposed. However, in the great majority of these cases the disease was very mild, with almost invariable recovery.

Ordinarily the protection given by typhoid vaccine does not last longer than one year. The vaccine is given at weekly intervals in three doses by injection under the skin. If the person remains in an area where typhoid fever is prevalent, a booster dose of typhoid vaccine is advisable each year. This should maintain the level of immunity at a relatively high efficiency.

Typhoid fever immunization is advisable at any age during an epidemic of the disease or during a catastrophe such as a flood or a hurricane where there has been, or is likely to be, contamination of the public drinking supply over a long period of time. Immunization is also advisable when there has been exposure to a known carrier of the disease. If a person lives in an area where there is continuous exposure to typhoid fever, it is wise to have periodic immunization against typhoid fever. For most people, however, vaccination against this disorder is needed only when travel is contemplated into an area where there is likely to be exposure to the disease.

Typhus Fever

During World War II the United States Army immunized its military personnel against epidemic typhus fever whenever there were troop movements to certain areas. The vaccine used consisted of a 10 per cent suspension of organisms causing the disease. Three injections of the typhus vaccine were given by injection under the skin at intervals of seven to ten days. This immunization was followed by booster doses every six months whenever the military personnel were in an area where typhus fever was present. Later on, the first immunization was reduced to two doses of vaccine rather than three.

Only sixty-four cases of epidemic, louseborne typhus fever were reported in the entire United States Army during World War II. No deaths occurred among these sixty-four patients. All the patients had been immunized against the disease. Army experience indicated strongly that typhus fever immunization was effective in preventing death and serious illness from the disorder. It was found that the chance of death was reduced to practically zero if a person had been adequately immunized at least two weeks before exposure.

The primary control of typhus fever, however, no longer depends upon vaccination of the individual. For example, in the city of Los Angeles after one year's intensive rat control work by the City Health Department, the number of typhus fever cases of the murine or endemic type (which is spread by fleas from infected rats to humans) fell to less than one third of what it had been during the previous year.

Sanitary measures, including the use of DDT powder, have been very effective in controlling epidemic or louse-borne typhus fever. This was shown in Naples when dusting of the entire population with DDT powder, shortly after World War II, put an abrupt and dramatic stop to an incipient epidemic of louse-borne typhus. Although vaccines are available for immunization against both types of typhus fever, this is no longer the primary measure of control over these diseases.

The international sanitary regulations pertaining to typhus fever are based upon the fact that epidemic typhus can be prevented readily by public health measures. Vaccination against typhus is no longer required under these regulations for travel in an area from which it is desired to keep out typhus fever.

Whooping Cough

For many years medical men debated whether vaccination against whooping cough actually protected the child against this disease. Gradually, however, information has accumulated which shows that there can be little doubt that immunization is a valuable procedure for infants and children.

One study of this problem, conducted by the British Medical Research Council, showed that vaccination against whooping cough reduced the incidence of the disease by about 78 per cent. When whooping cough did develop in the vaccinated group of children, the disease was less severe and of shorter duration. The conclu-

sion of the British Medical Research Council was that immunization against whooping cough does give substantial protection against the disease.

Most of the deaths from whooping cough occur in children under the age of one year. In a study by the public health officials of the state of New York, covering a five-year period, it was found that slightly more than 50 per cent of the deaths occurred in children under six months of age. This discovery has led to the modern practice of vaccinating against whooping cough at the age of three months.

It is common practice now to immunize against whooping cough in conjunction with poliomyelitis, diphtheria and tetanus. Injections of the multiple vaccine are given intramuscularly, usually in alternate arms, beginning at the age of three months. There is some variation in practice, but the three injections may be given at one-month intervals. Six to 12 months after the last of the three injections the child should receive his first booster shot of the multiple vaccine. He is then reasonably well protected until 15 to 18 months later when he should receive another booster shot.

Some physicians have reported the successful immunization of unborn babies against whooping cough by vaccinating the pregnant mother late in the stages of pregnancy. Laboratory studies indicated that the blood of the newborn babe contained protective substances against whooping cough. This, however, is not standard procedure.

Yellow Fever

The two most effective methods of control for yellow fever are vaccination and mosquito eradication. International regulations now call for the vaccination of all travelers who move from an area in which the disease exists to another region where the disease may develop. The current vaccine gives a high and effective level of immunity lasting about six years. Vaccination is not intended primarily for protection of the individual against the disease, but is required in international travel in order to protect against spread of the disorder from one area into another.

Persons holding a valid international certificate of vaccination or revaccination against yellow fever are exempt from quarantine measures. Hundreds of thousands of persons, mostly military personnel, have now been immunized against yellow fever.

The most commonly used yellow fever vaccine is known as the 17D strain, which is grown on chick embryos. The vaccine is given by injection under the skin in a single dose.

Thousands of cases of jaundice that developed in the early part of the war among American soldiers who had been vaccinated against yellow fever were found to be due to the presence of small amounts of human blood serum which had been added as a stabilizing agent to the vaccine. After the deletion of this human serum from the yellow fever vaccine no further complications of this type occurred.

A person contemplating travel in an area where he will be exposed to yellow fever should be vaccinated at least ten days before he leaves his own country. This means that steps should be taken for immunization against yellow fever at a still earlier date, since the yellow fever vaccine is not routinely available in most communities and the physician doing the immunization must obtain the vaccine from certain central points, or the patient must travel to these central areas to be immunized.

The recent spread of yellow fever in the jungle animals of Central America northward towards the United States raises the possibility that vaccination against this dreaded disease of the past may come to be of great significance even in this country. It should never be forgotten that yellow fever once occurred in epidemic proportions in the United States. As yet, however, no immediate problem exists with the disease in North America.

Questions

1. Would simultaneous immunization of every person in a population be an effective way of wiping out diphtheria? Why would such an attempt not be advisable?
2. Should all immunizations that are available for the prevention of disease be used routinely by an individual, or should they be used only on certain occasions?
3. Can the proved value of immunization for certain diseases justify this approach to the control of communicable disorders when an occasional severe reaction or even death may occur from the immunization?
4. What are the arguments in favor of the immunization of dogs rather than humans in the control of epidemics of rabies?
5. Why is immunization not an effective means of controlling all communicable diseases?

For Further Reading

1. Public Health Service: *Immunization Information for International Travel.* Public Health Service Publication No. 384 (revised annually), Washington, D.C., 1960.
2. World Health Organization: *Yellow Fever Vaccination.* New York, Columbia University Press, 1956.

Recommended Film

Public Health Service: *Rabies Control in the Community.* 16 mm., black and white, sound, 11 minutes running time, 1956. Obtain from Communicable Disease Center, 50 Seventh St., N.E., Atlanta 23, Georgia.

20

TUBERCULOSIS:
WORLD HEALTH PROBLEM

ALTHOUGH the number of deaths from this disease on a worldwide basis is not accurately known, it has been estimated for years that at least five million people die annually from tuberculosis. This figure has been greatly reduced in the last several years by treatment with antibiotics on an international scale.

Asia and South America are main reservoirs for the disease. It is estimated that in China alone about one million people die each year from tuberculosis. In India tuberculosis was described in the writings of medical leaders thousands of years ago. All over the world, through centuries of time, tuberculosis, the white plague, has been a major killer. Today it still ranks as one of the greatest health problems.

Tuberculosis in the United States

No one knows exactly how many cases of tuberculosis there are in the United States today. It is estimated, however, by experts in the United States Public Health Service and the National Tuberculosis Association, that there are about one million tuberculous persons in this country.

Despite the fact that about 1,000,000 persons in this country are known to have tuberculosis, the deaths from this disease have been decreasing in recent years because of a vigorous national effort to stamp out the disease. By 1958 there were only 12,361 persons who died of tuberculosis in the United States and fatalities from this disease have been declining so rapidly that health experts are now talk-ing about stamping out the disorder entirely with vigorous use of chemotherapy.

How Tuberculosis Spreads

Today tuberculosis spreads mostly by nose and throat discharges from a person suffering from an active stage of the disease. The disease is more likely to spread between members of a family than to others. In other words, if one member of the family has the disease, other members of the family, because of the close association, will have a higher hazard in exposure.

In one study it was observed that of 100 children suffering from tuberculosis,

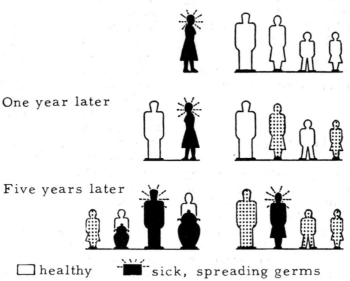

TUBERCULOSIS SPREADS IN THE HOUSEHOLD
A sick servant carries tuberculosis
into a healthy family

One year later

Five years later

☐ healthy   ▥ sick, spreading germs
▦ infected   ♟ death from tuberculosis

Figure 31.   How tuberculosis spread in one household. (Courtesy of Los Angeles Tuberculosis and Health Association.)

ninety had caught the disease from their mothers. In only ten cases was the father the source of the disease. Since the mother is much more likely to be closely associated with the care of small children, it is logical that she would be the source of the disease more frequently than the father, even though both of them might be infected with tuberculosis. It was also found that children below the age of five years who get tuberculosis almost invariably get it at home or from servants, neighbors or friends who visit the home.

VARIABLE SUSCEPTIBILITY

"Remarkably little is understood about the circumstances which favor infection. . . . It is not unusual for a nurse to serve many months on an active tuberculosis ward without becoming positive to the tuberculin test. But an entire roomful of guests at a Christmas party once was found to have been infected in a single evening by one visiting seaman, the only active case in the lot."

Office of the Surgeon General, 1960

Children above the age of five appear to get the disease from outside the home. It may be reasoned that if the child has not contracted the disease within the home by the age of five, the disease does not exist among the family members. In such case the infection is likely to be picked up from someone outside the family.

Symptoms of Tuberculosis

The symptoms of tuberculosis vary somewhat according to the degree of immunity possessed by the individual and the course of the disease. Most people have a fairly high level of resistance to tuberculosis. This is shown by the fact that less than 10 per cent of all those who are infected with the disease will die from it.

After a first infection with tuberculosis of the lungs there may be little or no evidence of the disease. Within three to seven weeks after the original infection there may be a few symptoms such as moderate temperature and a general feeling of indisposition. Usually no drug treatment is needed, although strict bed rest is advisable for a few weeks.

In the majority of cases, if there is no further infection with the tuberculosis, about the only effect of this first infection is a change in the tuberculin reaction. In other words, a person who has previously had a negative tuberculin test will now have a positive reaction. In a great majority of cases symptoms of this stage of the disease may be so mild as to pass unnoticed, or at least to escape diagnosis.

Most of the symptoms of tuberculosis arise in the reinfection type of pulmonary tuberculosis. The classic symptoms in this form of tuberculosis are as follows:

1. FEVER.   In the acute stage of tuberculosis of the lungs the usual experience is for the patient to have a normal or near-normal temperature in the morning and to have a gradual rise until between about 4 and 8 P.M., when the fever, which may range from 100° to 106° F., reaches its height. By the next morning the fever has diminished until the temperature is relatively normal, and then the rise in temperature is repeated throughout the day.

There is no standard pattern for the fever, since the body temperature will depend partly upon the degree or intensity of the infection. In mild cases there may be a slight afternoon fever only if the person engages in vigorous activity. This fever may disappear rapidly with rest, and the patient may be unaware that his temperature is elevated unless some measurement is made.

2. COUGH.   Cough does not usually occur in tuberculosis until there has been some breakdown in the body defenses in the lungs and there is accumulation of fluid and other materials which irritate the lining of the bronchial tubes.

The cough is likely to be very slight at

first and to be quickly relieved after the accumulated substances have been cleared from the chest or throat. In more severe cases the cough may be sustained, exhausting and painful.

3. SPUTUM. Sputum containing pus is brought up from the chest when a person has tuberculosis in a more advanced stage. Most of the sputum is likely to be brought up in the morning by clearing the throat and after some coughing. It must not be assumed, however, that a person has tuberculosis when he brings up some such discharge from the chest, since the production of sputum may be related to many other disorders and to sinus drainage.

4. BLOOD IN THE SPUTUM. The production of blood in the sputum occurs in about half of the acute cases of tuberculosis of the lungs. The amount of blood produced in the sputum is likely to be small and is due to the rupture of tiny blood vessels in the walls of tuberculous cavities in the lungs.

More extensive hemorrhages may occur in the lungs of tuberculous patients in more advanced stages of the disease. Even in these cases, however, the bleeding seldom results in death of the patient. In such instances the patient is likely to be badly frightened and to think that he is dying. Usually he will recover without the use of any special measures by the physician.

5. PAIN IN THE CHEST. Pain is not usually caused by tuberculosis of the lungs except indirectly. The lungs contain no sensory pain fibers, but severe pain may be experienced if certain complications arise from the infection, such as pleurisy or laryngitis. The pleura (the lining of the lung) is most likely to be involved if the tuberculosis infection is located in that part of the lung close to the lining.

6. LOSS OF BODY WEIGHT. In persistent, active tuberculosis of the lungs there

is likely to be sustained and gradual loss of body weight.

It must be emphasized strongly, however, that all the foregoing symptoms may be due to diseases other than tuberculosis. The modern diagnosis of this disease is not based solely on the observation of symptoms.

The Diagnosis of Tuberculosis

The diagnosis of tuberculosis is not easy. In Chicago, a city reputed to have the largest case-detection program in the world, more than one-half of the persons who died from tuberculosis in 1958 had had cases previously unknown to medical or public health authorities. During the year indicated, 203 out of 377 cases resulting in death had gone undetected.

Today tuberculosis is virtually never diagnosed solely on the basis of clinical findings. In other words, a person who has a persistent fever, cough, blood in the sputum, and loss of body weight is not judged to have tuberculosis, although obviously this disease will be suspected by the physician.

An actual diagnosis of tuberculosis is routinely made on the basis of several of five factors. These are as follows:

1. A POSITIVE TUBERCULIN TEST. With a negative tuberculin test the patient is not diagnosed as having tuberculosis, although symptoms and x-ray pictures may be highly suggestive. On the other hand, a positive tuberculin test does not indicate active tuberculosis automatically. Only 1 to 2 per cent of people who have a positive skin test for tuberculosis will have an active stage of the disease. The positive tuberculin test is more likely to indicate only that the person has taken tuberculosis germs into his body at some time during his lifetime. The chances are that he will have handled the disease

very well without ever having an active stage of the disorder. If the tuberculin test is negative, however, it must be assumed that the person does not have tuberculosis.

2. CHEST X-RAY. A specialist will be able to diagnose tuberculosis by chest x-ray in a majority of instances. Even he, however, can make mistakes for the reason that there are a number of other chest diseases in which the x-ray findings closely resemble those of tuberculosis. Histoplasmosis, blastomycosis, coccidioidomycosis and other diseases may give a chest x-ray picture that resembles that of tuberculosis.

Another reason why the chest roentgenogram alone may not be depended upon for a diagnosis of active tuberculosis is that it takes some weeks in a new case of tuberculosis before changes in the chest will be revealed by the roentgenogram. In other words, a person might have active tuberculosis in the very early stages and still have what appears to be a normal chest roentgenogram.

The chest roentgenogram, however, is one of the strongest weapons in the program to find tuberculosis. Its widespread use in mass surveys of populations has been relatively discontinued because of the concern over reduction of the amount of radiation for young people. Chest x-rays are far safer than many people realize, however. One scientist has calculated that a person could have 40,000 chest x-rays before reaching a hazardous point of radiation exposure.

3. POSITIVE SPUTUM. When sputum which has been obtained from a person suspected of having tuberculosis is properly stained and examined under the microscope, it may be possible to find tubercle bacilli. When the tuberculosis germs are found in the sputum by this means, a positive diagnosis of the disease can be made. However, it is not always possible to find these germs in the nose and throat discharges of people suffering from the

disease. This is because there is sometimes an intermittent discharge of the organisms, so that at one time the sputum may be free of the germs, but at other times may contain the tubercle bacilli. It is also possible that there might be only a few of the germs present in the sputum and that they would escape detection under the microscope.

Since very small children do not expectorate, it is not possible with them to make a diagnosis of tuberculosis by this means.

4. GASTRIC ANALYSIS. When the sputum is negative but it is strongly suspected that a person has active tuberculosis (or if the patient is a small child) a sample of the stomach contents may be obtained by means of the so-called stomach pump. After concentration of the stomach contents, by means of the centrifuge, and staining, a microscopic search for tuberculosis germs can be made. If tubercle bacilli are identified in the stomach contents, then a diagnosis of active tuberculosis can be made.

5. GUINEA PIG INOCULATION. Samples of the sputum or the stomach contents may be inoculated into a guinea pig or other experimental animal in an attempt to diagnose the disease. If, after a time, the animal remains healthy and there is no autopsy evidence of tuberculosis, then it must be concluded that the person does not have tuberculosis. On the other hand, even though the sputum may be negative and the chest roentgenogram doubtful, if the guinea pig test is positive, then a diagnosis of active tuberculosis must be reached.

Even if the x-ray films suggest active tuberculosis, if the disease cannot be confirmed by some of the above methods, then the diagnosis of tuberculosis is not made. A tentative diagnosis of "suspicious tuberculosis" may be recorded by the physician.

TUBERCULOSIS—WORLD HEALTH PROBLEM

The Tuberculin Test

Nuclear developments have brought about a revival of the importance of the tuberculin test in the discovery of tuberculosis. Because of the possibility that there might be excessive exposure to radiation from various sources, the chest x-ray is no longed used in surveys for the detection of tuberculosis on an indiscriminate scale. The chest x-ray is much safer than is generally realized, however, is still used, and is advisable for special groups in which there is a high expectancy of tuberculosis. In keeping with a general policy of reducing exposure to radiation as much as possible, public health authorities have turned once more to the tuberculin test as a screening method before x-ray examination in groups where there is a low expectancy of tuberculosis. Such a procedure not only reduces the exposure to radiation but also reduces the cost of screening programs.

The most commonly used type of tuberculin test is the Mantoux test, in which the test material is injected into the skin. If there is redness and swelling at the site of the injection within forty-eight to seventy-two hours, the test is judged to be a positive reaction. This does not mean that the person has active tuberculosis, but only that he has taken tuberculosis germs into his body at some time or another. The test is not dangerous, although it is slightly inconvenient and is sometimes disliked because it involves the use of a needle. The material injected into the skin contains no living tuberculosis organisms, so that it is not possible to get the disease from the tuberculin test.

The patch test has been used, especially with children, to escape the inconvenience and discomfort of the needle. In this test, filter paper or some other suitable material is saturated with undiluted tuberculin and dried. This substance is then applied to the skin by means of a strip of adhesive tape. A positive reaction is indicated by redness and a raised area of the skin, which attains its peak about the fourth day and persists several days longer before subsiding. The patch test is dependable, but not quite as accurate as the Mantoux test.

In England the patch test is known as the tuberculin-jelly test. The English technique is to rub the skin with very fine sandpaper after it has been cleansed with acetone, and then to apply the tuberculin jelly and cover it with adhesive tape. A study by the Medical Research Council revealed that a jelly containing 60 per cent of old tuberculin was as dependable as the Mantoux test. In general, however, the patch test has not been found to be as reliable as the Mantoux test.

A third and less commonly used tuberculin test is known as the Calmette ophthalmic test; it involves the addition of a 1 per cent tuberculin material inside the eyelid. If the conjunctiva becomes red and inflamed within twenty-four to seventy-two hours, it is judged that a positive reaction has been obtained. This test is not as widely used as the others, partly because of the fact that the eye tissues may become inflamed as a consequence.

The Heaf test has recently appeared as still another form of the tuberculin test. This is a multiple-puncture test developed by Frederick Heaf of Wales. In the Heaf test a metal device is used which operates by spring to cause six needles to be driven to a predetermined depth through a drop of tuberculin on the skin.

The skin of the forearm is first cleansed with acetone and then a drop of tuberculin preparation is placed on the skin. The metal device is then applied to the drop of tuberculin and the needles are released. The area is allowed to dry and no dressing is needed. The test is read 72 hours later, although a longer time can be taken.

The Heaf test can be used to test about 100 or more persons per hour. There is no pain associated with the slight penetration of the needles which do not need sharpening or replacement until after about 2,500 tests have been performed. The metal guns or lancets are sterilized after each use; this can be done rapidly. The Heaf tuberculin test was used by school and public health authorities in New York City with 61,000 pupils during 1958. It was found to be acceptable to both students and staff and more dependable than the patch test. The test compared favorably with the Mantoux test and was judged to be a satisfactory substitute for the latter test in mass tuberculin screening programs.

A person who has a negative tuberculin test does not have tuberculosis. On the other hand, a person who has a positive tuberculin test may or may not have active tuberculosis. In fact, in about ninety-nine cases out of 100 the person who reacts positively will not have active tuberculosis. Only about 1 per cent of the positive tuberculin tests are indicative of active tuberculosis.

The great value of the tuberculin test lies in its indication of exposure to active tuberculosis when the reaction changes from negative to positive in a person. In other words, when there is a positive tuberculin test in a person who has had previous tests that were negative, then there is clear-cut evidence that the person has been recently infected with tuberculosis. In such a case public health authorities will conduct a search to discover a source of the disease. This helps to prevent further infection of the patient as well as to protect others from possible illness.

The tuberculin test may have great value when it is used in conjunction with the roentgenogram. Occasionally a chest roentgenogram may give strong evidence of tuberculosis when the disease is not actually present. For example, fungus infections of the lungs have sometimes been mistaken for tuberculosis. Other chest diseases may also be confused with this disease. In one instance a fifteen-year-old schoolgirl was admitted to a sanatorium with x-ray evidence and diagnosis of tuberculosis. When it was discovered that the girl had a negative tuberculin test, additional studies were done that showed she was suffering from atypical pneumonia rather than tuberculosis; she was soon discharged from the hospital. If a tuberculin test had not been done on her, she might have remained for a long time for treatment of the wrong disease.

The World Health Organization has reported that the tuberculin test cannot be used in tropical regions for clearcut results in the detection of tuberculosis. In tropical lowlands it has been found that a large proportion of the tuberculin reactions are in an intermediate zone so that it is difficult to distinguish whether the results are clearly positive or clearly negative. World Health authorities have speculated that the population in tropical areas may be massively exposed to unidentified agents that produce cross reactions to tuberculin and thus confuse the picture so far as tuberculosis is concerned.

The Chest X-ray

The roentgenogram has great value in the discovery of active tuberculosis. It should not be assumed, however, that the detection of tuberculosis is the sole purpose of the chest roentgenogram. Studies show that other chest diseases outnumber tuberculosis, and important clues to their presence may be obtained by means of the chest roentgenogram. It may reveal such conditions as active tuberculosis, healed tuberculosis, pleurisy, pneumonia, heart disease, spinal deformity, cancer of the lung, other tumors of the lung, severe lung cavities, and still other conditions. Its value in the detection of disease has been well demonstrated in many communities of the United States.

Some hospitals now require a chest roentgenogram for every patient. This requirement is aimed primarily at the discovery of active tuberculosis, but is useful in finding other conditions also. Chest surveys of hospital patients have been found to be the greatest current source of the discovery of new, active cases of tuberculosis.

For proper interpretation, the chest roentgenogram must be examined by an expert, the average person would be unable to draw any conclusions from looking at it. The physician, however, and especially the tuberculosis expert, can draw significant conclusions from the x-ray films. It is not customary, however, to make a diagnosis of any specific disease directly from the x-ray film. Additional studies are required for the diagnosis of many diseases, including tuberculosis. When the chest roentgenogram is positive, then careful search is made for other signs of the disease. The sputum will be carefully analyzed for the presence of tuberculosis germs; a careful medical examination of the patient will be made. By combining the roentgenogram with a number of other diagnostic measures, it is possible to arrive at an accurate diagnosis in the majority of cases.

Tuberculosis Is Not Hereditary.

Tuberculosis is not a hereditary disease. On the other hand, it has been repeatedly shown that tuberculosis is more common in some families than others. This can be explained by the fact that members of a family are closely associated with each other. Since tuberculosis is a communicable disease, there is maximum opportunity for spread of the disorder among members of a family who live in the same house, eat at the same table, and do things together.

It is to be expected that once tuberculosis has entered a family, members of the family will be more likely to have the disease than persons in other families where there is no known case of the disorder. The results of certain studies have suggested, however, that there are families in which there is a low resistance to tuberculosis, and other communicable diseases.

Tuberculosis and Economic Status

A number of studies have given definite evidence of an association between tuberculosis and economic status. The lower the income and the greater the poverty, the higher the overcrowding within a family dwelling, and the greater the death rate from tuberculosis.

A twenty-year study in Edinburgh, Scotland, gave overwhelming evidence of the relationship between tuberculosis and overcrowding. Tuberculosis was found more frequently among families living under crowded conditions, and the death rate from this disease was higher in such groups. Another study, conducted in ninety-two large cities of the United States, showed a correlation between death from tuberculosis and low income.

One interesting study conducted in Buffalo showed, however, that deaths from tuberculosis among wives had not equalled those of their wage-earning husbands, although both lived in the same economic, social and home environments. Deaths from tuberculosis occurred among working husbands about twice as frequently as among their wives. Since it has long been known that rest is very important in both the prevention of tuberculosis and in recovery from the disease, the investigators assumed that the logical explanation of the difference between husbands and wives was that the husbands were required to do more strenuous physical activity on their jobs.

Tuberculosis Among Minority Groups

Tuberculosis in the United States is more prevalent among such minority groups as the Indians, Mexicans and Negroes.

Among American Indians tuberculosis

is a great health problem. In one ten-year study of more than 16,000 Indians on seven Montana reservations, the death rate from tuberculosis was found to range from six to ten times as high as that for the white population in the same state.

In San Francisco the infection rate for tuberculosis among the American-Chinese is several times as great as that of the white population in the same city.

Among Spanish-Americans and Negroes the same observation holds true. The infection and death rates for tuberculosis are higher than in the native white population.

Some authorities have attempted to explain this difference on the basis of hereditary differences between racial groups. Others believe that the discrepancy is due solely to differences in the social and economic environments of the minority groups.

Tuberculosis in Medical and Nursing Students

Tuberculosis has come to be recognized as an occupational hazard of student nurses and doctors. This is because it has been observed that in almost every class of medical or nursing students one or more will become infected with active tuberculosis during the course of study. This is not surprising since both the young nurse and the young doctor are exposed to a much greater extent to tuberculous patients than is the average person. In the general wards of most hospitals there are likely to be patients with active tuberculosis, which has led certain hospitals to require chest roentgenograms of all patients on admission in order to detect tuberculosis before there is exposure to others.

The medical profession has become much interested in this problem and is taking steps to prevent the spread of tuberculosis among both medical and nursing students. The hazard, however, does exist in greater proportion than in most other occupations.

Tuberculosis in Food Handlers

Periodic health examination of food handlers has fallen into disrepute because a person examined today may become ill tomorrow or the next day, and because the cost for discovering such diseases as typhoid fever is high. In New York City it was found that in a seventeen-year period of required stool examinations of food handlers it cost abouty fifty thousand dollars to discover each single typhoid fever carrier. The case is different with tuberculosis.

Because tuberculosis is a chronic disease lasting a long time and because there is particular hazard in regard to the spread of tuberculosis through food, many public health departments do require a periodic chest roentgenogram of all food handlers. The value of such chest roentgenograms is shown by the experience in Philadelphia. During a ten-month period, chest roentgenograms of 771 food handlers resulted in the discovery that slightly over 2 per cent had tuberculosis. In the first nine months after chest roentgenograms had become a requirement among Philadelphia food handlers, sixty-six active cases of tuberculosis were recommended for hospitalization from this group. Obviously, the removal of sixty-six active cases of tuberculosis would result, in time, in a substantial reduction in the spread of this disease through food.

Raw Milk as a Source of Tuberculosis

One of the important factors in the control of tuberculosis in the United States has been the consistent progress made in wiping out tuberculosis among cattle. As long as cattle infected with tuberculosis exist, the consumption of raw milk from these herds will spread this disease. Outbreaks of typhoid fever, scarlet fever, septic sore throat, food poisoning, paratyphoid fever, undulant fever, dysentery, diphtheria and other diseases have been caused by the consumption of raw milk in this country. Even though the danger from tuberculosis through milk has been declining because of the growing conquest of tuberculosis in cattle, it is still advisable to drink only pasteurized milk because of the possibility of contracting one of these other diseases.

Over a ten-year period it was shown conclusively that the vast majority of milkborne disease outbreaks are due to the drinking of raw milk. These reports show clearly that the risk of getting a disease from the drinking of raw milk is approximately fifty times as great as that from drinking pasteurized milk. Medical and public health experience has shown that proper pasteurization can and does prevent the spread of disease through milk.

In many countries where dairy herds are still infected with tuberculosis, the consumption of raw milk may be a principle reason for the high death rate from tuberculosis. Even in this country it must not be assumed that we have stamped out tuberculosis in our cattle completely. Most of the milk in the larger communities of the United States is pasteurized, but raw milk consumed in small towns is still a source of disease epidemics.

Treatment of Tuberculosis

The modern treatment of tuberculosis revolves around six main factors, as follows: (1) rest, (2) diet, (3) drugs, (4) surgery, (5) rehabilitation and (6) health education.

Despite the development of the modern miracle drugs, rest must still be considered a basis of all treatment for tuberculosis. Diet is also important, especially when there is some concomitant evidence of nutritional deficiency, such as nutritional anemia.

The development of the antibiotic drugs has greatly increased the effectiveness of medical treatment for tuberculosis. Currently, streptomycin, para-aminosalicylic acid (also known as aminosalicylic acid) and isoniazid are the three leading drugs in the treatment of tuberculosis, although other drugs have been found helpful in the disease. For the first time in the history of tuberculosis in the United States, chemotherapy gives promise of wiping out the disease.

Surgery no longer occupies so prominent a position in the treatment of tuberculosis as it did before the discovery of the antibiotic drugs. Surgery is still advisable in certain cases, however, particularly when there are various types of complications.

Rehabilitation, both occupational and physical, is an important measure in the treatment of tuberculosis. Frequently the patient who is recovering from this disease will not be able to return to the type of work in which he may have been engaged for years. If the success of treatment is to be maintained after the patient has left the sanatorium, frequently another line of work must be found. This involves both physical and occupational redirection of the patient. The learning of new skills so that the patient may follow a line of work he is physically able to do, may be as important as almost any other measure in prevention of relapses. In the modern tuberculosis sanatorium considerable attention is given to the retraining of patients whenever this appears to be advisable. Governmental agencies cooperate with the physician in placing the retrained worker in an occupational field that will not be detrimental to his health.

People who have been cured of active tuberculosis must learn to work within their capacities. The value of adequate rest and sound nutrition, as well as protection from exposure to tuberculosis, must be well understood by the patient. Frequently this involves extensive re-education of the patient in simple hygiene. Once a person has become infected with tuberculosis, it is imperative that he be removed from the source of the infection or that the latter be removed.

It has been shown that only about 3 per cent of the children who get tuberculosis will become reinfected with the disease after successful treatment if they are removed from the source of the infection. In other words, if active tuberculosis is arrested by proper medical treatment, the patient will not spontaneously have tuberculosis at a later time (in the great majority of cases) if he is not reinfected by someone who has the disease in an active stage. A spontaneous flaring up of tuberculosis is possible, however, in those who eat poorly and in those who do not obtain enough rest.

When a person gets tuberculosis early in life, removal from the source of infection, proper medical treatment, adequate rest, and a good diet are fundamental steps in prevention of a recurrence of the disease. Of these measures, rest and proper treatment and removal from others who have the disease appear to be the most important.

Drugs in the Treatment of Tuberculosis

The antibiotic treatment of tuberculosis has revolutionized the outlook on this disease. Many patients can be treated with these drugs without being hospitalized or sent to a sanatorium for months or years of bedrest and restricted activity. So spectacular have been the results of the modern treatment of tuberculosis with drugs that many health experts believe that with the passing of the older generation, in which most of the tuberculosis of today exists, antibiotics will so reduce the hazard of spread that the disease will vanish from the United States.

Three drugs have considerable value in treatment; streptomycin, para-aminosalicylic acid and isoniazid. Combinations of these drugs have greater value than any of the single medicines. Best results have

been obtained with a combination of isoniazid (a derivative of isonicotinic acid) and either of the two other drugs.

> "If the opportunity to end tuberculosis is not seized now, it may be lost indefinitely. Medications that are effective today must be applied broadly before the tubercle bacillus develops resistance to these drugs . . . otherwise . . . the disease may rise again . . ."
>
> *Office of the Surgeon General, 1960*

Streptomycin must be given by intramuscular injection, since it is not absorbed in sufficient amounts when given by mouth to have value against tuberculosis. It does not kill the tubercle bacilli in the body, but it does help in defending against the disease. Its greatest value, therefore, seems to be in its use in conjunction with other treatment. Another limiting aspect of treatment with streptomycin is that the tuberculosis germs are able to develop resistance to the drug. Bacilli which become resistant to streptomycin appear to be able to pass this quality along to their descendants; hence, it becomes more difficult with the passage of time to secure good results with streptomycin. When it is used in combination with some other drug, the results are much better.

Para-aminosalicylic acid, commonly known by the abbreviation PAS, and more lately by the shorter name of aminosalicylic acid, also has a suppressive, rather than curative, effect upon tuberculosis. This drug can be given by mouth. This drug is not more effective than streptomycin and is ordinarily used in combination with the latter to achieve best results. Para-aminosalicylic acid, in combination with streptomycin, appears to prevent the development of tubercle bacilli resistant to the latter drug in a much larger proportion of cases than when streptomycin is used alone. The drug is frequently helpful when streptomycin has failed to produce good results.

Great publicity has been given in the

newspapers and popular journals to the use of isonicotinic acid and its derivatives in the treatment of tuberculosis. The derivative isoniazid has given best results when used in combination with aminosalicylic acid (PAS) or with streptomycin as indicated in the foregoing paragraph. Although fevers disappear, appetites improve, and there is a gain in body weight as well as reduction in the number of bacilli present in the sputum, the drug does not cure all patients.

THE BEST DRUGS

"Isoniazid, streptomycin, and para-aminosalicylic acid remain the three best drugs . . . any regimen containing isoniazid is superior to others . . ."

Dr. Rea M. Schneider, 1960

Other drugs have proved useful in the treatment of tuberculosis, but have not been used extensively because of certain undesirable effects or because they have not proved to be as effective as the previous three drugs.

Surgery in Tuberculosis

Although surgery has now taken second place to the use of drugs in the treatment of tuberculosis, there are certain cases in which surgery may be very helpful.

Five surgical procedures are still used to some extent in the treatment of this disease: phrenic nerve paralysis, pneumoperitoneum, pneumothorax, thoracoplasty, and either lobectomy or total pneumonectomy. These technical terms are explained in the following paragraphs.

1. PHRENIC NERVE PARALYSIS. The crushing of the right or the left phrenic nerve results in paralysis of that side of the diaphragm, since it is by means of this nerve that the regular movement of the diaphragm is achieved. Since the diaphragm is involved in the breathing mechanism, this results in an elevation of the diaphragm by paralysis and a reduction in movement of the lung on the impaired side. The purpose of the operation is to reduce the activity of the lung, since, by resting the lung tissue, healing of tuberculous cavities occurs more rapidly.

Permanent paralysis, however, is not generally advisable in the treatment of tuberculosis. Hence the phrenic nerve treatment has been decreasing in popularity. In some cases, even though a temporary paralysis is intended, there may be a permanent impairment of the function of the diaphragm on the side on which the phrenic nerve was crushed. Temporary paralysis of the phrenic nerve is still advisable in the treatment of certain patients, but should be used in conjunction with other treatments.

2. PNEUMOPERITONEUM. This procedure causes a reduction in lung movements during respiration. In this treatment a quantity of air is introduced into the peritoneal space in such a way as to cause an elevation of the diaphragm and reduction of movement in the lung. The air pocket, however, is gradually absorbed over a period of time; hence, the air must be replaced at intervals if the lung is to be rested. The reduction in size of the air pocket can be ascertained by fluoroscopic study.

3. PNEUMOTHORAX. In this treatment, air is introduced into the pleural space on the side of the tuberculous lung. The purpose is the same as in the two preceding measures, namely, to decrease the movement of the lung during respiration. The effect is to bring about a partial collapse of the lung which is sustained for several years. There are a number of disadvantages to this type of treatment, and the trend is toward fewer and fewer measures of this type for the control of tuberculosis.

4. THORACOPLASTY. In this surgical operation several ribs are removed to bring about a collapse of the lung tissue in

order to rest the diseased area. This tends to result in a permanent collapse and is advocated only when other measures appear to be ineffective.

5. LOBECTOMY OR PNEUMONECTOMY. Lobectomy is the surgical removal of one lobe of the lung, which would obviously be the diseased portion. Pneumonectomy is the surgical removal of one entire lung. Such surgery is done only when all other methods of treatment have failed to cure the patient, or when there is good evidence that other procedures will not be satisfactory.

None of the foregoing surgical procedures for the treatment of tuberculosis actually destroys the tubercle bacilli that may be present elsewhere in the body; hence, the patient must be treated medically in the standard approved manner. Surgery, however, in selected cases may give just the margin of advantage needed by the patient to overcome his disease.

The Cost of Treating Tuberculosis

The cost of treating and curing tuberculosis increases greatly when the disease is diagnosed in its late stages. The earlier the disease is discovered, the more successful the treatment, the shorter the length of time the patient will have to stay away from his family, and the less expensive the treatment.

A study made by the National Tuberculosis Association has shown that when tuberculosis is discovered early, the patient will stay in the hospital for approximately six months. The costs of this hospitalization will vary from state to state, but the National Tuberculosis Association has found that the national average for non-federal hospital treatment for tuberculosis is $12.80 per day (1959). It cannot be expected that the patient will be completely cured after just six months in the hospital, however. Subsequent medical care takes many more months until a satisfactory cure is effected.

Costs have probably risen since this study was made.

Dr. Herman E. Hilleboe, Commissioner of Health in New York State, has estimated that more than 800 million dollars was spent during 1955 for the prevention, diagnosis and treatment of tuberculosis in the United States. In New York State alone nearly 50 million dollars was spent on tuberculosis in a single year. In 1958 Los Angeles County spent approximately 25 million dollars on its control.

The hidden costs of untreated tuberculosis in terms of social and economic penalties cannot be assessed accurately, but it is certain that they far exceed the money spent on the prevention and cure of known cases. Common sense tells us it is good to spend wisely in the search for undetected persons with active tuberculosis and to seek an early cure of those who are discovered. The spending of public funds in this direction is economical and necessary for the welfare of others.

The Recalcitrant Tuberculous Patient

A person with active tuberculosis is a menace to the community and especially to his own family. It might be assumed that such an infected person would welcome proper medical and sanatorium treatment. This is not always so, however. Some people fear the discomfort and inconvenience of confinement in a tuberculosis sanatorium more than the damage they might do to others. The public health officer has the legal authority to compel the person with active tuberculosis to seek treatment. If need be, the patient may be confined by law to a sanatorium.

Sometimes it is necessary to have a locked ward in order to handle patients with active tuberculosis who do not wish to obtain treatment. In a sense, then, the recalcitrant patient is actually imprisoned, although his term is being spent in a tuberculosis ward. The general practice is to give such people privileges when they demonstrate good behavior and willingness to continue with proper treatment.

The important point is that the community has a legal right to be protected against the person with active tuberculosis who does not want to seek proper treatment. Public health experience has indicated that forcible isolation of these patients does not develop a group of bitter, antagonistic persons. Most become cooperative in time.

Vaccination Against Tuberculosis

In the past few years much interest has developed in the prevention of tuberculosis by immunization with BCG vaccine. Although this method of control has been widely used in Europe, in conjunction with many other control measures, many public health and medical authorities in this country still consider it to be in the experimental stage. This subject is discussed more extensively in Chapter 19.

Questions

1. When a person who has active tuberculosis will not agree to proper treatment, is the community justified in compelling isolation in a sanatorium for adequate treatment?
2. Why does active tuberculosis in a family create a great economic problem for the group involved?
3. What factors give great promise that tuberculosis may be wiped out in the United States within a few generations?
4. What is the explanation of the recent dramatic decline in the death rate from tuberculosis in the United States?
5. What problems are faced by the person who has been successfuly treated for tuberculosis, so that the disease is in an arrested state?

For Further Reading

1. Cummins, S. Lyle: *Tuberculosis in History.* Baltimore, Williams and Wilkins Company, 1949.
2. Dubos, Rene, and Dubos, Jean: *The White Plague.* Boston, Little, Brown and Company, 1952.
3. Ferguson, R. G.: *Studies in Tuberculosis.* Toronto, University of Toronto Press, 1955.
4. Myers, J. Arthur: *Tuberculosis and Other Communicable Diseases.* Springfield, Ill. Charles C Thomas, 1959.
5. World Health Organization: *Tuberculosis.* New York, Columbia University Press, 1955.

21

FIVE VENEREAL DISEASES

FIVE VENEREAL diseases constitute the backbone of the problem of veneral disease in the United States. These five diseases are gonorrhea, syphilis, granuloma inguinale, lymphogranuloma venereum, and chancroid. Of these five diseases, syphilis and gonorrhea are by far the more important ones.

The discovery of the antibiotic drugs has made possible great progress in the field of venereal disease control. In 1948, for example, 338,141 cases of syphilis were reported in the United States. By 1959 only 119,981 cases were reported to the United States Public Health Service. Despite this great progress in recent years, by 1960 both syphilis and gonorrhea were on the rise again; the antibiotics had not eliminated them. Public health and medical authorities cannot wipe out venereal disease without the fullest cooperation of the general public.

> "One thing we all know to our sorrow; the gono-coccus and the spirochete are not inclined to take penicillin and die . . ."
>
> *T. Lefoy Richman, 1960*

The American Social Health Association has recently emphasized that the problem of venereal disease is still a serious one. More states and cities reported increases in early infectious syphilis in 1959 than for any previous year since 1953. It is estimated that not even one-sixth of the early infectious syphilis cases or one-quarter of the gonorrhea cases are being found and treated each year. In other words, there is a great reservoir of venereal disease that is serving to keep this problem alive.

Only by the most concerted effort can we keep this disease under control. Of special significance is the fact that venereal disease continues to increase in the teen-age population. Over one-half of those who receive treatment in public clinics are teen-agers and young adults.

Since there are no known methods of building up immunity to the venereal diseases, the problem has been approached primarily by three measures: (1) treatment based on finding an infectious case and following it until a cure has been achieved, (2) legal measures such as the requirement of premarital and prenatal blood tests and (3) education of the public regarding venereal diseases.

What Kind of Person Gets VD?

A study in 1960 by members of the Maryland State Department of Health gives an indication of the types of people who get venereal disease. In this study a 29-year-old man was diagnosed as having primary syphilis. An investigation of his sexual contacts during the previous few months led to the blood-testing of more than 300 persons suspected of being involved in a chain of infection. Out of this group, 44 previously unknown cases of syphilis were found. All of the patients in the outbreak were Negroes. Most of them were from the lower socio-economic level and very few had steady employment or had attended school regularly. The group had come from broken homes and had experienced crowded living conditions. Many had recent police records and social maladjustments were common. The majority were young; of the 44 infected persons, approximately 57 per cent were under the age of 20. Sexual exposure by prostitution, homosexuality, and incest accounted for some of the infections. All of the persons involved were highly promiscuous. Most of the 44 cases of syphilis were found in a stable, progressive community with good medical and public health facilities.

> ". . . There are indications that only one out of four venereal disease cases is brought to diagnosis."
>
> *Conrad Van Hyning, 1960*

During World War II, efforts were made by army medical authorities to find out what kind of person is likely to get venereal disease. For example, personal interviews were conducted with a group of 200 men infected with venereal disease who were in Army hospitals in Italy. The characteristics of this group of 200 men infected with disease were compared with a similar group of men who did not have venereal disorders. In addition, the records of about 4000 army patients were studied for further information on this question.

From this study the following conclusions were drawn:

1. Soldiers with relatively little education were more likely to contract venereal disease than were those who had finished high school or gone to college.

2. Men with repeated arrests in civilian life and records of punishment while in the army were more likely to get venereal disease than those with better records.

Rank	Kind of Group	Number Examined	Positive Number	Positive Percentage
1.	Jail inmates	12,001	2,370	19.75
2.	Domestic servants	37,185	4,350	11.70
3.	Relief groups (on charity)	22,937	2,101	9.16
4.	Barbers and beauticians	5,066	291	5.74
5.	Hospital patients	299,345	16,715	5.58
6.	Industrial employees	183,718	9,974	5.43
7.	Midwives	475	25	5.26
8.	Foodhandlers	37,647	1,862	4.95
9.	Miscellaneous voluntary exams	93,479	3,718	3.98
10.	Private patients	155,497	4,751	3.06
11.	Enlisted men	7,336	126	1.72
12.	Blood donors	4,686	80	1.71
13.	Expectant mothers	282,667	4,791	1.69
14.	Applicants for marriage licenses	741,088	10,168	1.37
15.	Life-insurance applicants	4,287	43	1.00
16.	Students	10,185	38	0.37
	Total	1,897,599	61,403	3.24

3. Single men were more likely to get these diseases than married men.

4. Heavy drinkers of alcohol were more likely to get venereal disease. Among the white patients studied, 9 per cent of the venereal disease group were heavy drinkers, whereas only 2 per cent of those who did not have venereal disease were heavy drinkers. The discrepancy was even greater among the Negro patients. In that group, 23 per cent of those with venereal diseases were heavy drinkers, whereas only 6 per cent of the nonvenereal group were heavy drinkers.

5. Men who visited professional prostitutes while in civilian life, and engaged in sexual intercourse outside of marriage, were more likely to get venereal disease than those who did not engage in these activities.

6. No significant differences in the type of religious affiliation was found between patients with venereal disease and those without this disorder.

A few years ago the American Social Health Association analyzed nearly two million blood test results and found that approximately 3 per cent of the total were infected with syphilis. The highest rates of infection with syphilis were found among jail inmates, domestic servants and people on relief. The lowest infection rates were found among students (who had the best record of all), life-insurance applicants, applicants for marriage licenses and expectant mothers.

College students have been found consistently to have the lowest infection rate of any of the groups studied so far as syphilis is concerned. The accompanying table gives more complete information on the prevalence of syphilis in various groups as revealed by the American Social Health Association study.

People in jails have been found consistently to have higher rates of venereal disease infection. In the San Francisco County Jail, a study of nearly 4000 prisoners over a period of two years showed that slightly more than 10 per cent had positive blood tests for syphilis. An additional 11 per cent gave a previous history of syphilis, and 21 per cent had a previous history of infection with gonorrhea. Blood tests on 10,000 prisoners at San Quentin revealed that slightly more than 9 per cent were infected with syphilis.

A study of 500 venereally infected females treated at the Midwestern Medical Center in St. Louis, Missouri, showed that the majority had attended school only until the fourth to ninth grades. The intelligence of the group was also well below normal. The median intelligence quotient for 340 white cases was 84, whereas the median intelligence for 160 Negro girls was just below 70.

The mistaken idea that some people have had that the college student is more frivolous than the person who does not go to college is not borne out by records of venereal disease. In fact, quite the contrary appears to be the case. College students stand out clearly the least infected of all groups so far as venereal disease is concerned.

Recent Public Health studies have revealed a high rate of infection with syphilis among homosexuals. Studies made in two major cities of the United States suggest that in some communities homosexual relationships among males have assumed an important role in the spread of syphilis. In one large community during the year 1959 a total of 196 cases of syphilis was diagnosed in the venereal disease clinics. Of this number, 170 were males. Among these men, 89 were homosexuals who had acquired syphilis exclusively through male contacts.

It appears that this problem segment of a community may be even more injurious to the remainder of the population than has been suspected. In the study indicated, the 89 men named 551 contacts out of whom 93 previously undiagnosed cases of syphilis were found by Public Health investigation.

The kind of person, then, who is most likely to get venereal disease appears to be the one who has had a limited education, is somewhat below normal in intelligence, has a record of criminal offenses, is a heavy drinker of alcohol and is sexually promiscuous or perverted.

It must not be assumed, however, that only this kind of person will get venereal disease. The army experience has suggested that 60 per cent of the young men in military service will or will not be exposed to venereal disease, depending upon whether or not there is wholesome recreation available and whether or not the vice conditions in nearby communities are well controlled. In the last analysis, the final decision must rest with the individual. When morals are high and character is well developed, there will be little inclination to be exposed to venereal disease.

Sources of VD

Almost all venereal disease comes from sexual relations with infected persons. Some venereal disease does come from other sources, however. Babies may be born with congenital syphilis if the mother has the disease and does not receive medical treatment during the prenatal period. Venereal disease is also spread accidentally in some cases, especially among doctors and nurses who may be treating persons with venereal disease. The percentage of cases spread in this manner is very small.

The transmission of gonorrhea from an infected mother to her child at time of birth used to be a fairly common event, and many babies were blinded for life because of disease acquired in this manner. For many years, however, it has been a legal requirement that the eyes of newborn babies shall be treated with a silver nitrate solution of proper dilution or with other satisfactory drugs. Since the inception of this medical practice, the number of babies born with gonorrhea has been greatly reduced.

Under exceedingly poor sanitary conditions and general lack of cleanliness, it is also possible for some of the venereal diseases to be spread in an asexual manner. The number of cases spread in this manner, however, must be exceedingly small.

If we exclude the babies born with venereal disease because of infection of the mother, it can probably be said that more than 99 per cent of all other cases of venereal disease are spread by sexual contact.

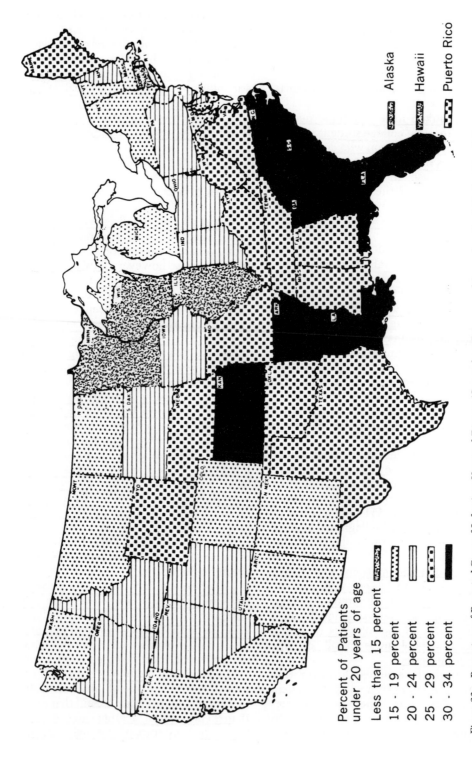

Percent of Patients
under 20 years of age

Less than 15 percent

15 - 19 percent

20 - 24 percent

25 - 29 percent

30 - 34 percent

Alaska

Hawaii

Puerto Rico

Figure 32. Percentage of Reported Cases of Infectious Venereal Disease (Gonorrhea, Primary and Secondary Syphilis Combined) Occurring Among Persons Under 20 Years of Age by State. Calendar Year 1958. (Committee on the Joint Statement: Today's VD Control Problem, 1960.)

Numerous studies have been made of the sources of venereal disease. Specific sources vary with the community. In the state of Washington a study of army and navy records showed that 52 per cent of the venereal disease acquired by men in military service in that area came from pick-ups; 24 per cent came from prostitutes encountered in the streets, hotels and brothels; 15 per cent came from "friends"; and 10 per cent came from wives. In this study, pick-ups and prostitutes accounted for about 75 per cent of the infections.

A wartime study in Cincinnati showed that about 80 per cent of the military forces infected with venereal disease acquired the disorder from "pick-up girls" or "friends." Medical examinations of these girls, many of whom were from fifteen to eighteen years of age, showed that more than 60 per cent had syphilis or gonorrhea, or both.

In another army study during World War II 68 per cent of the cases of venereal disease were acquired from so-called "pick-ups" and "friends" to whom the soldiers had paid no fee.

In a study of about 24,000 troops, on the other hand, 74 per cent of the total venereal disease infections were coming from houses of prostitution. When access to these houses of prostitution was made more difficult for the troops, the venereal disease rate dropped from eighty-three per 1000 men to fifty-four in one month and to thirty-one in two months.

Age Relationships

Venereal disease is essentially a problem of the young age group. Studies have shown repeatedly that the problem of venereal disease begins at a much earlier age than many people realize.

A study of 1077 girls treated for venereal disease in Florida showed that 427 were in the age group from fifteen to nineteen and that 377 were between the ages

of twenty and twenty-four, inclusive. Thus, nearly eight-tenths were between the ages of fifteen and twenty-four, inclusive. In this study it was also revealed that approximately 29 per cent of the infected girls had had sexual experiences before the age of sixteen.

In another study 2462 out of 16,642 cases of syphilis occurred in the age group from ten to nineteen, inclusive. Approximately three times as many cases occurred in the age group between twenty and twenty-nine, inclusive.

Since syphilis and other venereal diseases can be found even in the newborn child, it should be apparent no age group is immune to venereal disease.

Blood Tests

In the public mind, blood tests have become synonymous with the discovery of venereal disease. Blood tests do not exist, however, for all the venereal diseases. There is none for gonorrhea, chancroid or granuloma inguinale. Blood tests are of value in the diagnosis of lymphogranuloma venereum and syphilis and is the outstanding method for discovering syphilis.

The laboratory details of blood testing for syphilis are too technical to be described in a book of this sort. Although many people have heard of the Wassermann test, there are a number of other blood tests for this disease. The Kline, Kahn and Kolmer tests are probably the most widely known of the other blood tests for syphilis. The search for a faster, simpler and less expensive blood test goes on in the research laboratories constantly. The FPM (filter-paper microscopic test) and the Chediak blood test are examples of other techniques. These newer tests, however, have not achieved the degree of reliability obtained by the Wassermann, Kahn, Kline and Kolmer tests.

The RPR (rapid plasma reagent) test is one of the newer ones for the discovery of

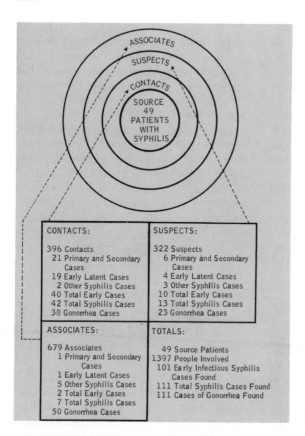

CONTACTS:

396 Contacts
  21 Primary and Secondary
      Cases
  19 Early Latent Cases
  2 Other Syphilis Cases
  40 Total Early Cases
  42 Total Syphilis Cases
  38 Gonorrhea Cases

SUSPECTS:

322 Suspects
  6 Primary and Secondary
      Cases
  4 Early Latent Cases
  3 Other Syphilis Cases
  10 Total Early Cases
  13 Total Syphilis Cases
  23 Gonorrhea Cases

ASSOCIATES:

679 Associates
  1 Primary and Secondary
      Cases
  1 Early Latent Cases
  5 Other Syphilis Cases
  2 Total Early Cases
  7 Total Syphilis Cases
  50 Gonorrhea Cases

TOTALS:

  49 Source Patients
1397 People Involved
  101 Early Infectious Syphilis
      Cases Found
  111 Total Syphilis Cases Found
  111 Cases of Gonorrhea Found

Figure 33. Cluster testing. (Committee on the Joint Statement: Today's VD Control Problem, 1960.)

syphilis that permits rapid and economical screening of large numbers of persons. For example, it has been used in El Centro, California, to screen large numbers of Mexican farm laborers who would be in the United States on a temporary basis. The success of the El Centro plan led to the establishment of other screening centers with the use of the RPR test on the border between Mexico and the United States. In this test three drops of serum or three drops of blood plasma are used with one drop of the antigen testing suspension. The reaction between these two substances indicates whether the person should be further tested or treated for syphilis.

The dependability of the blood test for syphilis depends upon when the test is given and which test is used. When a person first contracts syphilis, his blood test does not become positive immediately. Only after about eight or nine weeks will the test become dependable as a means of diagnosing syphilis. During the early stages of this disease, then, the blood tests are not reliable. In the early stages of syphilis the disease is diagnosed by the so-called darkfield microscopic examination. In this examination the syphilis organisms can be seen and identified.

Sometimes a blood test for syphilis can give a falsely positive result. By this it is meant that a person who does not have syphilis may be diagnosed as having it because of the positive blood test. This can happen when the person has any one of a number of other diseases, such as malaria or leprosy.

People who have been recently vaccinated against smallpox may exhibit a falsely positive blood test for syphilis. In one group of 133 volunteers who had been vaccinated for smallpox and were then examined for syphilis by means of blood tests within an eight-week period after vaccination, approximately 9 per cent showed some degree of misleading results as far as the blood tests were concerned. However, when four blood tests were done on these recently vaccinated people, only one showed a positive reaction on all four tests. Even in this one case the person did not have syphilis. The influence of vaccination on blood tests for syphilis is short-lived. Within a few weeks a repeat blood test will usually give the clear picture.

A diagnosis of syphilis is seldom made on the basis of one positive blood test. It is standard public health procedure to confirm one positive blood test by others. When blood tests are done at the proper time, that is, after changes in the blood have taken place and when the tests are properly done and confirmed by additional tests, then they are highly reliable. Under such circumstances the blood tests can be considered at least 98 per cent dependable. In other words, a positive blood test for syphilis is a reasonable indication that the person does have this disease.

The blood test for lymphogranuloma venereum is a distinct aid in the diagnosis of that disease. This is especially true when the blood test confirms medical observations. The test, however, is not as dependable as the one for syphilis.

Cluster Testing

One of the newer developments in public health procedures for the discovery of syphilis is known as cluster testing. This method of finding new cases operates on the principle that people who have already been found to have syphilis will know others whose habits of promiscuity may expose them to venereal disease, even though there has been no association between the persons involved. Under this plan patients with syphilis are asked to name others who, while not sex contacts, are thought by the patient to be having sexual experiences that parallel his own.

This method has revealed a larger number of cases of early infectious syphilis than other standard techniques and has now been adopted by 31 states and 51 cities, although in some communities and states physicians have not favored the cluster testing procedure; it is felt that it disturbs the delicate relationship between the private practice of medicine and the field of public health.

The effectiveness of the cluster testing technique is shown in an accompanying chart in which 49 patients with syphilis involved 1,397 other persons in whom 111 cases of syphilis and 111 cases of gonorrhea were found.

Syphilis

Syphilis is a disease which may exist in three different stages. All stages are caused by the same microscopic organism, the *Treponema pallidum.*

In the first stage of syphilis, which begins with a small sore at the spot where the syphilis organisms penetrate the skin or mucous membranes, there is soon a widespread dissemination of the organism throughout the body. During this first stage the germs are primarily in the body fluids.

In the second stage, the skin, mucous membranes and certain other parts of the body may give evidence of the disease.

In the third stage the germs are apt to be collected in circumscribed areas such as the brain or nervous system and blood vessels.

In a great many cases of syphilis no symptoms whatsoever may be apparent. A person who has been exposed to the disease is, therefore, not justified in assuming that no disease is present, since it may be well hidden. In medicine, syphilis has been

HOW SYPHILIS SPREADS

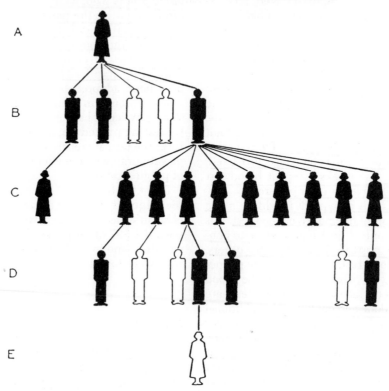

Figure 34.   A physician in a middle Western city asked the State Health Department to trace the source of infection in three cases of newly acquired infectious syphilis in his practice, all men (B). (Black figures represent persons examined and found infected; outline figures represent contacts examined, but not found infected.) The infection of all three was traced back to one woman, a prostitute (A). Then the inquiry turned to persons whom these men might have infected. It was discovered that one man had infected one girl, and another man nine girls, of whom six were under 18 years of age (C). Of these, four girls in turn infected four other men (D). In all, twenty-four persons were examined, and eighteen were found infected and placed under treatment. (Data furnished by the Minnesota Department of Health, Chart by the American Social Hygiene Association.)

known in previous years as the "great masquerader," because of the ability of *Treponema pallidum* to invade any tissue of the body and to produce symptoms characteristic of other diseases.

It used to be that infections less than four years old were classified as early cases. The old treatment with arsenic and bismuth gave best results when syphilis was in this early stage. Nowadays, an early case is one which has been diagnosed in days, weeks or months rather than years.

The discovery of the antibiotics has revolutionized the treatment of syphilis. The disease can now be cured in a remarkably short time. Whereas formerly the patient might be subjected to weekly injections of arsenic and bismuth preparations for a year or two, he or she can now be cured in a matter of weeks in the majority of cases.

Gonorrhea

Gonorrhea is an inflammatory disease of the mucous membranes of the sex organs or other tissues that may become involved, caused by the microscopic organism known as the gonococcus, or *Neisseria gonorrhoeae*. The symptoms of the disease depend largely upon the location of the inflammatory reactions. In the earliest stages the pelvic region of the body is the part most likely to be involved. The disease is spread by pus discharges from the infected sex organ of either sex.

Usually the disease starts from three to seven days after exposure. In some instances evidence of infection may arise as early as two days after, but seldom later than fourteen days after infection.

There is no immunity to the disease. When one infection is cured either spontaneously or by medical treatment, this does not mean that the person is protected against further infection.

When gonorrhea remains untreated, there is the danger of severe complications. The germs may settle on the heart valves and produce serious heart disease. The organisms may attack the joints of the body, with severe arthritis as a result. The eye tissues may become infected with serious impairment of vision. None of these complications is likely if treatment is sought.

The diagnosis of gonorrhea is sometimes difficult and time consuming, especially in the female. Studies by the Public Health Service have shown that even a combination of diagnostic approaches involving clinical information, smears and cultures from the suspected area and all other information allows, at best, a diagnostic accuracy of only 50 to 75 per cent for females with gonorrhea. Recently, however, fluorescent antibody methods have given more favorable results. In this technique, fluorescein-labeled antiserums are used for the detection of gonococcus. It has been found that the fluorescent antibody identification saves from three to nine days over conventional culture procedures.

Sulfa drugs and the antibiotics are especially effective in the treatment of gonorrhea. If penicillin treatment is started soon enough, cures may be achieved within several days.

Two complications have arisen in recent years regarding the control of gonorrhea. Some gonococci apparently are becoming relatively resistant to penicillin. It is possible that penicillin will lose some of its effectiveness against this disease as a consequence of the gradual evolution of a more resistant gonococcus organism. A second problem has arisen because of the increasing number of patients who are sensitive to penicillin. These people cannot be treated safely with this antibiotic.

Research is currently being conducted to find an effective substitute for penicillin in the treatment of gonorrhea. Great promise was reported in 1960 for synnematin B and oxytetracycline. Erythromycin propionate and erythromycin stearate have also been found to be useful, although not as effective as penicillin.

Granuloma Inguinale

Granuloma inguinale, a disease of the poor, the unclean and the promiscuous, has been described as one of the most loathsome of diseases. It begins as a swelling in the region of the sexual organs and then develops into sores and ulcers that spread slowly, covering the skin of the lower abdomen, the groin, the sex organs and even the buttocks. A strong, foul odor is associated with the disease. It is caused by a microscopic organism known as the Donovan body. Diagnosis of the disease is made when microscopic identification of the Donovan bodies is made from scrapings of the ulcerations.

It has been estimated that from 2000 to 10,000 cases of this disease have existed annually in the United States during past years. Fortunately, the discovery of streptomycin, Aureomycin and other antibiotics has given the medical world effective weapons against this disorder.

Injections of streptomycin daily for five to fifteen days have been effective in bringing about a cure of the disorder in most cases. Other antibiotics such as Aureomycin and Terramycin are also effective, but larger doses are needed for a longer time to bring about a cure. This disease has been especially prevalent among Negroes in the southern part of the United States.

Lymphogranuloma Venereum

Lymphogranuloma venereum is a venereal disease caused by a virus. It usually starts with an ulcer, but is not often recognized until swelling of the glands occurs in the regions of the body approximating the sexual organs. The virus spreads mostly through the lymphatic vessels and glands. Stiffness and aching is also apparent about the time that the swelling of the glands may be noticed. The swelling usually subsides after about three months, but drainage may go on for a longer time. The disease is more common among Negroes and is thought to be fairly prevalent in tropical regions.

Various complications may result when this disease is not properly treated. One attack of the disease does not give immunity.

The disease can be diagnosed by medical observation, blood tests, and confirmation by the Frei test. This is a skin test somewhat comparable to the tuberculin test. Although most cases occur from sexual intercourse, accidental infections can take place.

Chancroid

Chancroid, or soft chancre, is a disease which is primarily venereal in origin, but which does occur on contact with the bacillus which causes the disease. The disease may occur particularly among children, physicians or nurses through accidental inoculation. There is no immunity to the disease, and frequent attacks of the disorder may be experienced by any one person.

The disease is characterized by the formation of an ulcer, frequently with inflammation and swelling. It is the least important of the five venereal diseases described in this chapter and often responds to soap and water alone, according to some physicians.

The organism causing chancroid is known as *Hemophilus ducreyi*, or the Ducrey bacillus. When this organism is identified from smears or fluid obtained from the suspected sore, then a diagnosis of the disease is certain. The sulfa drugs are effective in achieving a cure. Treatment lasting for seven days with these drugs is usually sufficient to bring about a rapid cure. Some antibiotics are also curative.

Finding Venereal Disease

A great problem in the field of public health is that of finding the person with venereal disease, which is necessary in order to control the disease by medical treatment. A study by the Norfolk City Venereal Disease Clinic, covering more than 4000 cases of venereal disease, showed that there were ten main ways in which infected persons were found and brought under treatment. The ten case-finding methods, ranked in order of greatest to least efficiency, were:

1. SELECTIVE SERVICE EXAMINATIONS. Routine blood testing done on all males called up for military service was found to be the most effective way of discovering venereal disease in males. Obviously, this method would not be so productive of good results in the detection of venereal disease infections among women because

CASES OF SYPHILIS AND GONORRHEA AND RATES PER 100,000 POPULATION
REPORTED BY STATE HEALTH DEPARTMENTS
FISCAL YEAR 1948-1951[1]

Fiscal Year	Total Syphilis[2]		Primary and Secondary Syphilis		Early Latent Syphilis		Late and Late Latent Syphilis		Gonorrhea	
	Cases	Rate	Cases	Rate	Cases	Rate	Cases	Rate	Cases	Rate
1948	338,141	234.7	80,528	55.9	97,745	67.9	123,972	86.1	363,014	252.0
1949	288,736	197.3	54,248	37.1	84,331	57.6	121,931	83.3	331,661	226.7
1950	229,723	154.2	32,148	21.6	64,786	43.5	112,424	75.5	303,922	204.0
1951	198,640	131.8	18,211	12.1	52,309	34.7	107,133	71.1	270,459	179.5
1952	168,734	110.8	11,991	7.9	38,365	25.2	101,920	66.9	245,633	161.3
1953	156,099	100.8	9,551	6.2	32,287	20.8	100,195	64.7	243,857	157.4
1954	137,876	87.5	7,688	4.9	24,999	15.9	93,601	59.4	239,661	152.0
1955	122,075	76.0	6,516	4.1	21,553	13.4	84,741	52.7	239,787	149.2
1956	126,219	77.1	6,757	4.1	20,014	12.2	89,851	54.8	233,333	142.4
1957	130,552	78.3	6,251	3.8	19,046	11.4	96,856	58.1	216,476	129.8
1958	116,630	68.5	6,661	3.9	16,698	9.8	85,974	50.5	220,191	129.3
1959	119,981	69.3	8,178	4.7	17,592	10.2	86,776	50.1	237,318	137.0

[1]These data do not include migrant labor from other countries.
[2]Includes "Stages of Syphilis Not Stated."
From: Committee on the Joint Statement: Today's VD Control Problem. New York, American Social Health Association, 1960.

of the smaller number going into military service.

2. VOLUNTARY BLOOD TESTING. A good many persons will come in for voluntary medical examinations if they suspect possible exposure to venereal disease. This number is likely to increase greatly upon publicity and educational programs directed at uncovering hidden venereal disease cases.

3. EXAMINATIONS OF JAIL INMATES. As expressed elsewhere in this chapter, there is a higher rate of infection for syphilis and other venereal diseases among persons who are imprisoned for various crimes. It is a wise public health measure to have compulsory blood tests on all persons sent to jail. This is of value, not only to society, but also to the prisoner, who can then receive proper medical treatment during the period of confinement.

4. REFERRAL FROM OTHER CLINICS. In many people venereal disease is dis-covered accidentally when the person seeks medical care for some other condition. In such a case medical authorities often refer the infected person to the proper public health authorities in order to cure the disease.

5. CONTACT TRACING. Whenever a person is found with a venereal disease, it means that he has acquired that disease from someone else and that he may very likely have passed the disease on to others. Whether the infected person be male or female, the principle of contact infection and exposure still applies. It has long been standard public health practice to secure, if possible, the names of persons exposed to a person with venereal disease, or to obtain the name of the person from whom it is thought the disease was secured. When patients with venereal disease cooperate with medical and public health authorities, this method is valuable for finding others who have venereal disease and helping them secure proper medical treatment.

6. EXAMINATIONS OF FOOD HANDLERS. Whenever medical examinations are required of special working groups, some venereal disease will be discovered incidental to the broader examination. In Norfolk, examinations of food handlers were helpful in the discovery of syphilis and other disorders. Many communities, however, no longer require periodic health examinations of food handlers, but place stress on health education of the food handler. This method has been more effective in reducing the spread of disease through food.

7. READMISSIONS. Many persons with venereal disease may be reinfected after they have been cured of one infection. Sometimes patients stop medical treatment before a cure has been achieved because symptoms may have disappeared temporarily. In either case these persons may return for medical treatment. Readmissions thus become one of the standard methods of discovery of cases of venereal disease.

8. EXAMINATION OF INFECTED PERSONS. In Florida approximately 29 per cent of a large group of infected girls had more than one venereal disease. It thus becomes apparent that a search for more than one venereal disease should be made in any person found to be infected with syphilis. Such a search in the Norfolk experience turned up a number of additional diseases.

9. REFERRAL FROM PRIVATE PHYSICIANS. Many people who think they have venereal disease will go to their own physicians for treatment. Also, family physicians may discover venereal disease in a patient who comes in for other treatment. In either case the physician is required by law to report at least the number of such cases found, even though the name of the patient is not given. Many physicians will ask such patients whether they wish to obtain treatment by public health authorities in order to reduce the cost. Many patients may then desire to transfer to a venereal disease clinic for treatment.

10. PREMARITAL EXAMINATIONS. A number of states now have legal requirements of blood testing for syphilis before a marriage license can be issued or the marriage ceremony performed.

Mass Blood Testing

Mass blood testing of an entire population should be the most effective means of discovering new cases of syphilis. Since blood tests do not exist for all venereal diseases, this method would not bring to light all cases of these disorders. No state has yet made it mandatory that all persons in the population be examined for venereal disease. The closest approach to this has been the Alabama blood testing law for syphilis, which covers, however, only the age groups between fourteen and fifty years.

A pattern has been established for finding various types of illnesses in the population through mass roentgenograms for the discovery of tuberculosis. The enlargement of this approach into a multiphasic screening effort which can include a blood test for syphilis is a step in the right direction. These surveys are on a voluntary basis. Nevertheless, many cases of illness, including venereal disease, have been discovered by this mass approach.

The laws of many states now require a blood test for syphilis during the period of pregnancy. This prenatal regulation has resulted in the discovery of a fairly large number of cases of syphilis, many of which were unknown to the mother. Since the baby will be born free of syphilis if the mother receives treatment during the period of pregnancy, it is important to discover these cases. Widespread experience with the prenatal blood testing law shows that about 1 per cent of the women examined will have syphilis. It can be expected that this number will be reduced in the near future.

That education can be an effective means of discovering venereal disease has been shown in a number of instances. Efforts along these lines may consist in publicity campaigns and the transmission of knowledge about venereal disease in a short concentrated effort, or the educational approach may be extended over a longer time.

In the Mississippi delta plantation area, for example, an intensive educational and informational campaign which involved the use of films, pamphlets, lectures, radio broadcasts and newspapers, as well as mobile units of venereal disease teams, resulted in the discovery of 2073 cases of venereal disease at a cost of approximately twenty thousand dollars. The project was judged to be worth while by public health authorities because of its prolonged educational effect upon the people of the community.

The evidence of recent years seems to indicate that the venereal disease patient is much more willing to cooperate with medical and public health authorities than had been realized. The more widespread the education of the public, the greater the cooperation of all concerned in this problem.

A number of states have passed various laws intended to bring venereal disease under control. One of the outstanding examples of a legal approach to this problem is the Alabama blood testing program. This state law requires all persons between the ages of fourteen and fifty years to submit to a blood test for syphilis. Of the first 1,500,000 persons who complied with the law, 6.5 per cent were infected with syphilis. The number of cases of syphilis discovered and treated as a result of the first survey was sufficient to bring about a reduction of 50 per cent in this form of venereal disease.

Various cities now have laws that call for a medical examination to determine whether people who are picked up for vagrancy, prostitution or sex crimes are infected with venereal disease. These people may be held in jail until the examination for venereal disease has been completed.

The highest courts have upheld the legality of this procedure.

In general, the adoption of laws for the protection of the public health is considered to be a valid exercise of the police power of the state. Laws aimed at protecting the general population from venereal disease have received universal legal approval by the courts.

In Baltimore Dr. Nels A. Nelson and Virginia R. Struve, R.N., reported in 1956 on a study of 1220 children who were born to 423 *mothers who had syphilis.*

Every one of these pregnant women who received at least one full medical treatment for syphilis gave birth to a child who was free of the disease. Those mothers who were inadequately treated, for one reason or another, gave birth to babies with syphilis in nearly 6 per cent of the cases; whereas, among the mothers who received no treatment at all, approximately 13 per cent of the babies were born with syphilis. It was found in this study that if a woman received treatment for her infection she would give birth to a healthy baby *even if her blood test remained positive for syphilis.*

Other states have passed laws requiring blood tests for syphilis before issuance of a marriage license or performance of a marriage ceremony. These laws have been supported by the courts and have resulted in the discovery of many cases of venereal disease.

Emphasis on Character

Medical and public health leaders have been preoccupied with the discovery and treatment of venereal disease. In the minds of many of these health authorities, case-finding and medical treatment constitute the surest and most effective way to stamp out venereal disease. When the population is considered as a whole, this is undoubtedly the case. However, the value of character and moral precepts has been somewhat overlooked, especially in respect to individual control of promiscuity and venereal disease.

One of the strongest deterrents to exposure to venereal disease is the possession of an ideal that governs both present and future relationships with the opposite sex. A sense of moral responsibility and self-discipline coupled with a desire to enter into marriage on a clean and wholesome basis can be a powerful factor in the prevention of venereal disease. The decision rests with you.

Questions

1. What would be the difficulties encountered if an attempt were made by medical and public health authorities to wipe out syphilis in this country by simultaneous mass treatment with penicillin of all persons for several days?

2. Should more states follow the lead of Alabama in making blood tests of all adults a compulsory feature of the attempt to control syphilis?

3. What religious and moral objections, if any, can there be to curing a person who has a venereal disease?

4. What relationship, if any, might there be between crime and venereal disease in a community in which the latter was widespread?

5. Should persons with venereal disease who refuse treatment be confined in jail until cured of their disorder?

For Further Reading

Bowen, Carroll T.: *Handbook on V.D.* Coral Gables, Florida, University of Miami Press, 1952.

Recommended Film

1. Center for Mass Communication. *The Invader.* 16 mm., black and white, showing time 37 minutes, 1955. Rental or purchase from Center for Mass Communication, 1125 Amsterdam Ave., New York 25. A documentary film on syphilis.

2. Kansas State Board of Health and the U.S. Public Health Service: *The Innocent Party.* 16 mm., sound and color, 17 minutes, 1960. Kansas City, Calvin Productions, Inc., 1105 Truman Road; on loan from State Health Departments.

22

MALARIA

MALARIA is the greatest health problem the world has ever known. The study of malaria is therefore a learning experience in world affairs. To discover that this disease has been wiped out in the United States to the extent that it no longer constitutes a serious health problem is worth knowing, because we have shown thereby that malaria can be conquered. This disease is still the world's number one health problem (according to the World Health Organization), and there is always the potential threat that it may return to this country in full force unless our control measures are rigidly sustained.

On an international scale it had been estimated that malaria was killing *ten million people each year.* The widespread use of DDT in the control of mosquitoes caused this disease to change position with tuberculosis as the world's number two

THE MOSQUITO LEGEND

A Tale of South Viet-Nam

Once upon a time there was a happy young couple. They loved one another dearly. But Fate was envious of their bliss: one day, Death came and took the young wife away.

Overwhelmed with grief, the husband would not think of burying her. But the work of Death is the same for everyone, and her body began to return to dust. The sight was too much for the villagers and, rather than part from his wife, the young man chose to go away. He became a pariah rejected by everybody and went to live on the river, leaving his sampan only to fetch food from the nearest village.

Finally, because of his stubborn will to keep the object of his love, the Genii took pity on him. One of them appeared to him as he was drifting on the river in deep grief and despair. "It is my power to help you," the Genie said, "but you should know that it is not always wise to change one's destiny. You should learn to accept your fate. However, if you really want it, I shall make your wife live again . . . I hope you will not live to regret it."

The husband said that this was his fondest hope. He would never regret. Let it be done as you wish . . . the Genie said. He pricked the man's finger letting out a drop of blood which fell on the dead body of the girl. And lo, she was alive again, as beautiful and as fresh as ever.

The young couple decided to continue living on the river. But one night, coming back from the village where he had gone for food, the husband could not find his lovely wife. The sampan was empty. She was gone. He called for her but she did not answer. Yet he had not far to go to find her. She had left home to live with a man on a boat nearby. Her husband begged her to return, but it was of no avail. She did not want to come back. She would simply follow her will.

He tried to tell her how ungrateful she was. Was it not to him that she owed her second life?

Standing on the prow of the next sampan, the young woman answered him back, and they argued a long time. In the end she said she would have no more to do with him. He could have his drop of blood back.

She snatched a long pin from her hair and pricked her finger. A pearl of blood sprang out and rolled into the river. With it went the life that her husband had given back to her. Her body fell again into dust and drifted gently on the water. Slowly, the dust changed into tiny grubs, from which mosquitoes were born.

The husband then remembered the words of the Genie. He did not beweep his unfaithful wife. He married again and had many children, from whom we all descend.

As for the faithless one, she cannot overcome her anger and grief. She has been changed into a mosquito. She harasses mankind with her buzzing, thus expressing her sorrow, and she stings us, trying to steal back the drop of blood which would give her life again.

Source: World Health Organization, 1960

health problem. In May, 1956, however, when malaria moved back into position as the world's leading health problem, the World Health Organization first inaugurated a program for the total eradication of malaria from the earth. This decision was reached because it was becoming obvious that the malaria-bearing mosquitoes were developing resistance to various insecticides and that attempts to control malaria would ultimately fail unless the disease were stamped out soon.

CONQUEST AND CHALLENGE

"... World Health Organization has played a very important part in organizing and perfecting methods of combating málaria. The results have been spectacular, witness the fact that this disease has been practically eradicated in a group of countries whose population totals two hundred and eighty million people. But much more remains to be done, since the eradication program which is now being carried out is aimed at freeing more than a billion persons from malaria ..."

Daniel Bovet, 1960

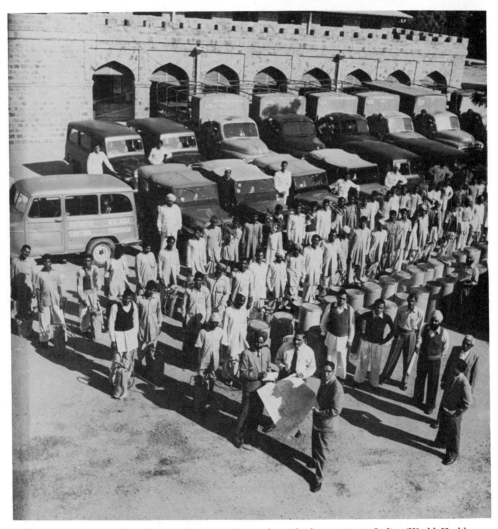

Figure 35. A single malaria-eradication unit stands ready for service in India. (World Health Organization.)

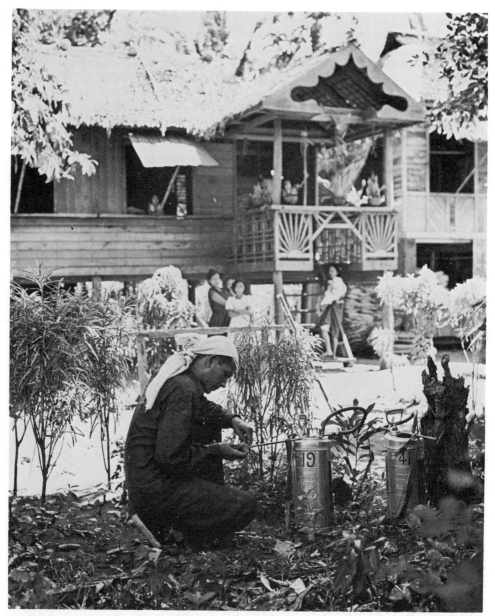

Figure 36. Preparation for the spraying of an entire village in the Philippines. (World Health Organization.)

The Spread of Malaria

Malaria is a disease spread by female mosquitoes of the genus *Anopheles.* Four different species of microscopic organisms are the cause of malaria. *Plasmodium vi-* *vax, P. malariae, P. falciparum* and *P. ovale.*

When the anopheles mosquito bites a person whose blood contains the organisms causing malaria, some of the germs are then transferred into the body of the mosquito, where they undergo certain changes over a period of time.

When an *infected Anopheles* mosquito bites a human being, he is apt to transmit malarial sporozoites. These organisms go through certain developmental phases in the human being and finally lodge in certain blood cells. Periodically the malaria organisms break forth from the cells and are spilled into the blood stream. These blood stream invaders may begin another cycle in their development and if so are then available for transmission if an *Anopheles* mosquito sucks up this contagious blood.

Diagnosis

The diagnosis of malaria is made on the basis of symptoms and a positive blood smear in which one of the organisms causing the disease is identified. The disease is not always easy to identify, since the examination of a single blood smear may afford detection of only 20 to 50 per cent of those persons infected. Even repeated blood smears may fail to identify the disease in some cases.

Symptoms

Malaria is a disease characterized by recurrence of chills and fever, enlargement of the spleen and anemia. Other complications may arise.

The patient with malaria usually becomes anemic because the malarial organisms develop within the red blood cells, which results in massive destruction of these cells.

The victim of malaria goes into a chill when great numbers of red blood cells burst and spill the malaria organisms into the blood stream. Fever begins during the chill and mounts rapidly, followed by a

drop in temperature within one to eight hours. The patient may have a severe headache and a fast heartbeat. He may suffer from nausea and vomiting.

According to the particular type of malaria that the person may suffer from, he has these attacks of fever and chills every 36, 48 or 72 hours—usually about every 48 hours—but there is much variation in these cycles.

Malaria usually involves the enlargement of the spleen which becomes sensitive to touch. This enlargement is because the cells in the spleen become filled with parts of red blood cells and parasites.

Treatment of Malaria

In the old days quinine was the principal drug used for the treatment of malaria; now it is used only if more modern drugs are not available. Primaquine, chloroquine, hydroxychloroquine and quinacrine are the modern drugs used in the treatment of this disease. These drugs can suppress the appearance of malaria while a person is traveling or living in a malarious area.

Effective drugs for the complete curing of malaria (after a person has been removed from the malarious area) are chloroquine and primaquine.

World Eradication of Malaria

By 1960 the World Health Organization was actively engaged in directing a massive attack against malaria in 92 countries and territories. However, the organization reported as of April 20, 1960, that 56 countries were making no concurrent effort to wipe out the disease. Ninety per cent of the cost of the program to wipe out malaria is borne by the countries in which the disease exists.

Dr. M. G. Candau, Director-General of

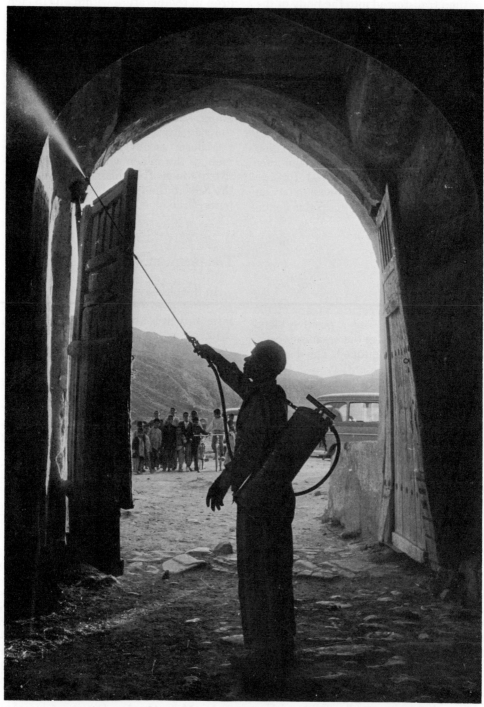

Figure 37.   Spraying of the inside of a building in Iran. (World Health Organization.)

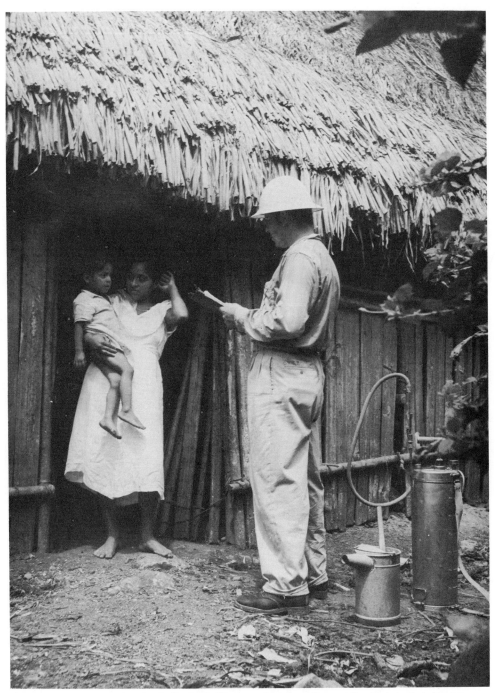

Figure 38.   A home is individually checked by a member of a malaria-eradication brigade in Mexico.
(World Health Organization.)

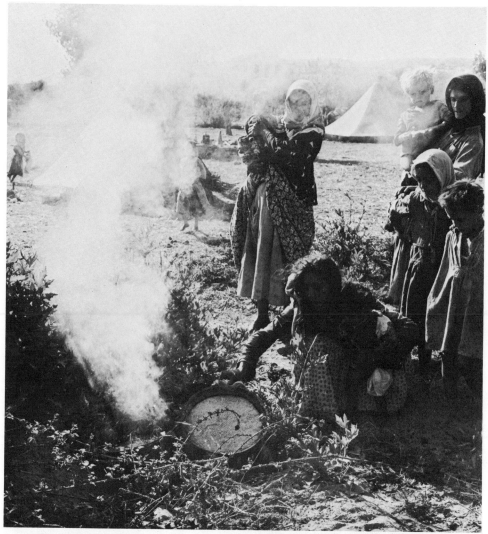

Figure 39.   Migrant families may carry malaria parasites in their blood. Greek nomads cooperating
with public health authorities are shown in this scene. (World Health Organization.)

the World Health Organization, has
pointed out that malaria is still a constant
threat to more than one billion people and
that it affects young children more severely than adults. In certain countries the
disease is held responsible for 10 to 15 per
cent of the infant mortality.

Although malaria is fast disappearing
from Europe there were still about fifty-
nine million persons in that area as late as

WIPING OUT MALARIA

"... The eradication campaign will utilize thousands of teams in the field, tens of thousands of
vehicles, and millions of tons of materials. Hundreds of millions of houses will be sprayed and
hundreds of millions of blood samples will be
taken during the course of the gigantic enter-
prise ..."

World Health Organization, 1960

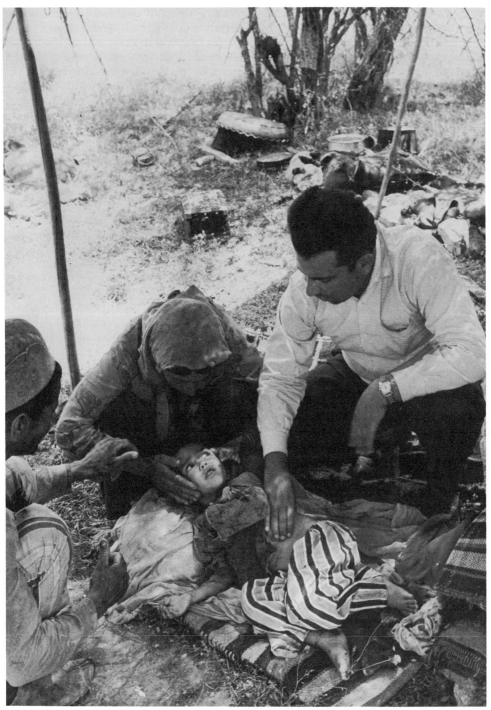

Figure 40. A child infected with malaria is examined in Iran. (World Health Organization.)

1960 who were exposed to the possibility of getting the disease.

During 1960 a panel of internationally famous experts in the field of malaria recommended that an eight-year campaign be embarked upon to eradicate malaria throughout the whole world. These experts believed that the job could be done at a cost of slightly more than one billion dollars.

Some time ago the fourteenth Pan-American Sanitary Conference approved a program for the eradication of malaria in North and South America. A recent analysis as to what has been accomplished toward this goal suggests that malaria can and will be eradicated from the Americas.

A good example of the manner in which efforts are made to eliminate malaria is in Mexico where control measures have been carried forward on a massive scale with military precision.

In 1955 more than fifteen million persons in Mexico were living in malarious areas. The control program began when the National Commission for the Eradication of Malaria, with fourteen zone offices in the malaria regions, was formed. Engineers located and numbered more than three million houses. Studies were made of each house and the surrounding area in preparation for massive spraying operations which began on January 2, 1957. Itineraries were drawn up for motorized brigades in the fourteen zones. All houses sprayed with Dieldrin were treated once each year, while houses sprayed with DDT were treated twice a year. By 1958 the Mexican public health authorities had 115 malaria-fighting brigades on foot, 178 in motor vehicles, 10 brigades in boats and 238 brigades on horses and mules. Military personnel were responsible for maintenance of the supply lines for the eradication program.

A large corps of malaria experts now operate a detection network involving doctors, nurses, pharmacists, mid-wives, school teachers and other volunteer community leaders for the discovery of cases of malaria and evaluation of results. Malaria teams are also making routine surveys to help evaluate the results of the eradication effort. Progress strongly indicates that malaria can and will be wiped out in Mexico in keeping with the objectives of the Pan-American Sanitary Conference and the World Health Organization.

The Economics of Malaria

The economic benefits of controlling malaria are enormous. Large areas of the world can be reclaimed to productive efforts when this disease is wiped out. The low vitality of large populations infected with malaria can be shifted to higher energy levels when infected people are treated and when malaria sources are destroyed in the environment.

The World Health Organization, in 1960, offered the following data to justify the expenditure of national funds for the control of malaria:

In Afghanistan, about one million peasants lived under the constant shadow of malaria, and some of the most fertile land could not be cultivated because of the ravages of the disease. The total cost of antimalaria operations from 1949 to 1959 did not exceed $750,000, whereas malaria was the cause of a yearly loss of earnings amounting to about $20,000,000.

In Ceylon, the disappearance of malaria has resulted in a saving of about $30,000,000 per year, that is, six times the total expenditure on the ten-year antimalaria campaign.

In India, the annual economic losses caused by malaria are in the neighborhood of $500,000,000. On the other hand, the total cost of a malaria eradication programme of several years' duration would not exceed $190,000,000.

In Mexico, where $175,000,000 worth of economic damage is caused every year by malaria, the total cost of the five-year eradication programme is expected to be about $20,000,000.

In the Philippines, the uprooting of malaria has made possible many projects which previously were out of the question such as construction of roads, opening of mines, and the building of houses and industrial premises.

In Thailand, it has been estimated that fifty million agricultural work days were lost each year on account of malaria. This equals a rice harvest of $15,000,000, whereas the cost of the malaria eradication programme from 1954 to 1958 was $500,000 per year.

Questions

1. If malaria has been exterminated in the United States why is it still one of the world's greatest health problems?
2. Is money spent on malaria control an expenditure or a saving? Why?
3. How does malaria affect the economy of a country?
4. Is it possible to eradicate malaria on a world-wide scale?
5. What are the things that might stop a country from wiping out malaria?

For Further Reading

Warshaw, Leon J.: *Malaria, the Biography of a Killer.* New York, Rinehart, 1949.

For Advanced Reading

Macdonald, George: *The Epidemiology and Control of Malaria.* New York, Oxford University Press, 1957.

Recommended Films

1. *Chills and Fever: Why?* 35 mm., color, sound, showing time 13 minutes, 1947. Atlanta, Georgia, Communicable Disease Center, Attn: Audiovisual.
2. *Clinical Malaria.* 16 mm., black and white, showing time 28 minutes, 1944. Washington, D.C., Bureau of Medicine and Surgery, U.S. Navy.

23

HEART AND CIRCULATORY DISEASE

HEART disease still ranks as the primary cause of death in the United States. Its prevention is a problem of many facets.

In some families there appears to be a major genetic tendency toward high levels of lipids (fatty materials) in the blood and it is now known that this is a major cause of coronary artery disease, strokes, and other conditions that impair health or cause death.

More and more evidence is accumulating that nutrition plays a significant part in the elevation of blood cholesterol, so that it may be possible to reduce mortality from heart disease by sustained attention to the diet, especially in the young and middle aged persons.

High blood pressure is a cause of stress for all arteries and this condition puts the heart under an abnormal work load that may result in heart disease, strokes and other injurious conditions. The reduction of blood pressure by drugs and other methods thus becomes a means of the prevention of heart disease.

Although over half a million people die annually with a diagnosis of heart disease in the United States, there is a growing realization in the medical and public health professions that heart failure is simply the reflection of other conditions that promote heart attacks. The real problem is therefore one of finding and preventing the basic causes of heart and circulatory failure.

NEWER CONCEPTS

"One of the most important changes that has taken place in medicine is the concept that we should no longer look upon disease of the coronary arteries as . . . heart disease, or strokes as . . . brain disease, or senile diabetes as . . . pancreatic disease, but that we should look upon most of these disorders as chance manifestations of a generalized process of atherosclerosis . . . What we treat in the heart or brain is the end-result . . . of a process that is more fundamental . . ."

Dr. I. S. Wright, 1960

There is no single cause of heart disease. One or several of about twenty different factors may be involved in a particular case of heart disorder.

Although most deaths from heart disease occur after the age of forty, and the five-year period of greatest fatalities is between seventy and seventy-four, deaths do occur at all ages. Heart disease, in fact, ranks fifth among the causes of death of school children, among whom it accounts for about 5 per cent of all deaths.

Some investigators of life statistics, however, do not consider heart disease the number one health problem in the United States. When the leading causes of death are compared in terms of the working years lost, accidents replace heart disease in the number one position. This is because most deaths from heart disease come in the later years of life, whereas the average age of death from accidents comes

much earlier; hence, there is a greater loss to society, to the family and to the individual when a person dies from an accident rather than heart disease.

Much progress has been made in the field of heart disease within recent years. Some types of cardiac disorders can now be cured, while others can be prevented because of modern developments in medicine and public health. The outlook is not as gloomy as it used to be.

Causes of Heart Disease

There are many causes of heart disease, and undoubtedly additional causes will be discovered in the future. At least twenty different sources of damage to the heart have been clearly revealed in medical and scientific studies.

THE AMERICAN WAY

"Atherosclerosis is now recognized as the earmark of the American way of life, since it already has been shown to afflict about 77 per cent of American males as early as in the 20–30 year age range."

Dr. Lester M. Morrison, 1960

Atherosclerosis is a basic disorder related to coronary artery disease. The coronary arteries, which supply blood to the heart itself, are weakened by the internal deposit of fatlike materials. In time, this weakness leads to structural collapse and hemorrhage or to impaired blood flow and clotting which may precipitate an acute heart attack. The role of diet in the elevation of blood cholesterol and the production of atherosclerosis has not been completely elucidated, but enough is known to suggest that long-term overconsumption of saturated fats such as those in butter, cream, eggs and meats is a major factor. Diet, therefore, may be one of the most important causes of heart disease. This is discussed more completely in a later section.

Rheumatic fever, which is discussed elsewhere in this book, is one cause of serious heart injury. High blood pressure is one of the outstanding causes of heart disorders because of the build-up of sustained and long-lasting resistance to the action of the heart. This results in an extra work burden for the heart which in time may result in serious disease.

Overweight is a common cause of heart disease, partly because of the high blood pressure with which it may be associated, but also because added work is created for the heart by the extra pounds the person carries. Syphilis is a cause of heart disease, although it was a greater problem in the past than in the last few years.

Developmental (congenital) defects of the heart constitute one of the main complications at birth. These often result in the early death of the child or adult. Bacterial infections and virus infections may create inflammation of the heart, and in some cases produce heart failure.

Severe anemia is occasionally a cause of heart disease, probably because of the deficiency of oxygen to the heart muscle itself as well as the extra burden of work which confronts the heart in supplying an adequate amount of oxygen and nutrients to all parts of the body.

Physical effort is sometimes a cause of cardiac pains in the condition known as neurocirculatory asthenia, although psychogenic factors are partly and sometimes primarily involved in this medical condition. Physical effort is also a cause of *pain* in the type of heart disease known as angina pectoris, but the cardiac *disorder* is not caused by the activity but by circulatory insufficiency under stress.

Tobacco has been reported as related to coronary heart disease as may be seen from the chart accompanying a later paragraph which shows that heavy smokers have a mortality rate more than twice that of non-smokers.

An overactive thyroid gland may also damage the heart, mainly because of increased metabolic activities throughout the body which place an added burden on the heart and result in a speeding up of the cardiac effort. An underactive thyroid gland may also produce heart disease.

Psychoneurotic heart ailments are fairly common and must be distinguished by the physician from organic heart disease. Sometimes the heart is damaged by mechanical injury, as in an automobile accident, with some penetrating wound to the chest wall. On some occasions deformities of the chest act as a damaging influence on the heart. The heart may also be damaged by toxic substances, by undernourishment, and in still other ways.

Symptoms of Heart Disease

When symptoms of heart disease occur, they are usually related to failure of the heart to do its job, to disturbances of rhythm, or an impairment of the circulation of the blood to the heart muscle itself.

When the heart fails to pump a sufficient amount of blood to the various parts of the body, there is apt to be congestion or fluid accumulation in the lungs, breathlessness, blueness of the face, swelling of body tissues and spells of difficult breathing.

A disturbance in the rhythm of the heart often causes great concern to the person involved. However, in the large majority of cases no disease will be found. The heart may appear to skip a beat on occasions, especially in the second half of life. Because the heart is then filled with an extra quantity of blood, the resultant contraction may give the impression that the heart is actually leaping out of the chest. In the great majority of cases, however, this has no particular significance.

When the heart rate is greatly increased, many people become alarmed, but there is no heart disease in at least 80 per cent of these cases, according to some authorities. Although consciousness of the beating of the heart is one of the commonest of all symptoms associated with this organ, it is also the least important.

When heart symptoms are associated with a failure of the blood vessels of the heart itself to supply an adequate amount of oxygen and nutrients to the muscle tissue of the heart, pain may result. Sometimes the blood vessels to the heart (the coronary vessels) may rupture and hemorrhage into the cardiac tissue. In such cases the pain may be exceedingly severe, so that shock is an immediate factor that must be treated by the physician. A very small hemorrhage would cause less severe pain and shock.

Chest pain in the region of the heart may come from many different causes. A sharp, stabbing pain which is aggravated by deep breathing is seldom if ever due to heart disease. Heart pain is more likely to be of a crushing or squeezing variety. If pain is increased by exercise or cold weather, it may be due to a cardiac condition, and a physician should be consulted. When the heart muscle itself is damaged by lack of oxygen and nutrients, intense nausea and vomiting may also accompany the pain.

At the National Heart Hospital in London it was found that about one in every three or four patients who came to the heart clinics was suffering from neurotic heart disease. In other words, these patients did not have real disease of the heart, but their symptoms were due to anxiety, especially about the heart. In these patients, fatigue, breathlessness, palpitation of the heart, dizziness, sweating, headache, and pain in the left chest were typical complaints.

Some authorities believe that almost 60 per cent of the patients who consult a heart specialist are suffering from an exaggerated anxiety about their hearts. Sometimes this anxiety is produced by the physicians themselves who diagnose heart disease because of harmless murmurs, irregularity of the rhythm or other signs or symptoms that are actually not related to heart disease. Improper or careless medical advice regarding the heart may cause patients to become unduly alarmed even when the heart is basically sound.

In one study of 175 persons who had been given a mistaken diagnosis of heart disease at some time in their lives, three physicians found that many of these patients who really did not have heart disease had been advised to restrict their activities, and 25 per cent were not working because they thought they had heart trouble.

Many of the mistaken diagnoses were based upon confusing physical signs such as murmurs, fast heart rates, and elevation of blood pressure. Others were given a diagnosis of heart disease on the basis of anxiety symptoms which gave rise to feelings typical of real heart disease.

A Boston physician reported a study of ten patients with chest pains that were characteristic of heart disease, but were caused by pressure on spinal nerve roots, a disease known as radiculitis.

A few words should be said about functional or innocent murmurs. A murmur is a gentle, rushing sound that the physician may hear when he listens to the heart with the stethoscope. Some infants are born with hearts that have a murmur during contraction. These murmurs can be distinguished by physicians and cardiac specialists from those that are caused by rheumatic fever or congenital heart disease.

It is important to know that many young people have temporarily such functional systolic murmurs during adolescence. Such people do not have heart disease and should not worry or restrict their lives because of such a fear. This problem is discussed in a subsequent section.

The Diagnosis of Heart Disease

Many different procedures are now used by the physician in the diagnosis of heart and circulatory disease. This is primarily because there are different causes of these disorders.

The diagnosis of heart disease usually starts with a careful analysis of the symptom descriptions that the patient brings to the physician.

Irregularities in the rhythm of the heart are not usually indicative of heart disease, but they should be reported to the physician for appraisal. Pain in the chest, pain in the arm, difficult breathing, and indigestion are sometimes symptoms of heart disease and, if persistent, should be investigated by the physician. All these symptoms frequently come from other causes than heart disease; hence, a person should not assume that he has a heart disorder in the presence of such symptoms.

In making a diagnosis of heart disease the physician will take a careful history and will appraise the chief complaint of the patient in terms of his findings with the stethoscope and by objective examination. It is becoming standard medical practice to ask the laboratory technician for a report on blood cholesterol levels in certain types of heart disease. The clotting qualities of the blood may also be examined. If the doctor suspects heart disease or wishes to rule out this possibility, he will ask the patient to submit to an electrocardiograph study. The interpretation of the electrocardiogram tracings is a technical matter. Usually the results of this study will give a clear indication as to whether or not the patient has heart disease.

Newer methods of determining the status of the heart have been evolved in recent years. Some of these are not in common use in the average doctor's office, although they may be available in major clinics, medical centers and leading hospitals.

In making his final decision, the physician assembles all the evidence and reaches a conclusion. From that point on, the patient should follow closely the advice of his doctor.

Blood Enzymes and Heart Disease

The study of blood serum enzymes is proving to be of value in the diagnosis, treatment and prediction of outcomes in the treatment of heart and circulatory disorders.

Although great attention has been given recently to studies on serum glutamic oxalacetic transaminase (SGOT), experts in the field of heart disease have used such studies for a number of years.

The determination of SGOT (serum glutamic oxalacetic transaminase) levels in the blood has value in the diagnosis of the form of heart disease known as acute myocardial infarction. The great majority of patients with this type of heart attack show a rise of SGOT above normal. The rise begins after about six to twelve hours and reaches a peak in 24 to 36 hours and is thereafter followed by a decline and return to normal after about five to six days. The magnitude of the increase in this enzyme in the blood is roughly proportional to the magnitude of the heart attack. Blood determinations of this enzyme are especially valuable when other diagnostic means are unavailable or controversial.

Digitalis and Heart Disease

In the popular mind, digitalis is the drug of choice for the treatment of heart disease. Actually this drug must be used with caution and only in certain types of heart disorders. It is not advisable for the normal heart or for many types of heart disease.

Digitalis is the drug prescribed by most physicians for congestive heart failure. In this type of heart disease the efficiency of the heart muscle has declined to such an extent that the heart is no longer able to pump the blood efficiently. As a result, back pressure is generated and blood tends to accumulate in the veins. This type of heart failure also results in the accumulation of fluid in the lungs. The legs swell because of the increased pressure in the veins and accumulation of fluid in the tissues nearby. The liver is usually enlarged. The fluid in the lungs causes the patient to have difficulty in breathing.

This type of heart failure is due to a loss of mechanical efficiency of the heart muscle itself. The effect of digitalis is to restore the efficiency of the heart muscle. Research shows that the efficiency of the heart muscle can be improved by about 45 per cent within about two hours when certain derivatives of digitalis are used. As the heart muscle improves, the heart is again enabled to pump out all the blood that comes to it. This overcomes the back pressure, and the fluid that has accumulated in the body tissues, lungs and liver, again enters the normal circulation.

Digitalis appears to reduce the mechanical efficiency of *normal* heart muscle and it is not advisable that this drug be given in many forms of heart disease.

Anticoagulants

Blood clots have been found to be the cause of much heart disease and circulatory failure, including strokes. It is said that approximately one million persons in the United States suffer from a heart attack each year. Almost one-half of these survive.

Recent autopsies have shown that a blood clot (thrombus) is responsible for the deaths of about 75 per cent of those who die from heart attacks. It is estimated that approximately two million persons suffer from strokes each year in the United States. *Approximately 80 per cent of these strokes are also associated with blood clots.*

This research shows the great importance of the clotting qualities of the blood in the precipitation of circulatory disorders, including strokes and heart attacks.

Anticoagulant drugs are powerful weapons against blood clots.

It has become widespread medical practice to use anticoagulant drugs such as heparin for the treatment of persons who have had heart attacks, strokes, loss of vision or other disorders due to the clotting of blood. The American Heart Association has shown that with the use of anticoagulants, deaths from heart attacks can be reduced by one-third and that complications among survivors can be reduced by four-fifths within the first few weeks after a heart attack of the coronary type.

Although there is some possibility that a person who is being given anticoagulants may suffer a severe hemorrhage because of the reduced ability of the blood to clot, the hazard from clotting in these patients is much greater than the hazard of hemorrhage. Under close medical supervision the danger of hemorrhage can be negligible.

Functional Heart Disease

Not all symptoms or signs relative to the heart are an indication that there is something structurally wrong with that organ. In other words, some people have heart symptoms when there is no organic heart disease.

Dr. Arthur M. Master of New York reported a study of 1000 patients with heart disease in which 382 suffered from functional heart disturbances. This large group of patients reported various symptoms and signs relative to the heart. Forty-five per cent had pain in the chest, 13 per cent reported occasional sudden speeding up of the heart, 13 per cent reported extreme muscular weakness upon effort, 5 per cent had premature heart beats, 4 per cent suffered from slight hypertension, 3 per cent had heart murmurs, and 3 per cent suffered from anxiety. Many of the patients had more than one of these symptoms or signs.

In those patients who experienced a

greatly increased heart rate, the rapid heart action was usually sudden in onset and often abrupt in its return to normal rate. In ten of the patients it was possible to establish the type of heart action involved by the use of the electrocardiograph. Nineteen of the patients had small hearts.

Some of the patients sought medical examination because of irregular beats or because of an unusual beat or thump of the heart.

Of the patients with anxiety and great weakness on physical effort, many were found to be nervous persons with cold, moist hands. It was found that this type of person often could not tolerate mental, emotional or physical strain as well as his associates.

Twelve of the patients had heart murmurs, none of which were serious or reflected organic change in the heart.

Many of the patients had miscellaneous functional disturbances such as shortness of breath, dizziness, fatigue, and a considerable concern or worry that their symptoms were caused by heart disease.

It is apparent from this and from other studies that a considerable number of persons may have signs and symptoms of heart disturbance without having a damaged heart. In other words, it is the way the heart works in these persons that creates the disturbance rather than any fundamental defect in the heart. Medical treatment of this type of heart disturbance is often unsuccessful. More research is needed into the causes of such disturbances and the methods that will bring best results in their alleviation.

The Heart Attack

The most serious type of heart attack is the one in which the blood vessels to the heart hemorrhage into the tissues or in which they no longer carry enough blood to meet the needs of the heart muscle. This may be because of a temporary constriction of the blood vessels, hardening and degenerative changes in the coronary arteries or a clot (thrombus).

In angina pectoris the problem is one of securing the necessary dilatation of the blood vessels to the heart so that sufficient oxygen and nourishment can again be supplied to the heart muscle. This relaxation of the blood vessels in the heart can usually be obtained with a drug such as nitroglycerin, which is given under the tongue. Relief from the pain, if this method of treatment is successful, may come within one or two minutes.

When a blood vessel to the heart has ruptured and hemorrhaged into the cardiac muscle tissue, there may be serious damage to the heart accompanied by severe pain and shock. In medical terms this damage to the heart is known as myocardial infarction. In semipopular terms such a heart attack is likely to be known as a "coronary." In this emergency one of the first necessities is to control pain. The reason is that the shock associated with pain reduces the likelihood that the patient will survive the heart attack. Pain may be treated by various drugs, but it may be necessary for the physician to use morphine to bring about relief from this type of heart attack. In some cases the shock of such an attack may be treated with blood plasma, but this is likely to be a dangerous procedure, since circulation of the added fluid may prove to be an additional burden for the damaged heart.

Anticoagulants to prevent complications from the formation of blood clots are very important in the treatment of myocardial infarction. As a result of their use substantial reduction in deaths from heart attacks may be achieved when the major problem is one of blood clotting. The use of anticoagulants for this purpose is discussed more fully in other paragraphs.

The provision of oxygen for a patient suffering from a heart attack may bring considerable relief and a better chance of survival.

Bed rest of two to four weeks is usually advised for any patient who has suffered a heart attack. A longer time may be needed if there has been more extensive damage to the heart muscle. Other forms of cardiac disease require special treatment.

Personality and Heart Disease

Two San Francisco physicians recently studied the possible relationships between heart disease and personality structures in three groups of men who were put in separate research categories because of differences in behavior patterns.

It was found that the men who had intense ambition, competitive drive and constant preoccupation with work deadlines and urgencies had seven times more coronary artery disease than the men in the other groups. This was true despite the fact that the diet, physical activity, age, height and weight of the men in the three groups were comparable. A much higher blood level of cholesterol was found in the intense, ambitious group of men.

These two investigators suggested that the behavior patterns of these hard-driving men were in themselves largely responsible for the higher blood cholesterol levels and possible hastening of clotting time, which might account for the much higher rate of clinical coronary artery disease. There is much truth in the basic concept that a heart attack is fostered and encouraged by the restless, hard-driving, ambitious habits of the person who has never learned to relax and enjoy life. Many persons need to develop a philosophy that will permit them to abandon the overactive life that hard work frequently entails. This becomes especially important in later years. In youth the heart can sustain great physical and emotional effort without damage. It is somewhat different during and after middle age.

Heart Disease and Working Capacity

The widespread idea that when a person has heart disease he is disqualified from working is false. Most patients with heart disease can continue working for a number of years. A study conducted by the New York Heart Association showed that of 2081 patients attending their clinics, 65 per cent were able to remain at work.

Adjustments in the work responsibilities of the patient with heart disease, however, may be necessary. At the Work Classification Unit of the Bellevue Cardiac Clinic an effort is made to appraise the physical capacity of the worker with heart disease. The physical demands of the job are then appraised and an effort is made to match the work that the patient has to do with his capacity for performing the work.

In a Cleveland study of 300 railroad workers with heart disease, it was found that 28 per cent of the men were still able to remain on the job after twelve years. In the light of this and other evidence it must not be assumed that a person with heart disease should quit his job. The basic assumption should be that with some modification in his work program he can continue to work as before.

The Michigan Heart Association offers a unique community service to housewives with heart disease. On approval of the patient's application for this service by a physician, an analysis is made of the daily work habits of the patient. Each detail of the work performed in the home is studied. Waste motion and useless trips are pointed out to the patient, and rearrangements in storage and work spaces may be suggested.

In one instance the changes suggested to a housewife in the preparation of one meal alone reduced the number of steps from 672 to 266, the number of times the patient stooped from 20 to 8 times, and the number of times the patient stood on tiptoe from 44 to 29 times. The total number of steps saved in preparing this one meal represented 61 miles in a year.

This patient and others like her have found a reduction in the work load and provision for more time to rest. The patient is able to do more for herself without feeling fatigue by the end of the day.

Instruction of this sort is not limited to the preparation of meals, but also includes bed-making, cleaning, dusting and other household tasks.

The Heart and Athletics

The effect of athletics and sports upon the heart has been studied by various groups. Some years ago an extensive investigation of this subject was made in Austria. After ten years of study and careful medical evaluation of the heart it was concluded that if the heart is normal to begin with, no amount of vigorous physical activity will damage the organ. On the other hand, it was found that if the heart is defective before participation in athletics is begun, the physical activity would damage the heart further. In general, this is in keeping with modern findings.

In one instance a study was made of the cardiac status of a group of high school participants in a 2½-mile cross-country race. The ages of the contestants ranged from fifteen to seventeen years. Upon physical examination no harmful effects upon the heart or blood vessels were found after the race. The electrocardiograms showed no evidence of heart disorders, though increase in heart size was found after the race as compared to the size of the heart before the race.

Although some investigators have found a slight increase in the heart size of athletes, this enlargement has been symmetrical and has been judged to be a normal expectation. On the other hand, the hearts of many athletes have not been made larger by running.

On the basis of current evidence it must be concluded that no positive evidence has been found that athletics is damaging to the heart if it is normal before the person begins strenuous activity.

Infections and Heart Disease

It has been known for many years that communicable diseases such as diphtheria, syphilis and streptococcal infections might damage the heart. More recently it has been found that when a mother has German measles during certain periods of pregnancy, the baby may be born with a developmental heart disease.

It has been shown also that inflammation of the heart muscle occurs after many communicable diseases of bacterial, virus and other origins. It has been thought that inflammation of heart muscle did not exist except as a result of rheumatic fever and diphtheria. A study at the Army Institute of Pathology during World War II, based on 1402 cases of inflammatory heart disease, has shown that the heart may be damaged by many different diseases such as scrub typhus, scarlet fever, syphilis, rheumatic fever, malaria, trichinosis, virus pneumonia, and tuberculosis. Typhoid fever, dysentery, mumps, gonorrhea, meningitis and infectious mononucleosis have also been incriminated as causes of inflammatory damage to the heart muscle.

Changes in the electrocardiogram reveal that in many acute infectious diseases the heart may be temporarily affected by the disease process. Later it may return to a normal status. In some instances, however, permanent damage to the heart may be done. It is now apparent that to control certain forms of heart disease we must secure more effective control over certain communicable diseases.

It can be expected that the development of the antibiotics for prompt and adequate cure of many infections will result in less heart disease due to this cause. One example of such a development is apparent in the treatment of subacute bacterial endocarditis with penicillin. In previous years this heart disease was always considered fatal. Since the advent of penicillin, massive treatment of the disorder with this antibiotic has had very good results. Patients with this hitherto fatal disease are now recovering.

In one study of the effect of virus infections upon the heart three physicians took electrocardiogram readings on forty-seven patients. It was found that in twenty-one cases there was evidence of a heart disturbance according to the electrocardiogram, although there were no signs of heart or circulatory disorders otherwise. These physicians suggested that the elec-

trocardiogram should be used more frequently during an acute virus infection in order to study the effects of the disease upon the heart.

Tobacco and Heart Disease

For most people tobacco does have an effect upon the heart and blood vessels. In the majority of patients the heart rate increases slightly after the smoking of one or two cigarettes, and the peripheral or superficial blood vessels contract sufficiently to increase the blood pressure to some extent.

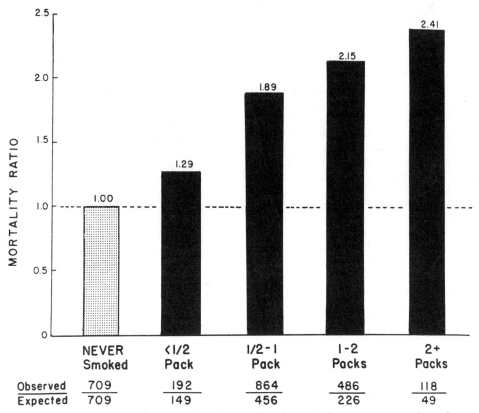

	NEVER Smoked	<1/2 Pack	1/2-1 Pack	1-2 Packs	2+ Packs
Observed	709	192	864	486	118
Expected	709	149	456	226	49

Figure 41. Tobacco and coronary heart disease. Mortality ratios for coronary artery disease by current amount of cigarette smoking. (Hammond, E. Cuyler: Smoking in relation to heart disease. Am. J. Pub. Health, *50*:20–26, March, 1960.)

The effects of tobacco upon the circulatory system are due to nicotine. Physicians have differed in their opinions as to whether or not nicotine is a cause of heart disease. Some feel that tobacco angina is a rare condition that may not exist at all. Others feel that there are some patients in whom it has been proved that heart attacks are caused by smoking of tobacco. Whether the attack is caused by constriction of the blood vessels and elevation of blood pressure or whether the small arteries of the heart itself participate in the constriction and thus reduce the flow of blood to the heart muscle is unknown.

It does seem apparent that in some persons nicotine will have marked effects upon the heart and that pain may be produced. Freedom from attacks after smoking is stopped appears to distinguish this type of heart disease from true angina pectoris. These cases are relatively rare, however, and possibly are restricted to people who are allergic to nicotine or other ingredients of tobacco.

Recent statistics suggest that there is a definite correlation between the smoking of tobacco and an increased mortality rate from coronary artery disease (shown on the preceding page). This does not prove, of course, that smoking by itself is the cause of the higher death rate from this type of heart disease, but the association strongly implies that a person with heart disease might do well to give up smoking.

Whether or not a patient with heart disease should be permitted to smoke tobacco is a matter for decision between the patient and his physician. Some doctors advise all patients with heart disease to eliminate smoking, while others permit the practice because of the psychological satisfaction it may bring the patient.

High Blood Pressure

Blood pressure varies with individuals, and at different times will change greatly for the same person. In general, if the systolic pressure is not above 140 mm. and the diastolic pressure does not go above 90 mm., most doctors consider the blood pressure normal. Studies on hundreds of thousands of college students indicate that for this group of the population, which is mostly under twenty-six years of age, the following blood pressures are typical.

The average *systolic* pressure for college men is about 122 mm. of mercury, while that for college women is about 110 to 115 mm. of mercury. The average *diastolic* pressure for college men is about 75 mm. of mercury, and for college women, about 70.

A person's blood pressure, even when normal, will vary with circumstance. At times it will rise to high levels for brief periods. This temporary fluctuation is called *transient* hypertension.

What Causes High Blood Pressure?

High blood pressure should probably be looked upon as a symptom rather than as a disease. What happens in most cases of hypertension, to put it most simply, is that the small arteries throughout the body have squeezed tighter, narrowing the diameter of the tubes. Since the same amount of blood has to crowd through this decreased space the result is increased pressure.

Any one of a number of factors may be to blame. Often there is no clear-cut, obvious cause to be found in the body to account for high blood pressure. This type of hypertension is called *essential hypertension*.

It may be caused, in part, by one or several of the following factors:

1. HEREDITY. A history of high blood pressure occurring early in life can often be found among the brothers or sisters of a person suffering from this disorder. This may be due to a family inheritance of a tendency to high blood lipids (fats). Some authorities have reported a strong genetic

factor for the development of high blood lipids.

2. FAULTY DIET AND OVERWEIGHT. Often overweight is associated with an increase in blood pressure. Sometimes a satisfactory loss of excessive weight is sufficient to lower the blood pressure to normal levels even though no other treatment may be attempted. A certain type of combined molecule of fat and protein in the blood may be responsible for obesity and high blood pressure.

3. HORMONES. The action of certain chemical substances formed in the body appears to be definitely involved as a cause of some cases of high blood pressure.

4. THE EMOTIONS. It is common knowledge that strong emotions may raise the blood pressure. Long-continued emotional stress, especially that due to anger, fear and resentment, may bring about a sustaining hypertension through excessive activity of the sympathetic nervous system. When nervous tension is maintained a long time, it seems to produce degenerative changes in the walls of the small blood vessels, causing them to be permanently thickened.

5. KIDNEY DISEASE. High blood pressure may occur when a kidney is diseased. Study has shown, however, that high blood pressure is seldom due to a damaged kidney, so that in the majority of cases other sources of the disease must be sought.

6. PHYSIOLOGIC CHANGES IN THE VOLUME OR QUALITY OF THE BLOOD. Theoretically, high blood pressure may be caused in humans by increases in the volume or viscosity of the blood. Erythrocytosis, a disease in which there is an increase in both the total blood volume and the number of red cells, is an example of this source of increased blood pressure.

Psychotherapy for Hypertension

Emotions can make you ill. When you feel anger, fear or resentment, various parts of the nervous system become overactive. Even the tiniest blood vessels may respond to emotional tensions by constriction and reduction of blood flow with an increase in blood pressure.

You cannot always relax merely by deciding that you ought to. When you cannot, it is plain common sense to seek help from a psychiatrist. Many emotional conflicts may have their beginnings in childhood troubles, which are often exceedingly hard to identify without expert guidance.

In addition to psychologic help, the tense, worried person should plan a way of living which gives him regular rest and vacation periods, mild exercise that is adapted to his physical condition, and sometimes a careful use of sedatives as prescribed by his physician to help relieve his uncomfortable symptoms. It is important, too, for such a person to break out of routines which fret and depress him, and to find activities which give him real satisfaction. This is not always easy, and it is often wise to seek expert guidance.

Salt Restriction in the Diet

Sometimes the elimination or reduction of salt in the diet of a hypertensive patient will bring relief through a lowering of the blood pressure. Moderate restriction of salt does not help much; salt must be as completely eliminated from the diet as possible. Foods must be selected which are naturally low in salt content, although they can be made more palatable with the use of salt-free condiments.

Low salt intake does not seem to benefit every high blood pressure patient. However, this is so easy a method of treatment that it is often advised by the physician.

Cholesterol and High Blood Pressure

Atherosclerosis is a disease of the blood vessels in which there are deposits of a cholesterol-like substance or substances in the walls of the aorta and other parts of the circulatory system. These concentrations of fatty substances appear to have much to do with high blood pressure and damage to the blood vessels and heart.

In February, 1950, Dr. John Gofman of the University of California and his coworkers found a method for detecting in the blood serum of humans a giant molecule of combined lipid (fat) and protein. It is this lipid protein that appears to be related to the development of atherosclerosis, for it is found in large amounts in the blood of people who have this disease.

Preliminary research data suggest that a low-fat, low-cholesterol diet will cause a reduction of these giant molecules in the blood; hence, this type of dietary adjustment may be an important step in the prevention of hypertension and disease of the circulatory system.

A high blood concentration of these combined giant molecules is apparently not the only factor in development of circulatory disease. Studies show that when the walls of the arteries are damaged or changed in some manner, calcium may be deposited and cholesterol precipitated in the walls of such vessels, regardless of blood concentrations.

Drugs and High Blood Pressure

The treatment of high blood pressure with antihypertensive drugs is described as a medical procedure that is still in its infancy. It is already possible, however, to help from 60 to 70 per cent of the patients with high blood pressure through the use of drugs.

The drugs that have been most useful in lowering blood pressure are the Rauwolfia derivatives, hydralazine hydrochloride, chlorothiazide and its derivatives, bretylium tosylate, guanethidine sulfate and the ganglion-blocking agents.

All of these drugs which can reduce high blood pressure are not without their com-plications and side effects. The ganglion-blocking agents, for example, often cause constipation, dryness of the mouth, impotence and so on. Both bretylium tosylate and guanethidine sulfate produce mental changes and the latter drug also produces a very troublesome diarrhea. Chlorothiazide is one of the drugs that has been widely used in recent years in the United States for the reduction of high blood pressure. This drug results in substantial dehydration of the body, which helps greatly in the reduction of high blood pressure.

Some of the side effects among patients treated with Rauwolfia preparations for high blood pressure are nasal congestion, drowsiness, nightmares, overeating, irrational behavior, and depression.

The tranquilizing drugs in some cases have been very effective in the reduction of high blood pressure but they are not completely safe and should be used only under the guidance of a competent physician. Over a long period of time the tranquilizing drugs would seem to have a greater value in the reduction of hypertension when they are given to patients suffering from associated tensions which would aggravate the blood pressure, even if such tensions were not the basic cause of the elevation.

Drugs for high blood pressure must be taken only under the guidance of a physician if the health of the patient is to be safeguarded.

Surgery for High Blood Pressure

For some patients with high blood pressure, surgery offers great hope. For certain carefully selected patients a definite and prolonged drop in the blood pressure can be expected as a result of the surgical removal of parts of the sympathetic nervous system (sympathectomy).

For whom is a sympathectomy strongly advisable? For the patient with malignant hypertension, if kidney or heart damage is not too extensive; for the patient who is not helped by other forms of treatment and whose blood pressure is very high, especially if the diastolic pressure is extreme.

Patients for surgery should be selected very carefully so as to avoid putting them through an operation which does not improve their condition. It is possible to predict, with a fair amount of success, whether the blood pressure *can* be lowered, and several tests for this purpose exist. These tests are technical and need not be described here.

The most striking result of surgery for high blood pressure has been the improvement in heart conditions. Improvements in kidney function have resulted as well. Eye conditions which would have resulted in blindness have been so greatly relieved for some patients that vision has returned to normal. Patients who were totally disabled for long periods have been restored to normal earning capacity.

The discovery and use of new drugs for the treatment of hypertension has reduced substantially the need for surgery. These drugs were discussed in earlier paragraphs.

Heart Surgery

It used to be thought that surgery had no place in the treatment of heart disease. This is no longer true. Especially since 1926, cardiac surgery has developed into a lifesaving and life-extending service. The first heart disease to be corrected with a high degree of success by surgery was constrictive pericarditis. In this condition a fibrous sheath or covering due to tuberculosis and other conditions so restricts the heart that it elevates blood pressure, creates fatigue, and ultimately causes death. Surgery is able to remove constriction to the point where the patient can make a considerable recovery.

Surgery has also been successful in the repairing of certain kinds of congenital defects of the heart. Sometimes this has meant the rerouting of certain blood vessels or the closing of certain openings which should not be present. The publicized "blue baby" heart operations represent surgery of this sort that prevents the mingling of oxygenated with nonoxygenated blood by the correction of structural defects.

In recent years successful efforts have been made to impart a new blood supply to the heart in coronary artery disease and angina pectoris by transplantation or imbedding another artery (such as the mammary artery) in the heart muscle. This so-called Beck operation has been reported as safe and effective. Not only is there relief of cardiac pain, but the improved cardiac circulation lengthens life, especially if the operation is done early in the course of coronary artery disease.

Heart surgery is now a well developed specialty that is becoming more and more accepted by both the general public and the medical profession.

Taking Care of Your Heart

Taking care of the heart is a complex problem, because there are so many different causes of heart disorders. The most effective means of preventing heart disease is to live a wholesome life without becoming unduly concerned about the heart. In other words, a person should avoid developing a special worry about that part of the body.

There are certain things, however, that make good sense. When a person is establishing his eating habits he can try to develop a taste for oils instead of the fats that are hard at room temperature. A diet low in saturated fats may control the blood cholesterol level with subsequent reduction in the likelihood of coronary artery disease. Sound eating habits over a period of years may lengthen life and reduce the chances for heart or circulatory diseases.

When a person has an infectious disease, he should seek medical care promptly and have the condition treated. The longer the disease goes without proper medical care, the greater the likelihood that the heart can be damaged. If a person has high blood pressure, he should seek medical care, and work to bring this pressure down, because by so doing he will spare his heart the possibility of serious damage. A person who tends to put on extra pounds should watch his diet and, if possible, reduce his body weight to below the average for his age group during the latter half of life. People who are especially disposed to rheumatic fever should be particularly careful to seek medical care promptly for sore throats in order to reduce the allergic reactions and complications that may ensue if the disease goes untreated. Disturbances in basal metabolism, if detected, should be properly treated by the physician. This, too, may prevent heart disease. The use of toxic or injurious substances should be avoided, since the heart can be damaged by these. A well rounded diet containing an adequate supply of the vitamin B complex will make for a healthier heart as well as for better health in general.

The adaptation of work and recreation to the capacity of the heart is another means of protecting this organ and preserving health. The development of a philosophic attitude toward life, which permits greater relaxation and less concern about values, can decrease tension and in many cases lower blood pressure, with subsequent reduction of the work load on the heart.

Any symptoms of heart disease should be reported promptly to the physician for analysis and advice. On the other hand, care should be taken to avoid the development of a neurotic attitude toward the heart. Such an attitude may have a serious influence on one's life even when one has a normal, healthy heart.

Atherosclerosis and Heart Disease

In atherosclerosis, yellow, fat-like and sometimes mushy deposits of material are laid down in the walls of the arteries. When these arteries are a part of the circulatory system of the heart, the blood vessels are weakened and may rupture. If this occurs, hemorrhage into the muscle of the heart produces the heart attack known as coronary heart disease. When the blood contains a high level of cholesterol there is greater likelihood that this fat-like material will play an important part in the damaging deposits established in the blood vessels.

In studies of populations whose diets are high in animal fats, atherosclerosis is found to be high. Some investigators have found that a high blood level of cholesterol is associated with three to six times as much coronary heart disease in middle-aged men. The same association has been found in high blood pressure. Other abnormalities that increase the possibility of coronary heart disease are overweight, diabetes, heavy smoking, sedentary living and possibly psychologic stress.

It has been shown that blood levels of cholesterol can be reduced by diets low in the cholesterol type of fats or by the use of oils (such as olive oil) instead of fats in the diet. Diets in which oils are used are reported to be palatable, pleasant and varied.

Although the cholesterol content of the blood does not appear to be the only factor in the production of coronary heart disease, it is the only one that we can do something about at the present time. Our lack of knowledge about the other factors handicaps their control.

Fats differ in their effects upon the amount of cholesterol in the blood and therefore in their effects upon the blood vessels of the heart. The so-called saturated fats appear to be the ones that do the damage. These are the fats that are usually hard, or solid, at room temperature, such as meat fats, butter, margarine and cooking fats. The fat in milk is a hard fat, too, but is apt to escape notice because it is finely dispersed throughout the liquid. Fish oils, seal oil, olive oil, peanut oil and corn oils are the opposite kind of fats that do not harm the walls of the blood vessels, according to Dr. Louis N. Katz and Dr. Norman Jolliffe.

Life Expectancy and Heart Disease

The number of years that a person may expect to live after the onset of heart disease depends upon the kind of disease involved.

A group of doctors in Rochester, Minnesota, recently reported their observations on 6882 patients who had angina pectoris who were examined at the Mayo Clinic over a period of eighteen years.

The average age at the time of diagnosis was fifty-nine years. Within the first year after diagnosis 15 per cent of the total group had died. Thereafter about 9 per cent died each year. However, 58 per cent had survived for five years, and 37 per cent were still alive after ten years. The highest survival rate was among those patients who had angina pectoris, but who showed normal electrocardiograms.

In another study of 1700 patients 59 per cent of the women and 51 per cent of the men with heart disease had lived beyond the age of sixty years. Most of the patients were still alive at the time of the study, but of those who had died, the average length of survival after onset of the disease was slightly less than five years.

In a study of 500 patients with heart disease it was found that the average survival time was about ten years following the initial diagnosis of the disorder.

Averages, however, do not tell the whole story. Many of those who adjust their ways of living to the capacity of the heart can be expected to reach the normal life expectancy.

SOME COMPARATIVE CHOLESTEROL VALUES* OF FOOD

Food	Approximate Ratio
1. Fresh milk	1
2. Codfish	2
3. Salmon	2
4. Chicken (dark meat)	2
5. Duck	3
6. Chicken (light meat)	4
7. Breast of veal	4
8. Lean beef	4
9. Pork spareribs	4
10. Pigeon meat	4
11. Beef (medium fat)	5
12. American cheese	6
13. Swiss cheese	6
14. Veal shank	6
15. Shrimp	6
16. Heart	6
17. Tuna fish	6
18. Tripe	6
19. Crab	6
20. Sardines	8
21. Monterey Jack Cheese	8
22. Oysters	9
23. Sweetbreads	11
24. Butter	11
25. Beef liver	13
26. Calf liver	14
27. Beef kidney	16
28. Whole egg	18
29. Lamb liver	24
30. Egg yolk	80

*The ratio of 1 for milk represents approximately 25 milligrams of cholesterol per 100 grams of moist food. All other ratios are multiples of this base; thus in terms of the stated weight Swiss cheese would have six times as much cholesterol as whole milk. Obviously the amount of food eaten by a person would determine his cholesterol intake, as well as the amount of the substance in a given amount of the food.

Mended Hearts, Incorporated

A few years ago, in Boston, a small group of patients who were alive because of heart surgery met and incorporated under the above title. In 1955 a total of 400 such patients with 350 relatives and

friends attended the meeting. This group
visits persons who are anticipating or recovering from heart surgery to give encouragement and living evidence of the
success of this lifesaving operation. The
slogan of "It's great to be alive and to help
others" guides the members of Mended
Hearts, Incorporated, into a social service
that is highly personal and encouraging to
cardiac surgery patients. Heart disease is
not the fatal condition that many people
believe it to be.

Questions

1. Should people with heart disease be encouraged to
   lead a normal life?
2. When is rest actually undesirable for a person with
   heart disease?
3. Is it possible that a person with heart disease might
   actually live longer because of his disease? If you
   think so, explain why.
4. Why does most heart disease occur in old age?
5. How can a person whose heart has stopped beating
   be brought back to life?
6. What are three things that a person can do to prevent or control heart disease?
7. How is the personality involved in high blood pressure?
8. Is high blood pressure more hazardous than low
   blood pressure? How can the two be compared?
9. How is eating related to heart disease?

For Further Reading

1. Brams, William A.: *Your Blood Pressure and How
   to Live With It.* Philadelphia, J. B. Lippincott
   Company, 1956.

2. Gofman, John W.: *What We Do Know About
   Heart Attacks.* New York, G. P. Putnam's Sons,
   1958.
3. Gofman, John W. and E. Virginia Dobbin: *Dietary
   Prevention and Treatment of Heart Disease.* New
   York, G. P. Putnam's Sons, 1958.
4. Marvin, H. M.: *Your Heart: A Handbook for Lay-
   men.* New York, Doubleday and Company, 1960.
5. Mozes, Eugene B.: *High Blood Pressure.* Philadelphia, J. B. Lippincott Company, 1959.
6. Mozes, Eugene B.: *Living Beyond Your Heart Attack.* Englewood Cliffs, N. J., Prentice-Hall, 1959.

For Advanced Reading

1. Moyer, John H.: *Hypertension.* Philadelphia, W. B.
   Saunders Company, 1959.
2. Rosenbaum, Francis F. and Belknap, Elston: *Work
   and the Heart.* New York, Paul B. Hoeber, 1959.

Recommended Films

1. American Heart Association and the National Heart
   Institute: *A Report to the Nation.* 16 mm., black
   and white, sound, showing time 29 minutes,
   1960. Communicable Disease Center, Atlanta
   22, Georgia, Attn: Audiovisual.
2. American Heart Association: *Pump Trouble.* 16
   mm., color, sound, showing time 14 minutes,
   1954. Rent or purchase from American Heart Association Film Library, 13 E. 37th St., New York
   16.
3. *The Doctor Examines Your Heart.* 16 mm., black
   and white, showing time 11½ minutes, 1955.
   Bray Studios, Inc.

24

CANCER

CANCER is a disease of cells. Its origin is most often in tissues which habitually renew themselves such as the skin, the linings of the digestive tract, organs of the reproductive system, the lungs and the liver. For reasons yet unknown, the cells which normally reproduce themselves in a controlled manner in these tissues suddenly proliferate, forming large continually growing tumors. Individual cells from these tumors may find their way into the blood stream or the lymphatic system and are carried to other parts of the body where they continue to reproduce and grow, interfering with the normal body processes of other tissues. This is called metastasis. Usually, unless treated by radiation, chemotherapy or surgery, the malignant cells continue to grow until their interference with body processes causes the death of the patient.

317

As a college student you are quite safe from cancer at this time. Between the ages of 15 and 24 only 7 women and 10 males will die of cancer out of every 100,000 persons each year; the chances are approximately one in 10,000. For older members of your family, and for you in the future, the risks are much greater. In the ages from 55 to 64 years approximately 340 women and 446 men out of every 100,000 will die from cancer within the space of a year. By learning about cancer now you may save the life of some member of your family, or your own.

Because about 40 per cent of our population is now over the age of forty years, cancer has become one of the foremost public health problems in the United States. Even though we may expect in the next generation or two an even larger proportion of old people in our population, the problem of cancer is not entirely hopeless. A tremendous program of research is currently being conducted in all aspects of the problem. It is to be expected that more progress in the control of this disease will be made in the next twenty years than in all the previous years put together.

CANCER CURES

"Many people do not realize how much progress has been made in treating cancer. Despite the serious problem it presents . . . half of all cancer patients could be saved with maximum cooperation between the public and the medical profession."

Dr. John R. Heller,
Director of the National Cancer Institute, 1960

About 270,000 persons per year die from cancer in the United States. This death toll is increasing at a rate of about 3 per cent annually, mostly because of a steady and continuing increase in the number of older people in our population. On the other hand, about 25,000 persons are now being cured of cancer each year, and probably 50,000 others are having death postponed by proper treatment.

The chances of obtaining a cure are tremendously increased if there is an early diagnosis of the disorder. This places an important responsibility on the individual to know enough about the early signs of cancer so that he will be prompted to seek medical attention while the disease can be arrested.

CONQUEST OF CANCER

". . . The question is no longer *whether* cancer will be conquered, but *when* it will be conquered."

Dr. Pierre Rentchnik, Geneva, 1960

Your responsibility is to learn enough about cancer so that you are no longer frightened by it.

The Seven Danger Signals

So far as the possibility of cancer is concerned, there are seven danger signals that should prompt a person to consult his physician.

The seven danger signals are:

1. Any sore that does not heal.
2. A lump or thickening in the breast or elsewhere.
3. Unusual bleeding or discharge.
4. Any change in a wart or mole.
5. Persistent indigestion or difficulty in swallowing.
6. Persistent hoarseness or cough.
7. Any change in normal bowel habits.

A study by the National Opinion Research Center reveals the findings from detailed interviews of 500 family doctors in regard to their attitudes toward the American Cancer Society's education of the general public on the "seven danger signals." It was concluded that the average physician strongly endorses this educational campaign.

As many as 44 per cent of the doctors felt that some fear was generated by cancer education even though they approved of the program, but only 7 per cent suggested less emphasis on the cancer education programs. On the other hand, 56 per cent of the doctors believed that no harm whatsoever was done by cancer education.

No one should make the mistake of diagnosing cancer in one's self on the basis of any of these seven danger signals. This would be a very foolish mistake. All these signs or signals *could* mean cancer, but in the majority of cases other explanations are usually found by the physician. The sensible conclusion for anyone to make is that these signs should not be neglected. Going to a physician for advice on the possibility of cancer should result in either peace of mind from learning that there is no cancer, or proper medical or surgical treatment with the likelihood of cure.

The Diagnosis of Cancer

The diagnosis of cancer is based upon one or more of the following procedures: (1) biopsy, (2) x-ray, (3) microscopic examination of body fluids and (4) blood studies.

Biopsy is the examination, under a microscope, of tissue taken from the living body. By this means the pathologist or physician is able to tell whether the individual cells of the tissue are those of a cancer or whether they represent normal, healthy tissue. The accuracy of cancer diagnosis by biopsy ranges in general from 90 to 100 per cent.

The surgically removed specimen from the suspected part of the body is usually frozen and then examined under the microscope. It is often possible in the better hospitals to secure a decision on the tissue within a very brief time. In the meantime the patient may be prepared for surgery in case the biopsy report is positive for cancer. Such a procedure means that the malignant growth can be removed with the greatest possible speed.

A biopsy may also be done on a tumor or other tissue, which is removed just as though it were a cancer. In this case, biopsy may confirm the wisdom of having removed the cancerous tissue or it may be a reassurance that no further likelihood of cancer remains since none existed in the first place.

X-ray examination of the patient is important when cancer of the stomach or other internal malignancies are suspected. Diagnosis of cancer is seldom made on the basis of x-ray evidence alone, but it may be helpful since certain tumors do show up on the x-ray film. In some types of cancer the x-ray evidence may be almost diagnostic in itself. In cancer of the prostate gland, for example, there is sometimes a spread of the disorder to the bones of the spinal column. The density of bone may be so altered as to suggest strongly that cancer of the prostate exists. The x-ray may also give important clues to cancer of other body structures.

In some hospitals and clinics, as well as in the offices of some private physicians, it is now a routine procedure to secure samples of certain body fluids for special staining and examination under the microscope. By this means cancer cells can be detected with a high degree of accuracy. About 95 per cent of the cancers of the uterus or cervix can be detected by this means. The same procedure is now used for examination of fluids discharged from the lungs when cancer of this structure is suspected. Cancer cells in the urine, sputum and stomach may also be detected in this manner.

Although there is no simple blood test for the discovery of cancer in its early stage, special blood studies are often helpful in the diagnosis of certain types of cancer. For example, a certain enzyme in the blood (phosphatase) is often increased in cancer of the prostate gland and cancer of the bone. Persistent low blood sugar is sometimes suggestive of a malignant tumor of the pancreas gland. Other malignancies may also be suggested by certain biochemical changes of the blood.

Fundamental to all the foregoing means for detecting cancer is the observation and judgment of the physician. Many cancer cells have typical characteristics that can be recognized easily by the physician if the cancer is located in a part of the body that is accessible to gross examination. Nevertheless, the physician seldom makes a diagnosis of cancer on the basis of observation alone. When a cancer is suspected, he will want to confirm or refute the suspicion by use of one or more of the methods described.

The Value of Early Diagnosis

Theoretically, all cancers can be cured if they are found early enough. From the practical standpoint, however, a certain amount of time is needed for the development of a cancer, and the insidious onset may cause delay in recognition and the seeking of medical advice.

It is still the patient who is primarily responsible for delay in the diagnosis of cancer. A study of this disease at a leading hospital showed that the patient was responsible for the delay in 32 per cent of the cases; the physician alone was responsible for delay in approximately 28 per cent. It is apparent that both the individual patient and the physician carry responsibilities for the early detection and diagnosis of cancer.

Approximately 50 per cent of all cancers develop in a part of the body that can be examined directly by the physician, so there is definite hope that if a person has a thorough medical examination regularly, cancer can be discovered in an early stage. Malignancies of the throat, thyroid gland, breast, skin, prostate glands, uterus and rectum can all be examined directly by the careful physician.

If treated late, all cancers are potentially fatal, although delayed treatment may be successful in some cases. Striking differences between the curability of cancer when it is treated after early diagnosis and

its curability when the disease is moderately advanced have been found consistently in all modern medical and surgical experience with this disease. The value of early diagnosis of cancer is shown in the accompanying table.

TYPE OF CANCER	Percentage Rate of cure where the diagnosis is:	
	Early	Late
Breast	78	36
Uterus	70	35
Lips	90	15
Skin	95	40
Rectum	40	3
Bladder	55	5
Large intestine	85	14

World Health Organization, 1960

There are variations in the length of time until death when cancer goes untreated. Cancer of the esophagus is rapidly fatal. When cancer of the mouth, stomach, larynx or prostate gland go completely untreated, about 50 per cent of such cases result in death in about one year. About 90 per cent of the patients with lymphomas and leukemias (malignancies of lymph tissue and blood, respectively), as well as those with cancer of the bladder, will die within five years after the onset of the malignancy if no treatment is obtained. Cancer of the breast, on the other hand, is the least malignant of the leading types of cancer, according to Dr. Michael B. Shimkin of the National Cancer Institute. Shimkin found that without any treatment whatsoever, approximately 20 per cent of those with breast cancer would be alive five years after the beginning of signs or symptoms of the disease. On the other hand, this means that if such cancer is totally untreated, 80 per cent of the breast cancer patients will have died within five years.

A study reported in 1956 on the survival of a group of 2065 persons in whom cancer had been diagnosed at an earlier date showed that approximately 33 per cent were still alive after five years. This figure was reached after adjustment of the statistics to rule out the normal, expected deaths that would have occurred in the group during this time.

More significant than the total survival percentage is the information that this study, and others like it, gives in relation to specific kinds of cancers. For example, 100 per cent of the women and 87 per cent of the men with skin cancers were still alive. Eighty-six per cent of the men with cancer of the lip were still alive. Some 51 per cent of the women with cancer of the uterus were still living, as were approximately 46 per cent of those with breast cancer.

It is strikingly clear from medical experience that cancer can be cured in a high percentage of cases when there is an early diagnosis of this disorder. Late diagnosis greatly increases the hazard of cancer. When no diagnosis is made, or when no medical treatment is obtained, the disease is eventually fatal.

Cancer of the Digestive Organs

Each year about 90,000 persons in the United States die from cancer of the digestive organs and the associated peritoneum (the membranes lining the abdomen and enveloping the digestive organs).

Cancer of the stomach is of great importance in this group of malignancies. Although many theories exist, its cause is unknown.

There are no symptoms by which cancer of the stomach can be recognized in the early stage. Loss of appetite, loss of weight, pain, anemia, blood in the stools and the vomiting of blood may all be signs of cancer of the stomach, but these seldom occur in the early stages of the disease. In fact, some evidence suggests that cancer of the stomach may be present for at least twenty months before such signs and symptoms appear.

The most effective means for discovering cancer of the stomach is the use of the x-ray or fluoroscope. In the hands of a trained specialist the x-ray picture of the stomach gives important evidence of cancer when this disease is present.

The only worth-while treatment for cancer of the stomach is surgical removal. One of the most comprehensive studies of the value of surgery in treatment of cancer of the stomach has been made by physicians at the Mayo Clinic. Over a period of forty-three years there were 9620 patients operated on for cancer of the stomach at the Clinic. The greatest loss of patients occurred among those in whom cancer was found when the disease was too far advanced for surgery to be of much help.

Not all patients operated on for cancer of the stomach in the Mayo study had the disease. It appears that of the number operated upon *who actually had cancer of the stomach,* only about 14 per cent were alive five years after the cancer had been removed. However, of the 86 per cent who did not survive for this period of time, 56 per cent were lost because the disease was too far advanced at the time of operation.

The use of the gastroscope, a device for inspecting the interior of the stomach, is often a valuable aid in diagnosis. The examining physician can actually see the inside of the stomach and may even take pictures of the interior. Obviously there are many cases in which this can be of real assistance in interpretation of x-rays of the stomach. A combination of the two diagnostic procedures often gives a better chance of proper diagnosis.

Cancer of the stomach can be cured if detected soon enough. As many as 50 per cent of the patients operated on for this disease may survive five years or more if the disease is recognized before it spreads to surrounding lymph nodes. As one physician has put it, the strongest forces to overcome are inertia and neglect. Cancer of the stomach can be and is being cured frequently.

Cancer of the Breast

About 25,000 persons die from cancer of the breast annually in this country. It is the leading form of malignancy in women, and The American Cancer Society reports that approximately 52,000 women are found with cancer of the breast each year.

It has been shown that a very high percentage of cancers of the breast can be treated successfully if treatment is begun in time. If the disease is detected before it spreads under the arms, 90 per cent of the patients receiving treatment can be cured.

Cancer of the breast occurs approximately twice as frequently as any other type of cancer in women. About 4 per cent of all adult women suffer cancer of the breast, although it is rare before the age of twenty-five years.

Inspection and examination of the breast by the physician is essential for early diagnosis of cancer. There are certain signs, however, that may be observed by the patient. Though these do not always indicate cancer, they should not be neglected, but should be investigated by a competent medical authority.

A discharge from the nipple, for example, must always be considered somewhat abnormal, even though it may not indicate cancer. Milk is often discharged from one or both breasts, but this is harmless. A discharge of pus from the nipples is likely to be a reflection of infection or abscess.

A discharge of blood should always be investigated promptly. It must not be assumed, however, that a bleeding nipple means a sure diagnosis of cancer. Dr. Ian MacDonald of Los Angeles has reported a study of 183 women with bleeding nipples. Nearly 60 per cent of these women did not have cancer, although they did have harmless tumors. In this study only about 4 per cent of cancers of the breast caused bleeding. In the New York Presbyterian Hospital only 1 per cent of the breast cancer cases were accompanied by a discharge from the nipple.

In other words, cancer of the breast does not usually cause an abnormal discharge, but any discharge should be carefully investigated by a physician, since this may indicate a malignant tumor (cancer).

NIPPLE DISCHARGE
"The significance of nipple discharge lies in the insignificance with which it is regarded."
Dr. Edward F. Lewison
and Dr. Robert G. Chambers

Erosion of the nipple is one of the important signs of cancer. It is especially diagnostic of the cancer known as Paget's disease. Not all erosions of the nipple are due to cancer, but that a specific erosion is not should be made certain in any individual case by a careful medical examination. The percentage of cancer in such cases is so high that microscopic examination of the tissue removed is necessary. Fortunately this type of cancer is less malignant than other forms, and cure may be obtained even when the erosion has involved a rather large surface of the skin over the breast.

The presence of a lump in the breast should impel any woman to consult a physician. The most common condition that may cause such lumps, however, is not cancer, but chronic cystic mastitis. This is a change in the breast brought about by endocrine or glandular activity. These lumps usually represent thickened breast tissue and cysts. The great majority of such cysts will not develop into cancer. The diagnosis is fairly simple, and the patient may be treated and then reassured.

Many physicians, as well as the American Cancer Society, now favor self-examination of the breasts by all women, since by this means early symptoms of cancer may be revealed. Instructions on self-examination of the breast may be obtained from the family physician or from a film entitled "Breast Self-Examination," produced by the American Cancer Society and the National Cancer Institute.

Surgery, radiation and chemotherapy are all useful in the treatment of breast cancer.

Although no drug or chemical has yet been found to cure this disorder, the chemotherapeutic agents have been found to be very useful in the treatment of breast cancers that cannot be operated on, or are too far advanced to be cured. In these cases sex hormones and cortisone have sometimes been found to be helpful, but certain newer drugs such as thio-TEPA have been found to lengthen life and to make the patient more comfortable by relieving pain and restoring, for months or years, the capacity to work at home or in business. Thio-TEPA may be injected directly at the site of a malignant tumor and may also be used in the bloodstream to prevent the spread of cancer cells to other parts of the body.

Surgery is still the most effective means for the curing of breast cancer, especially if an early diagnosis is made.

Radical mastectomy is a type of breast surgery that calls for complete removal of the breast and the lymphatic glands associated with this tissue. This includes removal of the lymphatic glands under the arm as well as in other parts of the chest wall. This type of complete surgery carries the best possible chance of cure.

Sometimes patients do not understand that the smaller the breast cancer, the more important it is to have a radical mastectomy. Complete removal of the breast and the associated glandular tissues in such a case can give almost 100 per cent cure. Radical mastectomy is an extensive surgical operation calling for removal of the skin over the breast, removal of certain muscles, dissection of the underarm area and removal of all these tissues in one block. It is necessary to remove certain muscles because only by this measure can the lymph glands hidden beneath be located and removed. Since cancer of the breast spreads to other parts of the body through these lymphatic glands, it is necessary to remove them in order to guarantee a better chance of cure.

From 90 to 95 per cent of the women who have cancer in one breast will never have the disease in the second breast. A careful search for malignancy must be made regularly in the second breast, however, to catch the few cases that may occur, no matter how long a time has elapsed since the disease was treated in the first breast.

To summarize, cancer of the breast can be detected early and can be cured. The most effective cure is that type of surgery known as radical mastectomy. More than 30,000 mastectomies are performed each year in the United States.

Breast Nursing and Cancer

Laboratory research with experimental *animals* in recent years has shown that a factor may exist in breast milk which has a relation to the development of cancer.

It has been found possible to breed both cancer-resistant and cancer-susceptible strains of mice. In one experiment, when the offspring of cancer-resistant mice were nursed by mothers with high susceptibility to breast tumors the number of cancers grew from 5 per cent to approximately 78 per cent in a single generation. In another experiment, when the offspring of cancer-resistant mice were removed at birth and nursed only on cancer-susceptible mice the percentage of mice with cancer rose from 5 per cent to 44 per cent.

On the other hand, when the offspring of highly cancerous mice were removed from their mothers at birth and then nursed only on a strain of mice that had high resistance to breast cancer, the percentage of cancers in the nursing mice fell from about 69 per cent to 55 per cent.

It has not yet been substantiated that the milk of human mothers who are susceptible to breast cancer will increase the number of malignant tumors in their children. More research is needed on this subject. Some investigators feel, however, that if there has been an unusual prevalence of cancer of the breast in the women of a family, it might be preferable for the children to be bottle-nursed rather than fed at the breast.

More research is needed on this subject before sound conclusions can be drawn so far as humans are concerned. It does appear that *in animals* there is convincing evidence that breast milk may improve the resistance to cancer or lower the resistance to the disease, according to whether the nursing mother is herself of a cancer-resistant strain of animals or is from a cancer-susceptible family.

Cancer of the Uterus

Among college women the incidence of invasive cancer of the cervix or uterus is small, being present in only about 5 out of every 100,000 women in the age group between 20 to 30.

In succeeding decades the finding of cancer of the uterus rises so rapidly that the American Cancer Society recommends that women over the age of 30 or 35 years should be routinely examined by a physician for this type of cancer.

Cancer of the uterus is the second leading cause of death from malignancies among women. Each year about 15,000 women die from this type of cancer in the United States. Probably 10,000 of these could be saved by early diagnosis.

Because this is an internal type of tumor and because signs and symptoms of the disease are virtually absent in the early stages, most cancers of the uterus are discovered by pelvic examination. Since most cases are found only in the obstetrician's office in pelvic examinations associated with pregnancy, childbirth, and pelvic diseases and disorders of various kinds, there has been an effort to establish cancer prevention clinics on a national scale for the pelvic examination of women in good health.

The American Cancer Society has rec-ommended that the office of every physician should be looked upon as a cancer detection center, since many more patients will visit the doctor's office than will attend the cancer detection clinic for examination. The Society does favor the continuation of cancer detection clinic programs, however.

Many physicians who specialize in the treatment of pelvic disorders in women now make the microscopic examination of uterine or vaginal discharges a routine procedure in the search for early signs of cancer of the uterus. By this diagnostic method it is possible to identify cancer cells when they are properly stained and observed under the microscope. It has been shown that this method of discovering cancer of the uterus affords the earliest possible diagnosis and permits a cure of the disease in better than 90 per cent of the early cases.

Cancer of the Prostate

Cancer of the prostate is one of the most frequent kinds of malignant growths in men. Each year there are close to 14,000 deaths from this disease in the United States.

In the early stages there are few symptoms of the disorder. As the disease develops, cancer tissue from the diseased prostate gland spreads to other parts of the body.

Cancer of the prostate occurs mostly in older men. A reduction in urinary output, the presence of pain, and advancing age are some of the factors that may lead the physician to suspect this disease. Blood studies help in the diagnosis of cancer of the prostate, since the acid phosphatase usually rises in the blood, although this biochemical change is not always present.

Although the chance of obtaining a cure of cancer of the prostate is relatively small, medical and surgical treatment today can lengthen life considerably. The progress of the disease can be stopped by hormone treatment, removal of the prostate gland by surgery, and x-ray irradiation of the prostatic region and the testicles. By hormone treatment alone the length of life may be extended as much as three to seven years. If the disease occurs in a person past the age of sixty or seventy years, this increase in the length of life represents a considerable medical service.

A study of 1560 patients with cancer of the prostate gland was reported by Dr. Thomas L. Pool and Dr. Gershom J. Thompson, of Rochester, Minnesota. These physicians found that maligancy of the prostate gland can seldom be detected early enough for anything but conservative treatment. This is not discouraging, for approximately 40 per cent of the patients in this group were still alive five years after surgery of a conservative nature. In some cases castration and use of the hormone diethylstilbestrol by mouth were strikingly beneficial. These specialists concluded that a spirit of optimism regarding the treatment of cancer of the prostate can be justifiably maintained. Though permanent cures may not be obtained, life can be considerably lengthened and pain can be controlled, so that patients with cancer of the prostate can live useful lives in freedom from suffering.

Cancer of the Lung

During the past twenty-five years or so, autopsy studies throughout the world have shown a phenomenal increase in the number of deaths due to cancer of the lung. During 1958 in the United States there were 36,116 deaths from cancer of the respiratory system reported, and mortality from this cause is increasing rather than decreasing.

There are no early symptoms of cancer of the lung that can be distinguished from those causing the common respiratory diseases. There are no characteristic physical signs of the disease.

Symptoms or signs arise only after cancer of the lung has been present for some time. At the Lahey Clinic in Boston an analysis of the symptoms and signs of cancer of the lung in 157 cases showed that 93 per cent of the patients had cough, 54 per cent experienced pain or chest discomfort, 53 per cent brought up sputum from the chest when they coughed, 44 per cent spat up blood, and 14 per cent showed wheezing.

None of these symptoms or signs would permit the physician to make a diagnosis of cancer of the lung without verification by other means. Any of them, however, should cause the physician to suspect that cancer of the lung might be present, just as he would suspect tuberculosis and a variety of other diseases of the chest.

The best chance for detection of cancer of the lung in an early stage rests with the periodic x-ray examination of the chest. Cases found in this manner may be in an early enough stage so that surgical cure can be achieved. Patients cured of lung cancer have lived for more than seventeen years in good health.

The microscopic examination of sputum or other material produced from the chest may give verification of suspicious findings from the x-ray. Cancer cells in the discharged tissues or sputum from the lungs can be recognized under the microscope if they are properly stained. The Papanicolaou manner of staining the cells or tissue fragments is one of the most dependable methods.

The bronchoscope can also be inserted into the bronchial tubes to a certain distance for examination of a suspected tumor in that area. A telescopic lens may assist the examining surgeon in getting a better view of the bronchial tissues. In early cancer, however, it may not be possible to recognize the disease by means of the bronchoscope.

Surgical exploration of the chest in suspected cases of cancer of the lung may be advisable. Chest surgeons feel that cancer of the lung is such a fatal type of disease that suspicious shadows on the x-ray film of the chest are sufficient verification of the need for exploratory chest surgery. If it is confirmed by this means that the patient has cancer of the lung, the malignancy can be removed in the same operation.

Air pollution is suspected of having a relation to the cause of cancer of the lung. The increase of smog in industrial communities, with its heavy pollution of the air, is thought by many physicians to be an important cause of lung cancer. Studies in various parts of the United States, in Europe and South Africa tend to give support to this viewpoint.

CANCER AND MOTOR EXHAUST GASES

". . . Exposure in urban motor traffic is a significant factor in lung cancer incidence . . . driving mileages above 12,000 per year are associated with a lung cancer hazard fully twice that of driving mileages below this level . . ."

Dr. C. A. Mills, 1960

In recent years the smoking of tobacco has also been suspected of causing cancer of the lung.

The American Cancer Society study of the smoking habits and lung cancer deaths of 188,078 men from fifty to seventy years of age was reported in June, 1955, to the American Medical Association. At that time four main conclusions appeared justified, according to the directors of the study. These four conclusions were:

1. The lung cancer death rate was more than three times as great for smokers of two packs of cigarettes daily than for smokers of one pack or less daily.

2. Lung cancer death rates are high among cigarette smokers and very low among nonsmokers.

3. Lung cancer is a rare disease among men who have never smoked at all.

4. Among smokers of two packs of cigarettes daily the deaths from lung cancer were twenty-seven times as great as among those men who had never smoked regularly.

The association of smoking and cancer of the lung is discussed more fully in the chapter on tobacco and health.

Once the diagnosis of cancer of the lung has been made the surgery is relatively safe. One group of surgeons has been able to remove individual lobes of the lung or whole lungs diseased with cancer at an operating mortality of less than 4 per cent. Thus, 96 per cent of the patients who submit to surgery for cancer of the lung survive the operation. The chance for recovery from the cancer depends upon how early the diagnosis has been made and how soon the surgical treatment has been obtained.

Leukemia

Leukemia is a malignancy (cancer) of the blood-forming organs. It is a type of cancer in which the white blood cells show an abnormal increase and infiltration of other tissues, such as bone marrow, spleen and lymph nodes.

Acute leukemia occurs most frequently in children under the age of five and is one of the leading causes of death in this age group, although it can occur at any age. Chronic, or more slowly developing, leukemia is most frequently found after the age of fifty. About 12,000 persons die from this disease each year in the United States.

There is no definite cure for any type of leukemia, although life may be extended and the disease held in remission for a while by such drugs as 6-mercaptopurine, methotrexate, thio-TEPA, myleran, TEM, nitrogen mustard, urethane and others. The drugs themselves frequently cause toxic reactions. Hormones such as corticotropin and cortisone are also helpful for some weeks or months. X-rays and radioactive phosphorus help, but all types of leukemia are fatal, and no real cure has yet been found.

Cancer of the Bladder

About 3 or 4 per cent of all the deaths from cancer in the United States are due to cancer of the bladder. As with other cancers, there is usually no pain associated with cancer of the bladder. The first symptom is usually blood in the urine, although this may not be apparent until the urine is examined under the microscope. Often this is the only symptom of cancer of either the bladder or the kidney.

Blood in the urine, however, may come from a number of other causes such as kidney stones, various types of infections that affect the excretory system, injuries to the kidney or bladder, tuberculosis and other disorders. Obviously, any blood in the urine should receive prompt medical investigation.

Untreated cancer of the bladder is rapidly fatal. In one study of sixty patients who had this disease, but did not receive medical or surgical treatment, the average lapse of time between the onset of symptoms and admission to the hospital was nine months. The time between beginning of symptoms and death was only thirteen months. Only about 10 per cent of such patients will be alive after five years if no treatment is obtained.

Is Cancer Hereditary?

It has been reported by a University of Pennsylvania medical research team that cancer of the breast does not run in families. This group made an investigation of cancer in a group of 12,000 persons over a period of eight years and found no evidence that breast maligancies were inherited.

In this research a group of 200 women who had cancer of the breast were compared with another group of 200 women without cancer of that part of the body in respect to the number of relatives with the same disease. In all, 12,000 relatives of the two groups were studied. There was no evidence of the inheritance of breast cancer.

At times it appears that cancer definitely runs in certain families. This does not prove, however, that cancer is hereditary. Such an occurrence could happen entirely by chance. It may also be that certain families are more cancer-susceptible than others. This would still not prove that cancer can be hereditary. On the other hand, it does appear certain that retinoblastoma, a specific cancer of the eye, is hereditary.

Studies in human genetics have also revealed some families in which cancer has been widely prevalent. In one family of four generations, gastrointestinal cancer was found to be widespread. Members of the second generation had cancers on a widespread scale; more than 40 per cent had the disease. This family is being studied to see whether a definite hereditary factor can be found for cancer.

In another family, cancer occurred in both breasts in a mother, two daughters and in a grand-daughter. In each instance the development of the cancer was identical, and it was located in exactly the same sites. Members of the family stated that other relatives had been known to have cancer, but this was not definitely proved.

It has not been proved that cancer is hereditary in human beings. On the other hand, it has not been adequately proved that the disease is not hereditary. All that can be said at this stage is that not enough evidence is available to draw a definite conclusion.

Treatment of Cancer

There are now three accepted methods of treating cancer: surgery, radiation, and chemotherapy.

Surgery is the oldest method and often the most successful. If a malignancy can be completely removed from the body before it has spread to other tissues, an assured cure has been achieved. Surgery is used for the diagnosis of cancer as well as for treatment, and cancer prevention can often be achieved by the surgical removal of pre-cancerous growths. Surgery has other uses in the management of cancer (such as the extension of life) even when the malignant growth may not be removable.

Radiation has been used in the treatment of cancer for about 50 years. It is reported by the National Cancer Institute that about 6 out of every 10 cancer patients are now treated by radiation. X-rays and radioisotopes are the principle forms of radiation used in the treatment of this disease.

Chemotherapy, or the drug treatment of cancer, is the newest method of treatment, but none of the drugs have been reported as giving complete cures, although they have lengthened life, relieved pain and stopped the growth of some malignancies. About 50,000 chemicals a year are tested for possible value against cancer. Of this number about 1 in 1,000 is given further attention after an initial screening.

Some of the more important chemicals that have been found to have value in the treatment of various kinds of cancers are thio-TEPA, nitrogen mustard, TEM, methotrexate, urethane, chlorambucil and myleran.

Cancer Quackery

Perhaps because cancer has been and is one of our most difficult medical problems, there has been much quackery in this field. This is extremely unfortunate because the inadequate treatment of cancer often results in the death of the patient; whereas, if a reputable physician had been consulted, the life of the patient might have been saved.

The medical profession has conducted a vigorous campaign against cancer quacks for more than a generation. Nevertheless the problem of incompetent advice and dishonest treatment for cancer is still a problem today.

Medical and public health journals, as well as court records, give frequent examples of quackery in this field. In Louisiana, for example, on July 31, 1952, the United States Court of Appeals ruled against the Hoxsey Cancer Clinic because of interstate shipment of two colored liquids intended for use in the treatment of cancer.

After listening to five nationally known cancer specialists and about fifty physicians and pathologists as well as twenty-five defense witnesses, the Court concluded that the Hoxsey remedies did not cure cancer.

It was testified that the drugs used in the two colored liquids were a laxative, potassium iodide, extracts of prickly ash, red clover blossom, alfalfa and lactated pepsin, a flavoring used to disguise the unpleasant taste of potassium.

Despite this court decision the Food and Drug Administration still found it necessary on April 4, 1956, to issue a public warning against the treatment of cancer by the Hoxsey method. The Administration pointed out that the Hoxsey treatment would cost the patient four hundred dollars plus sixty dollars in additional fees, and would yield nothing of any value in the cure of cancer. Quackery in the field of cancer is difficult to control.

Questions

1. Is it better or worse to avoid the development of a fear of cancer by letting a person remain in ignorance of the disease?

2. Who has the major responsibility for the early detection of cancer: the patient or the doctor?

3. Why is the cancer quack an especially dangerous element in our society, and what should be done about this kind of person?

4. Why is it said that theoretically every cancer can be cured, and under what conditions would this be true?

5. On moral and philosophical grounds, would a physician ever be justified in failing to do all he can to keep the patient alive who is in perpetual pain from an incurable cancer?

3. Crile, George, Jr.: *Cancer and Common Sense*. New York, Viking Press, 1955.

4. Public Health Service: *Treating Cancer*, Publication No. 690, Washington, D.C., Superintendent of Documents, 1960.

For Further Reading

1. Butler, Brancelia: *Cancer through the Ages: The Evolution of Hope*. Fairfax, Va., Virginia Press, 1955.

2. Cameron, Charles S.: *The Truth about Cancer*. Englewood Cliffs, N.J., Prentice-Hall, 1956.

Recommended Film

American Cancer Society: *Breast Self-Examination*. American Cancer Society, 521 W. 57th St., New York. (This film should be shown to female audiences only, preferably with a guest physician on hand for discussion.)

25

HEALTH IN

MARRIAGE AND PREGNANCY

IN 1960 there were approximately forty million married couples in the United States.

The greatest marrying age for both men and women is between twenty and twenty-five years, but almost as many women are married *after* as *before* these years, and more men.

A study of 600,000 marriages made by the National Office of Vital Statistics has revealed that *at the time of marriage approximately 93 per cent of the grooms and nearly 70 per cent of the brides were twenty years of age or older.* If you are under twenty years of age, it is not to be expected that you should be married. The statistics are all against it.

Once a person is married, the chances are overwhelmingly in favor of that person's remaining married for a good many years. National statistics show that 92 per

Per Cent Married Among Females 1958	
Age	Per Cent*
14–17	5
18–19	34
20–24	69
25–29	86
30–34	89
35–44	87
45–54	79

* Rounded to nearest whole number.

From: Bureau of the Census

cent of the women who have married before the age of forty-four are still married at that age. *A continued reduction in the death rate has been an important factor in keeping families intact.*

Good Health Is Basic

Ideally, two people planning marriage should have perfect health. Ideal conditions, however, rarely exist. If one partner has a communicable illness, he may transmit it to the other. If one partner has a hereditary disease, it may be passed on to the children. If the husband is chronically bedridden, it becomes necessary for the wife, who may be untrained, to earn a living; if the wife is hospitalized for a long period, the strain upon the husband may be great. The result of any of these conditions may be a deep emotional disturbance for the couple.

LOSS OF HUSBANDS AND FATHERS

"... each year thousands of wives are left with a heavy burden due to the untimely death of their husbands. Last year alone, about 100,000 children were orphaned by the death of fathers under age 45 ... After the husband's 45th birthday, family responsibility lessens rapidly as the children marry or leave the home for other reasons."
Metropolitan Life Insurance Company, 1959

Diabetes is a hereditary disorder. If diabetes should be present *on both sides* of the contemplated marriage, even though neither of the prospective marriage partners actually has the disease itself, then it is possible that as many as 25 per cent of their children may have diabetes. In such an instance, wherein both the prospective marriage partners would be known as carriers of diabetes, the actual number of children who would have the disease would vary according to circumstances. If the children of this union lived long enough, and especially if they suffered from overweight, then about 25 per cent could be expected to have diabetes.

On the other hand, if diabetes is known to be present *on only one side* of the planned marriage, it is unlikely that any of the children will actually have the disease themselves, although all of them would be carriers of the disorder.

Most mental illnesses are probably not hereditary, although some authorities believe that the severe depressive states are inherited in about 80 per cent of the cases. By "depressive states" is not meant variations in ordinary moods, but severe depressions. A tendency toward them is more likely to be due to heredity than any of the other common mental illnesses.

Rheumatic fever, it is believed, is due to heredity in the sense that the person who has an allergic reaction to streptococcal infections of the throat is more liable to get rheumatic fever. It is the allergic state which is inherited.

Epilepsy is not hereditary, but a brain wave pattern is inherited, and some patterns are abnormal in that they make the individual more likely to suffer epilepsy.

Communicable disease is an obvious hazard to marriage. Disease is spread by the intimacy of man and wife. Moreover, a marriage begun under such circumstances carries a burden. Some states have passed laws making marriage illegal between persons with certain communicable diseases, such as tuberculosis and venereal disease.

In the case of tuberculosis not only is the wife or husband endangered, but entire families may be infected and even wiped out if the disease is active.

A chronic illness of long duration may use up a family's entire savings and bring on heavy indebtedness. Illness is costly. Moreover, living in a home in which someone is gravely ill has its emotional hazards. Responsibility for the care of the sick places restrictions upon normal activity, which exact a price. The husband of an invalid wife may resent ceaseless medical bills; the wife who has to go out and earn a living for her husband may rebel against the burden, while the patient himself may feel bitterly that he is an undeserved load upon his wife instead of being her support.

Good mental health is absolutely essential for success in marriage. It is not the mere absence of mental illness that is important. It is even more vital that persons who are stable and reasonably well adjusted should know enough about the principles of mental hygiene to be able to contribute to the integrity of the family throughout its duration.

The Rh Problem in Marriage

An example of a potential health problem about which people who are contemplating marriage and parenthood should be informed is that of the Rh factor.

The Rh factor can be defined as one or more of a group of substances found in, or on the surface of, red blood cells. The Rh factor received its name because it was first observed in the red blood cells of Rhesus monkeys. The first two letters of this species of monkey have been used ever since to designate the comparable factor in humans.

About 15 per cent of all pregnant women are Rh-negative, according to medical studies, which means they do not have the Rh factor present in their red blood cells. When these women marry Rh-positive men (those who do have the Rh factor in their red blood cells) there is a possibility of serious damage to the unborn child when the woman becomes pregnant, providing the coming child inherits the Rh-positive type of blood cell. This happens in about 75 per cent of the children born of an Rh-positive husband and an Rh-negative wife.

The Rh-positive baby who is carried inside an Rh-negative mother may sensitize the mother to the Rh factor. The mother then produces in her blood serum antibodies against the Rh factor of the red blood cells of the unborn baby. In a physiologic, immunologic way, the mother turns against her baby. Her antibodies may destroy or damage great numbers of the red blood cells of the unborn baby. When this happens the health of the baby may be seriously impaired or he may even die before or shortly after birth. Usually it takes one or more pregnancies for the mother to become sensitized to the Rh factor, hence the first baby born to parents with an Rh incompatibility is usually healthy and undamaged. By the time of the second baby the mother may be sensitized to a point where she begins producing antibodies. The second baby thus may or may not be injured. By the time of a third child, antibodies may be produced in such abundance that there is serious danger to the child.

It is possible for a woman who is Rh-negative and who had had a previous blood transfusion with Rh-positive blood to become sensitized even before her first pregnancy. In that case the first child may be adversely affected by the mother's antibody production.

There is no sensitization and no hazard to the baby if the mother is Rh-positive, even if she is married to an Rh-negative husband. There is also no complication if both husband and wife are Rh-negative or if both are Rh-positive. In other words, they have compatible Rh blood types.

There is little that can be done to protect the baby during the mother's pregnancy, but once the baby is born blood transfusions in the hospital can replace the greater part of the damaged red blood cells so that there is greater chance of survival and good health.

Most men and women have Rh blood types that are not incompatible. Studies show that approximately 90 per cent of those who marry will not be troubled with this problem. It makes sense, though, to find out where your marriage stands before your baby runs the hazard of being damaged by different blood types of father and mother.

At birth the baby who has been damaged by the antibodies of the mother is apt to be jaundiced, to suffer from progressive anemia, to show swelling and enlargement of the liver and spleen and to suffer from hemorrhage. Such a baby will have a difficult time living or escaping permanent damage if it does survive, unless it is treated in the hospital by exchange transfusions. In this type of blood transfusion part of the baby's blood is withdrawn and replaced by undamaged blood which then mingles with the baby's remaining blood supply. Successive transfusions of this type gradually exchange the baby's blood for fresh, healthy blood until he is able to manufacture his own undamaged red blood cells.

It can be seen that it is very important to know in advance whether your baby is apt to be damaged by antibodies produced in the mother's blood because of an Rh incompatibility with the unborn infant. It may mean the baby's life.

Marriage Itself Is Healthful

Fewer married people have mental breakdowns than unmarried people and married people live longer. Of course this can be because the healthier and more stable people are most apt to marry, but it can also represent the results of better nutrition, emotional satisfaction and other advantages of a happy marriage.

Twenty Things To Know

Today many young people prepare for careers, but neglect preparation for taking care of a family. The truth is that to make a success of marriage is probably the most important thing you can do. It demands that you bring to the job as much of the accumulated experience and wisdom of your elders as you can absorb. It is not easy to have a superior marriage.

Just *how* should one prepare for it? Nobody can give you one sure-fire formula. But from the *health* standpoint a possible course in preparation for marriage might include the following 20 topics:

1. HEALTH QUALIFICATIONS FOR MARRIAGE. Anyone contemplating marriage should know why some illnesses make marriage inadvisable, either temporarily or permanently.

2. VENEREAL DISEASES. Because the venereal diseases are associated almost entirely with sex relations, it is important that anyone contemplating marriage should know something about the magnitude of this problem and how it can be handled in regard to prevention and treatment. This problem is discussed in another chapter.

3. MENSTRUATION. Both the husband and the wife should have an understanding of the normal menstrual period and problems associated with it, as well as the symptoms of abnormalities of menstruation and their significance.

4. BIRTH CONTROL AND ASSOCIATED PROBLEMS. Some people have religious scruples against birth control, but even when these do not exist, instruction in the details of birth control is the responsibility of the private physician rather than the school. However, any course in preparation for marriage can discuss health reasons for birth control and the broad public health aspects of the matter.

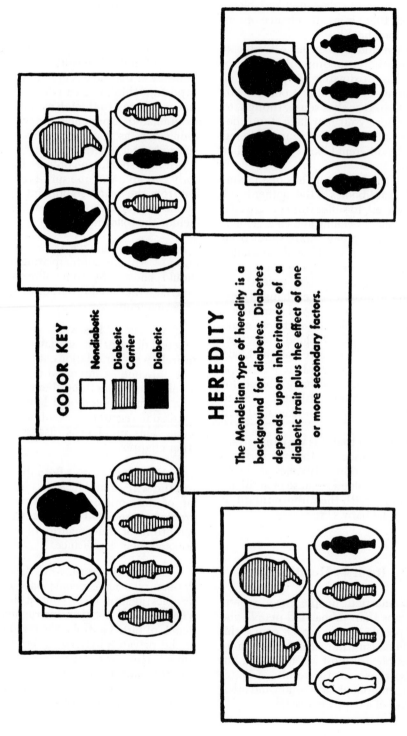

COLOR KEY

☐ Nondiabetic

▦ Diabetic Carrier

■ Diabetic

HEREDITY

The Mendelian type of heredity is a background for diabetes. Diabetes depends upon inheritance of a diabetic trait plus the effect of one or more secondary factors.

Figure 42. Diabetes is a hereditary disorder that prospective marriage partners should know about. (Courtesy of Eli Lilly and Co.)

Heart disease, syphilis, active tuberculosis, diabetes, kidney diseases and mental disorders are among some of the conditions accepted by physicians as making birth control desirable. Whether or not a married couple is justified in using birth control methods is a matter of religious beliefs and conscience as well as of health and economics.

5. PRENATAL CARE. Proper medical care during pregnancy is important to both the mother and the child, and hence to the husband indirectly, since his happiness is bound up with the welfare of his wife and children.

6. CHILDBIRTH. Childbirth is a normal process and, for the overwhelming majority of women, without unusual danger or complication. The idea that it is an excruciating ordeal is a false one that has almost reached the proportions of superstition, and must be erased by the truth.

YOUNG MOTHERS

"Most babies are born to relatively young mothers. This is advantageous to both mother and child. Not only are the hazards of maternity lowest among younger women, but the chances are very high that they will live to rear their children to maturity."

Metropolitan Life Insurance Company, 1959

---

7. DISEASE AND PREGNANCY. The effects of such disorders as German measles, diabetes, tuberculosis, venereal diseases, and so on, on the unborn child should be well understood by both partners to a marriage if proper medical steps are to be taken.

8. LEADING CAUSES OF INFANT DEATHS. Knowledge of the leading causes of infant deaths can help parents prevent fatalities by cooperation with medical authorities and by control of conditions which cause such deaths.

9. LEADING CAUSES OF MATERNAL DEATHS. Knowing the causes of mortality for mothers in pregnancy can be of great help in prevention of illness or death in childbirth.

10. INFANT AND CHILD CARE. A vast amount of information is needed by both parents in regard to infant and child care. Breast versus bottle feeding, schedules, crying babies, rest, discipline, need for affection, and so on, are only a few of the many problems associated with bringing up a child.

11. CHILDREN'S DISEASES AND THEIR PREVENTION. Parents should have at least a rudimentary idea of what to expect in the way of children's diseases and how to protect the child against them.

12. IMMUNIZATION IN INFANCY AND CHILDHOOD. Children can be protected against certain diseases, such as whooping cough, diphtheria, tetanus, poliomyelitis, smallpox, and others, and no conscientious parent would knowingly fail to give his children such protection.

13. JUVENILE DELINQUENCY. The mental health of childhood and the role of the family are overwhelmingly important in the prevention of juvenile delinquency. Parents must understand not only their responsibilities, but also how to exercise them for the welfare of all in the family.

14. MEDICAL CARE FOR THE FAMILY. It has been said that a great number of people are "medically indigent," meaning that their incomes are too low to enable them to afford all the medical help that is needed. A number of hospital plans and a variety of health insurance policies exist by which this protection can be made available to families with modest incomes.

15. HOME NURSING. Information on first aid, home nursing, medicines, when to call in a physician and associated problems, is important to the health of the family and at times may save a life.

16. HOME ACCIDENTS.   It is wise to become acquainted with hazardous areas in the home and to know the leading causes of accidents in the family, since as many people are killed annually in the home as on public highways.

17. FAMILY NUTRITION.   The wife who prepares meals should be well grounded in the selection and preparation of food to provide the maximum benefits in nutrition for her family. She should also understand the tensions and anxieties that may be created at the table by too much emphasis upon the eating habits of family members. For purposes of cooperation, the husband should understand the principles of good nutrition.

18. HEALTH PROBLEMS OF OLDER MEMBERS OF THE FAMILY.   Increasingly, as modern science prolongs life, it is important for people to become aware of the health problems of older people and how to care for them. The chronic diseases of age, menopause and mental hygiene are some problems of the aged.

19. MALADJUSTMENTS IN MARRIAGE. Knowledge of the causes of marriage failures, and ways in which to smooth out and bridge over incompatibilities between man and wife, help people to save marriages which might otherwise end in divorce.

COMMUNICATION AND UNDERSTANDING
"Most people, in fact, never learn to know their own feelings and how to handle them well enough to play a crucial role in other people's lives ... there is no right side or wrong side in marital disagreements—*just different sides ...* we must stop looking for the *right* and the *wrong* ... let us try to understand our different feelings."

Robert A. Harper, 1958

---

20. MENTAL HEALTH.   The great majority of marriage problems develop out of mental health problems, and such difficulties do not start with a marriage ceremony, but in childhood. Prevention, therefore, lies in preventing emotional disturbances in childhood, which necessitates improving the home atmosphere.

Probably the most immediate effects can be produced through a good program of instruction in the basic principles of mental hygiene, for marriage is basically a problem of understanding human beings.

In-laws and Mental Health in Marriage

When a young couple marry, they face the task of setting up an entirely new family unit. Ideally, it should be completely independent of interference by in-laws, for the roles of wife and husband are vastly different from the roles of daughter and son. Essentially, perhaps, the difference is that as a child you *take;* as a married adult you have to *give.* As a child, much thinking is done for you; as an adult, you must think for yourself and others.

Marriage requires adjustment on the part of two young people to a life situation that has changed for them. They must become independent and self-reliant. The marriage requires adjustment on the part of their in-laws as well: they must unlearn their former vigilance to protect their children, and learn new habits of remote self-control.

Many divorces have had as their immediate cause interference on the part of relatives. Overpossessive parents of overdependent young people are especially guilty of wrecking marriages.

Legal Reasons for Divorce

The causes for divorce which are recognized by law vary from state to state. In some states, for example, only adultery is recognized legally as sufficient reason for dissolving a marriage. The result is often collusion to build a case for divorce, in which the divorcing parties work together to fake an incident of infidelity. Some states have a narrow range of legal causes; other states a broad range.

On a national basis there are nine major *legal* reasons for divorce, as follows: (1) mental cruelty, (2) desertion, (3) adultery, (4) neglect to provide, (5) habitual drunkenness, (6) insanity, (7) fraud, duress or mistaken identity, (8) bigamy, and (9) impotence.

Health Reasons for Divorce

Either mental or physical illness could be the underlying explanation of any of the nine foregoing legal causes for divorce. It is especially apparent, however, that poor emotional or physical health is involved in mental cruelty, habitual drunkenness, insanity and impotence. In other words, divorce statistics support the conclusion that health is important to a successful marriage.

1. MENTAL CRUELTY. Mental suffering, the emotional disturbance arising out of a marriage that is unhappy, can seriously affect physical health. Most courts now recognize this fact. A great variety of emotional conflicts can exist between a married couple, but the term "mental cruelty" is so broad and so abstract that almost any sort of emotional conflict can justifiably be labeled with it. As a consequence, mental cruelty is used more as a cause for divorce than any other reason. Women use it more than men; it is more easily accepted as proof against a man than against a woman. Perhaps a tradition of chivalry is the explanation of this trend.

In a sense, the charge of mental cruelty in a divorce suit is an indication that one or both partners in a marriage have not understood the simple principles of human relations. In other words, there has been a failure to recognize and meet the basic emotional needs of the individual. One or both mates have not known enough about

mental hygiene to establish a happy marriage. Both mental health and mental illness are discussed in other chapters.

2. HABITUAL DRUNKENNESS. A lot of bad publicity comes to a couple seeking divorce on this basis, especially if they are prominent enough to be newsworthy; so if the claim of drunkenness is used in court, it probably is the actual truth. For the court to grant a divorce for this cause, drunkenness must be proved as habitual. Occasional sprees are not sufficient reason to dissolve a marriage. In some states no spouse can divorce a mate who was a heavy drinker before the marriage, because it is taken for granted that the habit was known about and accepted when the vows for better or worse were taken.

Though the exact cause of alcoholism has not been clearly defined, the medical world now looks upon the alcoholic as a sick person who is in need of medical and psychiatric help. This problem is discussed at greater length in other chapters, although it can be pointed out here that the alcoholic has both a harder time getting married and a more difficult time staying married than the person who drinks moderately or not at all.

3. INSANITY. Insanity is universally recognized as an obstacle to a successful marriage; all states will allow a marriage to be dissolved or annulled if one mate was insane at the time of the marriage. If insanity occurs after the marriage, the situation is considered different, and divorce may or may not be granted.

The term "insanity" is a legal definition of mental illness and is not a medical word. The point is, however, that the law recognizes that actual sickness of the mind is not conducive to a successful marriage and is willing to release the sound partner from the responsibilities and obligations of such an unhealthy union.

4. IMPOTENCE. Impotence, or the inability to function sexually, is a legal basis

for divorce in two thirds of the states, but sterility (inability to make pregnant, or to become pregnant) is not recognized as a ground for divorce. In cases in which the latter is the actual reason for divorce, it is usually hidden behind another charge, such as mental cruelty.

Impotence is sometimes psychogenic in origin. In such a case, psychiatric treatment is necessary, but may or may not be helpful, depending upon the severity and nature of the mental illness. Sometimes impotence is due to disease, accident or glandular deficiency. In such cases medical treatment may be able to bring about an improvement in the condition.

Pregnancy and Childbirth Are Safe

Pregnancy is 99.96 per cent safe for the mother, according to the most recent public health statistics. This means that the average woman can face the prospect of having several babies with virtually 100 per cent assurance that her health and life will not be at stake. Having a baby is a safe, normal experience which can and should be anticipated with confidence and composure.

It is, of course, a sensible thing for the young wife to establish early in her marriage, or even before, that there are no complicating reasons why she cannot have a baby. Such assurance can come from the premarital examination, which, from the health standpoint, ought to include an obstetrical analysis as well as a general health survey.

Diagnosis of Pregnancy

The diagnosis of pregnancy is not always easy, especially in the early stages. Some symptoms of pregnancy may be observed by the woman herself, such as the absence of an expected menstrual period. This is not a positive indication, for the menstrual period may be delayed by emo-

tional disturbance or physical illness. Some women, moreover, are irregular in their cycle.

Other indications of pregnancy, coming a little later than the missed period, are the nausea of morning sickness (which occurs in about 50 per cent of cases), frequent urination (which comes in the second and third months) and certain changes in the breasts.

Medical diagnosis can confirm pregnancy by examination of the pelvis for typical signs, and by laboratory tests. Still later the mother can feel the "quickening," the flutter of movement made by the fetus. After a while the doctor, through his stethoscope, can hear the sounds of the baby's heart and his movements.

In doubtful cases the physician may call for certain chemical tests in which a small sample of the urine may be injected into a frog or other animal. If ovulation or certain other changes take place in the test animal a diagnosis of pregnancy in the patient may be made by the physician.

How Long Is a Pregnancy?

Because of frequent inability to date the exact time of fertilization, a common method of estimating the date of birth of an expected child is to calculate 280 days after the beginning of the last menstrual period. Another method of figuring the birth date is by Naegele's rule: add seven days to the onset of the last menstrual period and count backward three months. That will give you the month and day of the expected arrival.

Medical Examinations During Pregnancy

When the fact of pregnancy is established, it is of vital importance that a careful medical examination be made. The doctor will take a *medical history*, recording data about previous pregnancies, menstrual history, surgical conditions, what diseases the woman has had, and much other information. He will also make a *physical examination,* taking pelvic measurements and looking into the condition of the heart, lungs and other organs. He will have *laboratory tests* made, including urinalysis, blood tests and vaginal smears. He will record the weight and blood pressure, which are very important criteria of the mother's health during pregnancy.

The pregnant woman should have a medical examination once a month for the first six months, twice a month for the next two months, and weekly during the last month.

OBSTACLES TO PRENATAL CARE

Approximately 7,000 Los Angeles city mothers delivered at ... County Hospitals ... received inadequate prenatal care ... the principal reasons given were as follows: (more than one reason given by some mothers):

Cause	Per cent
Did not feel care was important	25
Care of children	25
Lack of information about free clinics	19
Work	10
Fear of doctors and clinics	8
Did not desire the pregnancy	8
Illness	7
Miscellaneous	34

Los Angeles City Health Department, July 1, 1960. (Swayne, Ross and Edgerly)

Complications of Pregnancy

The vast majority of prenatal periods are completely without any serious complications. In fact, the great majority of women could go through pregnancy and even delivery without anesthesia or medical care, but it is wiser to obtain the latter as a form of insurance against the slight possibility of mishaps.

The odds are overwhelmingly in favor of a normal pregnancy terminating in successful delivery, so far as the mother's health is concerned. This fact has not been as widely appreciated as it deserves to be. Too many civilized people have thought of having a baby with awe and dread. Primitive people, on the other hand, have made very little of childbirth, accepting it as a normal part of everyday life.

For the tiny minority who do have serious problems, prenatal visits to the doctor and hospital delivery of the baby are insurance against trouble. The examining physician usually can detect, in advance, signs of possible difficulty, and can take measures to safeguard against them. He can, moreover, teach the pregnant woman to look for symptoms which indicate some sort of abnormality.

Nausea during the first three months is normal and need cause no worry unless it is very excessive and accompanied with vomiting. About one-half of all pregnant women do experience nausea.

Vaginal bleeding is not usual and should be reported immediately to the physician. It may be caused by something not connected with the pregnancy, but attention must still be directed toward its solution.

Pain in the abdomen is not a usual occurrence during pregnancy. If pain does occur, the physician should be told in order that he can trace it to its cause and institute proper treatment.

Such matters as *rapid gain of weight, persistent headaches, visual disturbances* and *excessive shortness of breath* should also be reported. *Toxemia* is a very serious condition for the pregnant woman. However, its warning signs of excessive weight gain and increased blood pressure can be detected by the doctor, who will know what to do about it.

AIR TRAVEL DURING PREGNANCY

"A study of abortion in 1,000 women aged 16 to 42 years, traveling by air during World War II, revealed no correlation between abortion and flying. Air travel is not harmful to a normal pregnancy regardless of the duration of the pregnancy ... Physicians generally agree that a woman with an uncomplicated pregnancy is not sick ...

Aerospace Medical Association, May 28, 1960

Swelling of any body parts and *diminished output of urine* are also symptoms to be reported at once to the doctor. *High blood pressure* and *albumin in the urine,* as well, are important signals which the doctor will check automatically at the regular prenatal visits.

Disease and Pregnancy

Should a woman ill with a disease have a baby? The average woman, naturally, does not plan to have a baby while she is ill. Sometimes, however, a woman will catch a disease after she has become pregnant, or she may disregard the consequences of illness in childbirth in the first place. When this occurs, all possible measures must be taken to protect the baby from the mother's illness as well as to treat the mother herself.

Tuberculosis is not hereditary. But the baby who remains in close association with a mother who is tuberculous is in great danger of infection. For that reason it's important to remove the infant from the mother immediately after birth.

If the mother is permitted to bear the baby, treatment for tuberculosis must, of course, continue; obstetrical care should be given in the same hospital. If the patient is not at a hospital, but living at home, it is necessary to give her domestic help as well as medical care.

Syphilis is not hereditary. But it is possible for the unborn baby to catch the disease through the placental membranes of the infected mother if she is not treated in time. Treatment in the early months of pregnancy will protect the baby from having the disease when born.

German measles is a hazard for the unborn child. Numerous studies since 1940 indicate that a high percentage of defects occur in babies born of women who had German measles during their first three months of pregnancy. Some of the commonest defects are cataracts, heart disorders and deaf-mutism, but almost any type of defect may be present. Many of the infants are poorly developed and have feeding problems. However, when the onset of German measles comes during the last six months of pregnancy, studies show that there seem to be no effects upon the infant.

THE MENTALLY RETARDED CHILD

"Between 3 and 4 per cent of all children born in the United States will ... be ... mentally handicapped ... Possible causes are certain prenatal conditions ... inadequate maternal diet, viral diseases such as German measles, exposure to radiation ... inborn errors of metabolism ... injuries at birth ... encephalitis or meningitis, poisoning by heavy metals, vascular accidents, and skull fractures ... care may well prevent the unborn child from becoming one of the mentally handicapped."

Therapeutic Notes, June, 1960

It is not advisable for women with serious *heart disease* to become pregnant. The death rate for pregnant women with heart disease may be as much as five times that of the rate for normal cases. Obstetricians differ on how to handle such pregnancies when they do occur. Some specialists in this field believe that the deliveries should be by cesarean surgery, while others believe that the normal birth should occur.

An *abnormal rise in blood pressure* of a pregnant woman is a warning sign to be heeded. Normally, blood pressures do not change much during pregnancy. When the pressure does rise excessively, there is a possibility of toxemia.

Women who have had one normal pregnancy have better than a 90 per cent chance that subsequent pregnancies will *not* be troubled by high blood pressure.

Deaths Due to Pregnancy and Childbirth

For every 10,000 live births in the United States, only four maternal deaths occur. This is one of the best maternal records in the world. Major causes for these deaths are hemorrhage, infections and toxemias. Infections as a cause of death from pregnancy have been declining in importance for the past few years, owing mostly to the discovery of the antibiotics with subsequent reduction in so-called childbed fevers.

The best guarantee against the complication of hemorrhage is for the expectant mother to have her baby delivered in a good hospital under competent medical care. In the hospital the physician has the equipment, supplies and trained personnel for stopping the hemorrhage and giving whole blood or plasma, which is the most effective treatment for the life-endangering shock that results from extensive blood loss.

Toxemia is a serious generalized condition which is best controlled by prompt delivery of the baby. Once the baby is born, the mother's symptoms subside rapidly unless the birth has been delayed too long. The careful attention of a physician in an acceptable hospital is the best guarantee that the mother suffering from toxemia will receive proper and lifesaving care.

Defective Babies

In the last few years much has been learned about the reasons why some babies are born with defects or abnormalities.

Most of the research on this subject was stimulated by the discovery, in Australia, that mothers who get German measles during the first three months of pregnancy are apt to give birth to a much higher percentage of babies born with defects. We now know that the embryologic tissues of the unborn baby may be damaged in many ways.

The time of injury to the tissues of the unborn child is a major factor in determining what kind of defect the baby may have at birth. Perhaps the time of injury is even more important than the kind of injury. Research has shown that if the embryonic tissues are injured up to seven weeks after conception a baby may be born with a cleft lip, but that if the injury to the tissues occurs between seven and

twelve weeks after conception, the baby may have a cleft palate. Since injury to the embryo may occur over a period of time that overlaps the seven weeks period it is commonplace to find that when a baby is born with a cleft lip that he may also have a cleft palate. Studies suggest that this defect may occur in only one case out of about 800 births.

The tissues of the unborn child may be injured by a severe deficiency of oxygen, such as when the mother suffers from a severe anemia; from a deficiency of vitamins such as riboflavin and vitamin A; from diseases such as German measles and a number of other virus infections; from radiation during the prenatal period and from excessive treatment with such drugs as cortisone during the prenatal period. Genetic factors may also be responsible for the presence of certain defects in babies at birth.

> **RADIATION DURING PREGNANCY**
>
> "The most radiosensitive period in human beings is probably the embryonic stage from day 18 through day 38. After the embryo is about 40 days old . . . gross fetal defects can occur only with larger doses of X-ray."
>
> *Roberts Rugh, Ph.D., 1958*

Research continues to substantiate the very great importance of the diet during the prenatal period. What the mother eats may well determine whether or not her babies will be normal.

A little more than one per cent of the babies who are born alive in the United States each year have some type of significant physical defect. Another way of looking at this problem is to recognize that 99 per cent of all babies born alive do not have such defects. Still, it is estimated that the total number of congenital defects in the United States each year is about 250,-000. Although most babies are born without abnormalities, the occurrence of birth defects is sufficiently great that the pregnant woman has just cause to give thought and attention to her health during the period of pregnancy in order to produce a normal baby.

Questions

1. Can a person with active tuberculosis justify marriage to a person in good health?

2. Should a marriage ever be dissolved because of an incurable illness?

3. Should a young married couple with epilepsy on one side of the family be encouraged to have children?

4. Why should a prospective mother have an obstetrical examination before pregnancy is established?

5. What religious arguments against the practice of birth control should be respected and observed?

6. Is the medical termination of a pregnancy ever truly justifiable?

7. What religious, moral and legal reasons are there for abolition of the "abortion racket"?

For Further Reading

1. Byrd, Oliver E.: *Family Life Sourcebook*. Stanford, California, Stanford University Press, 1956.

2. Duvall, Evelyn M.: *Facts of Life and Love*. New York, Association Press, 1956.

3. Fishbein, Morris, and Kennedy, R. J. R.: *Modern Marriage and Family Living*. New York, Oxford University Press, 1957.

4. Hall, Robert E.: *A Medical Guide for Pregnant Women*. New York, Doubleday and Company, 1960.

5. Heardman, Helen: *Relaxation and Exercise for Natural Childbirth*. Baltimore, Williams and Wilkins, 1959.

6. Jacobson, Paul H.: *American Marriage and Divorce*. New York, Rinehart, 1959.

7. Landis, Paul H.: *Your Dating Days*. New York, Whittlesley House (McGraw-Hill), 1954.

8. Parker, Elizabeth: *The Seven Ages of Woman*. Baltimore, Johns Hopkins Press, 1960.

26

INFANT AND CHILD CARE

PARENTS can be confident of their baby's survival, especially if he or she has been born at full time and is free of any handicapping defects or injuries. In this case the baby has very close to a 100 per cent chance of survival. In a sense, babies are tough and, with reasonably good care and medical attention, will live through even serious sicknesses.

Premature Births

Of the small percentage of babies who do not live beyond their first year, most die from causes arising from premature birth. (A baby who weighs less than 2500 grams (5½ pounds) at birth is regarded by most physicians as premature.)

343

"During April . . . 583 children were seen in the *Well Child Conferences* . . . during June and July 376 children were seen . . . Thirty-seven per cent of the children seen had an identified health problem."

Dr. Helen M. Wallace, Dr. Evelyn Hartman,
Dr. Vernon Weckwerth, M.S.,
and Dr. Eunice Davis, 1958

Not all the causes of premature birth are understood. Tuberculosis is a common cause. Syphilis also is a cause, though prenatal blood testing laws and proper treatment are eradicating this disease among expectant mothers. Other causes are complications of pregnancy, such as toxemia, and diseases of the mother such as severe anemia, undernourishment, overwork and tumors.

The premature baby may lack ability to regulate body temperature, owing primarily to failure of skin reflexes. In consequence, the baby overheats easily or chills easily.

The baby may lack protective immunity to infectious diseases. If so, even a mild infection can prove fatal.

The baby may suffer from nutritional deficiencies, such as inadequate storage of minerals and vitamins, incomplete development of enzyme systems, a diminished tolerance for foods or weakness of nursing muscles.

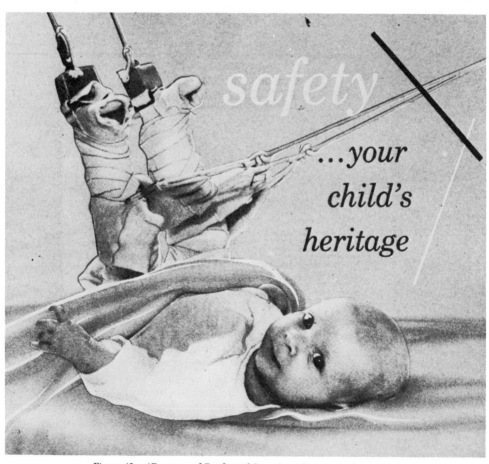

Figure 43. (Courtesy of Prudential Insurance Company of America.)

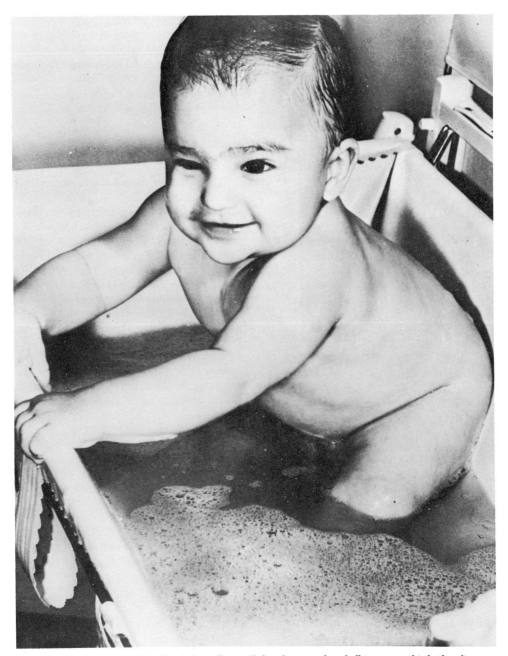

Figure 44. Soap may float but baby will not. If the phone or door bell interrupts his bath—disregard the call or take baby with you. (Courtesy of Prudential Insurance Company of America.)

The baby may have difficulties in breathing or in the circulation of the blood, or may be handicapped in other ways by incomplete development.

PREMATURE INFANTS

". . . premature infants . . . carry differences and handicaps beyond the neonatal . . . 500 premature infants . . . were shorter and lighter, had two to three times more physical defects and 50 per cent more illness than full term infants . . ."

Dr. Hilda Knoblock, Dr. Benjamin Pasamanick,
Dr. Paul A. Harper,
and Rowland V. Rider, D.Sc., 1959

Prevention of Deaths from Prematurity

Obviously, the best way to prevent infant deaths from prematurity is to prevent prematurity in the first place. Proper prenatal care and good obstetrics help to do this. When the premature birth does occur, the task then is to prevent complications.

Delivery should, of course, be in a hospital where emergency facilities are ready at hand. If possible, the mother should do without anesthesia, or at least should not request heavy sedation or excessive anesthesia, for drugs may make it difficult for the premature baby to start breathing after birth. The infant should be kept in an incubator if that is feasible; if not, a special crib should be provided, and temperature and humidity kept uniform.

Efforts should be made to provide rigid protection against communicable diseases. Before the mother is permitted to take the baby home, similar standards of careful control of temperature and safeguards against infection should be provided. This isn't always possible.

The premature baby requires special feeding care. He is often too weak to nurse from the mother. If fed too much, he may regurgitate and inhale the vomit into his lungs and be in danger of suffocation. He needs vitamins and minerals, calcium and phosphorus, and especially protein.

It is wrong to assume, however, that premature babies have just a slim chance to live. The fact is that about 85 per cent, if they are given proper care, survive as normal, healthy, intelligent babies. Some of the world's great men were born prematurely, among them Sir Isaac Newton, Charles Darwin, Victor Hugo, Jean Jacques Rousseau and Voltaire.

Illness of Infants

Though many data have been published on infant deaths, not nearly so much statistical information is available on the illnesses to which infants less than one year old are subject. The United States Public Health Service has issued a report, based on five surveys of family illness, which lists the most prevalent physical disorders of babies. The percentage figures in the accompanying table express the chance of any baby's getting the listed disease during his first year of life.

The two major groups of infant disorders are respiratory and digestive, and the younger the child, the more serious the illness is apt to be for him.

Type of Illness	Per Cent Chance of Getting the Disease in the First Year of Life
Colds and "running nose"	35
Bronchitis	16
Digestive diseases except diarrhea . .	14
Diarrhea and inflammation of the intestines	13
Whooping cough	9
Influenza	8
Ear and mastoid diseases	7
Defects present at birth and early infancy	6
Measles	5
Pneumonia	5
Teething and gum disorders	4
Eczema	4
"Sore throat"	4
Chickenpox	3
Injuries from accidents or violence	2

Respiratory Illnesses

Babies do have some general immunity to disease transmitted to them through the placental membranes of the mother. Such protection lasts from four to six months; it is, however, an incomplete immunity, and should not be relied upon to protect the baby against infections.

Whooping cough, if the child is neither immunized against it nor treated for it, is a highly dangerous disease for infants. About 95 per cent of babies under the age of one year who have no protection against whooping cough will die if they get the disease. According to studies by the New York State Department of Public Health, about one-half of these deaths from whooping cough occur in the first six months of life. This means that parents and physicians *must immunize against this disease at the age of three or four months* if additional lives are to be saved. This has been the conclusion of the New York authorities.

Parents have several ways of protecting their babies against respiratory infections.

First, babies should not be carelessly exposed to adults or other children suffering from colds, coughs and "runny" noses. This is especially important for the very young baby, since, in general, the younger the baby, the more serious the infection, because of the lesser powers of resistance.

Second, infants should be immunized (vaccinated) against whatever diseases the family physician or local public health officer may recommend. Usually it is wise to immunize against whooping cough, poliomyelitis, diphtheria, smallpox and tetanus. If an infant has been exposed to measles, it is important to immunize against this disorder, even though such protection is only temporary. The older child may be permitted to have a mild case of measles through partial immunization, depending on the judgment of the physician involved.

Third, parents should call a physician promptly if the baby gets a respiratory infection, especially if fever is obviously present. The discovery and widespread use of the antibiotics have saved the lives of many infants and will save many more.

Digestive Illnesses

Digestive disorders in babies come from two primary sources: feeding difficulties and infections. Of the two, intestinal infections with diarrhea are by far the more serious.

Repeated studies have shown that flies have much to do with spreading diarrhea in infants and children. Community programs of sanitation are most important in reducing diarrheal diseases, but such partial measures as the screening of homes, use of the fly swatter, and protection of the baby's food from flies can also help.

Parents must realize that diarrheal infection in infants is a serious disorder for which medical aid should be sought. Fortunately the use of antibiotics and fluids can do much to restore good health to the infant.

Feeding practices are important from the viewpoint of both digestion and infection. In this respect special attention should be given to the advantages of breast feeding, although bottle feeding is necessary in many cases and has some advantages also.

Breast Feeding

Some 14 per cent of mothers of newborn babies are unable to nurse them, according to one study of 4622 cases. In some 30 per cent additional cases, both breast and bottle feedings were required. But the majority of these mothers, 56 per cent, were able to give their babies sufficient breast milk by the end of the tenth day

> **NURSING**
>
> "... Every mother, if she can do so, should make a determined effort to nurse her own child ... failure in modern women is ... due largely to psychological and cultural causes ..."
>
> *Dr. Frank Howard Richardson*

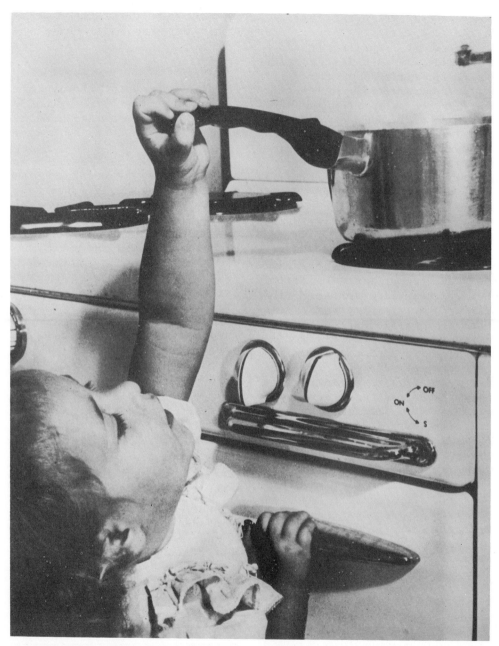

Figure 45.   Hot, scalding fluids should always be out of the reach of toddlers. Turn all handles of
pots and pans to the back of the stove. (Courtesy of Prudential Insurance Company of America.)

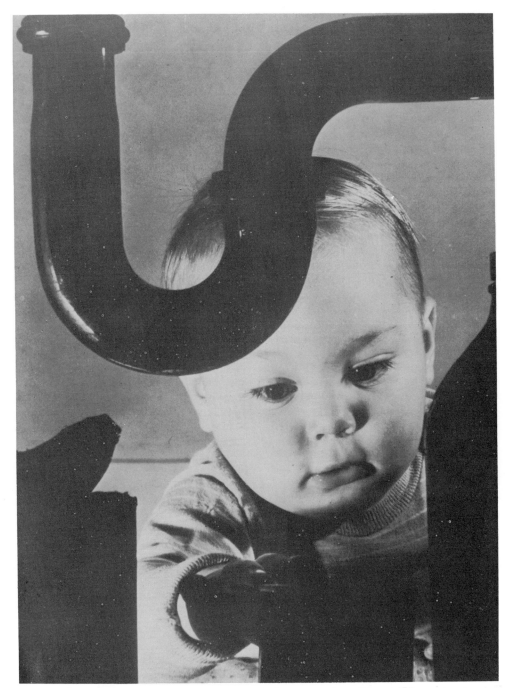

Figure 46. Death lurks under the kitchen sink and in low storage closets. Keep medicines, ant paste, lye and similar items out of reach. (Courtesy of Prudential Insurance Company of America.)

Unless there is good reason to the contrary, all mothers should nurse their babies at the breast rather than at the bottle, for the following reasons:

Breast feeding helps the mother recover physically from the delivery. Stimulation of the breast by nursing has a physiologic effect on the mother's uterus, causing it to shrink faster. This shrinking helps to control bleeding from the uterus. Since this is one of the potential hazards of childbirth, anything that assists in controlling hemorrhage will help protect the mother.

Breast feeding, morever, saves work. The mother is enabled to bypass the kitchen drudgery involved in preparing formula, boiling milk, sterilizing bottles and washing dishes. Reducing a mother's labor is help in protecting her from getting too tired, which, in turn, is a safeguard against the emotional disturbances to which a worn-out young mother is prone. Another advantage is the fact that breast milk does not cost anything. This may be important in families on a limited budget.

Breast feeding is best for the baby. The Infant Welfare Society of Chicago has reported two studies comparing deaths of babies among large groups of bottle-fed, partially bottle-fed and breast-fed babies. These studies show that of infants who died approximately 65 per cent were bottle-fed on artificial milk, whereas 28 per cent were fed partly on bottle and partly at the mother's breast. Only 7 per cent of the babies who died had been completely fed at the mother's breast.

It should be pointed out that most babies *can* feed on artificial milk or cow's milk and do very well on it. Of the groups of infants in this cited study, only four deaths occurred out of every 1000 babies, irrespective of how they were fed. There should be no feeling on the part of any mother, therefore, that if her baby must be bottle fed, his life is endangered. That isn't so.

Breast milk is practically sterile, which goes a long way to protect the baby from food infections. This is a very real advantage. Some authorities believe that the dreaded diarrhea of the newborn, which on occasion has taken as high as 30 per cent of the babies in a hospital nursery, is a virus disease spread by poor artificial feeding techniques.

Evidence indicates, furthermore, that there is less skin disease among infants fed at the breast. One study on this subject showed that babies fed on the bottle had seven times as much infantile eczema as did breast-fed babies. Infants fed partly at the breast and partly on the bottle had twice as much infantile eczema as did babies who were wholly breast fed.

Still another argument which some physicians advance in favor of breast feeding is that the milk of every mammal is specific for its young: nature provides in the breast of the mother the best possible food for the infant.

Breast feeding appears to be most important during the first three months of life. After this period it declines in importance, so that, even though a mother may not be able to nurse her baby throughout the later period of infancy, she may have gained most of the advantage for herself and her baby by nursing him for even one or two months.

Breast milk tends to decline in quality after about six to nine months, so that further breast feeding is usually not advisable, although some mothers have been known to breast-feed their children for two or more years.

> **BREAST FEEDING**
> ". . . satisfactory breast feeding is by far the simplest and best of all the methods of infant feeding. The difficulty is that many mothers do not find breast feeding satisfactory . . ."
>   *Frank E. Hytten, M.B., 1959*

Some mothers are not able to nurse their babies, even though they desire to do so. There are two primary reasons why this may be so. First, the breasts may be injured in the early days of feeding so that nursing becomes such a painful experience for the mother that it has to be abandoned. Second, the presence of high milk pressure in the breasts may lead to a rapid decline in milk production because of mechanical compression of the cells which secrete milk. In order to keep such a mother from "drying up," the breast pressure must be rapidly lowered. In such cases the use of the breast pump may be necessary.

Behavior Problems in Children

Most young mothers and fathers do not understand how to interpret the behavior of children. A mistake made by many parents is that of being so conscientious about the raising of a child that anxiety and tension become common characteristics of family life. Often this tension and concern does not lessen until the parents have a second or third child.

A first child is often like a book of life which the parents read and gain greater understandings of childhood behavior. Many a parent has realized with later children the mistakes they have made with earlier ones.

Children can be expected to misbehave. The responsibility of the parent is, first, to interpret the behavior of children correctly, and, second, to know what to do about this behavior. Much behavior of children needs only to be understood. Other behavior needs constructive action by the parents if children are to develop socially acceptable habits.

BEHAVIOR PROBLEMS

"The attitude toward emotional disorders in children should be the same as that toward physical illness. Neither physical nor emotional maturation occurs without some irregularities . . ."

Stuart M. Finch, M.S., 1958

Many children are restless and overactive. Some are apprehensive and easily worried. Others develop small habits that may reflect the presence of tension in the family. Some develop reactions that call for intelligent consultations by parents with experts on the behavior of the children.

Much behavior that annoys and distresses parents is relatively normal for the age group involved and will disappear as the child gets older. Some behavior is more serious and should not be ignored by the parents. Some behavior exhibited by children between the ages of six and twelve years is listed in an accompanying table.

BEHAVIOR OF 482 CHILDREN BETWEEN THE AGES OF 6 AND 12 AS REPORTED BY MOTHERS

Rank	Behavior	Per cent
1.	Overactivity	49
2.	Fears and worries	43
3.	Food intake, greater or less than normal	36
4.	Restlessness	30
5.	Nightmares	28
6.	Nail-biting	27
7.	Nose-picking	26
8.	Bed-wetting	17
9.	Biting, sucking or chewing objects	16
10.	Picking sores	16
11.	Grinding teeth	14
12.	Loss of temper daily or more	11
13.	Chewing or sucking lips or tongue or biting inside of mouth	11
14.	Unusual movements such as twitching or jerking	12
15.	Thumb or finger sucking	10
16.	Stuttering	4

From: Dr. Rema Lapouse and Mary A. Monk, Ph.D. An epidemiologic study of behavior characteristics in children, Am. J. Pub. Health, *48:* 1134–44, Sep., 1958.

Why Babies Cry

The new parent, especially if he or she is a tense person, may suffer considerable emotional distress when the baby cries. Friends are apt to point out, soothingly, that crying is normal, crying is the way the newborn fellow gets his exercise, crying is

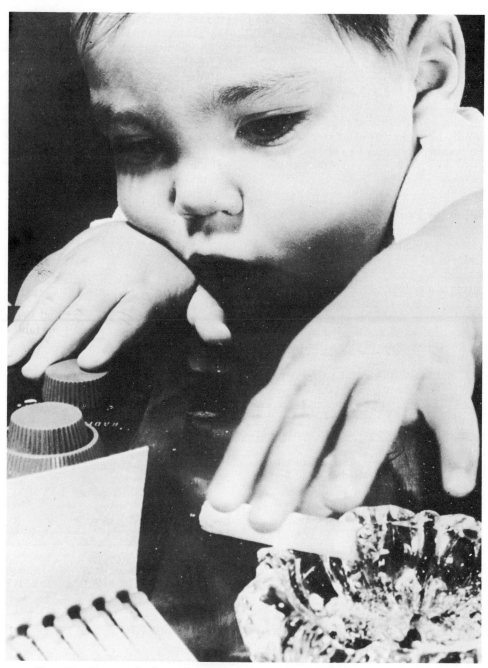

Figure 47. Gas stoves, bonfires and open fires are potential funeral pyres. Keep matches and cigarette lighters out of reach. Party candles and flimsy costumes invite disaster. (Courtesy of Prudential Insurance Company of America.)

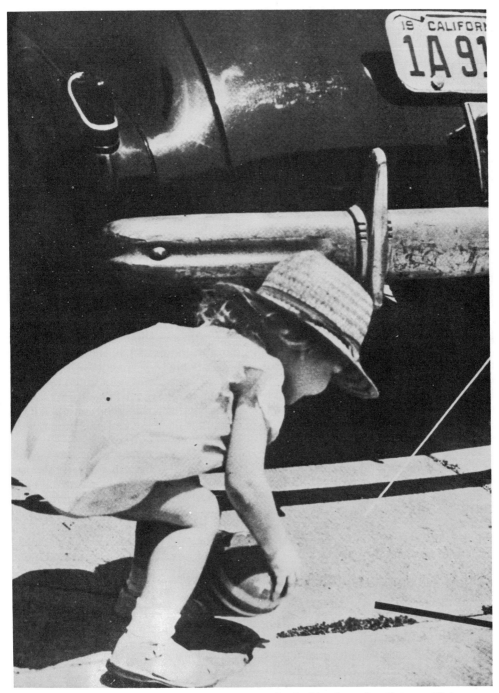

Figure 48. Your car does not have eyes . . . use yours when backing the car from the garage. Do not kill a child because of failure to look. (Courtesy of Prudential Insurance Company of America.)

just practice in vocalizing, but this is apt to be little consolation to worried parents.

Babies cry for reasons. It is up to the parents to discover what these reasons are and to take steps for the correction of disturbing influences regardless of whether they are mild or serious. Excessive crying is a signal for some sort of action on the part of parents.

Hunger crying is usually vigorous and all-out and fairly continuous. It may occur just before or after a meal—after, if the portion was too small to meet demand. This crying is easily controlled by adequate feeding.

A wet diaper may be a cause of disturbance. The baby should be changed on signal, since a wet diaper may cause a skin rash. If the signal is not heeded and the diaper is not changed, the baby may give up crying for such service and simply endure the wet diaper, though he will not like it.

Crying may be in reaction to various types of discomfort or pain, such as that caused by a safety pin sticking the baby, by a diaper that is too tight, by uncomfortable posture or some other factor. It is wise, when the infant complains lustily, to search for some source of irritation or discomfort.

The baby may cry because he has been clothed too warmly or covered with so many blankets that he is uncomfortable. On the other hand, he may have kicked off his covers and be lying wet in a cold room. Incidentally, a baby is more apt to suffer from excessive heat than from cold.

Colic may be the cause of continued crying. Colic refers to sharp pains in the abdomen. Various causes may be to blame, though the commonest are swallowing air because of fast or overlong nursing and the failure of the parent to bring relief by "burping" the child. Always, after a feeding, the baby should be placed against the adult's shoulder in a vertical position and his back patted until he discharges the air he swallowed with his meal.

Colic may be responsible for extended crying spells that last for hours. The baby may cry through the whole period between one feeding and the next. This next feeding will not relieve his pains, and may, in fact, add to his later discomfort. Some babies may have only occasional attacks of colic; others may have regular attacks every day between certain hours in relation to feeding habits.

The cause of some colic seems to be related to the nervous system of the baby.

A colicky baby is apt to get along better if the household is a tranquil one, and if he is handled very gently. For severe colic a physician should be called, but the parents' primary efforts should be devoted to prevention of the disturbance.

Crying may result from the pain of anal fissures caused by hard stools (feces) in which the bowel movements tear the rectum.

If the infant cries on moving his bowels, and blood is found in the stool or diaper, an anal fissure should be suspected. It is more common with bottle-fed than with breast-fed babies. Giving the infant more water to drink may help soften the stools enough to relieve the difficulty of passage, but a physician should be consulted if the condition does not respond promptly to such simple measures.

Fretful crying may result from nutritional deficiencies, especially if there is a lack of vitamin C, which may result in infantile scurvy. Babies suffering from this disease are apt to lie very still in their cribs, because movement is painful. This is because the joints become sore and painful from the bleeding of ruptured blood vessels, which may become very fragile unless there is enough vitamin C in the diet.

Infant scurvy is still fairly common, although the widespread practice of adding vitamin C to the baby's milk has greatly reduced the number of cases of this disease. Sometimes the scurvy develops even when the vitamin C has been added to the baby's bottle. Usually this happens when the mother has been adding the vitamin to milk before the baby's formula has been boiled. Since heat quickly destroys vitamin

C, the result is that the baby gets little or none of the vitamin, in spite of the mother's conscientious work. The vitamin must be added *after* the milk has been heated.

Sometimes the baby may cry because of an anatomic condition which requires surgical correction if his life is to be saved. An example of this type of emergency is the strangulated hernia. A great many babies are born with an inguinal or umbilical hernia. In many cases the hernia will heal spontaneously, but if it persists longer than six months or so, the chances of a natural healing are greatly reduced. Such hernias may escape detection by the mother, since they often protrude only when the baby cries. The danger is that the segment of intestine which comes through the opening of the wall of the abdomen may become caught or twisted in such a way that its normal blood circulation is interfered with. When this happens, the hernia is strangulated, and gangrene may result; then a surgical operation is necessary to save the baby's life. The alert parent who is able to rule out most other causes of crying may or may not suspect a strangulated hernia, but if medical aid is sought because of persistent crying, the baby's life will be saved.

Various infections may cause a baby to cry. Thrush, or "sore mouth," causes crying usually at nursing time when the infant has to use his mouth. When the baby is ill from any infection, he will be fretful and easily irritated to outright crying.

The detection of fever, suspected or proved, is usually the clue to realization that the baby is crying from an infection. In this regard it must be remembered that a baby's temperature should not be taken by mouth, since he may break the thermometer by biting, with subsequent injury from the broken glass and possible swallowing of some mercury.

Infant temperatures should be taken by rectum with a rectal thermometer, and the mother should remember that the reading will be about one degree higher when taken in this manner, as compared to the oral temperature.

The baby may cry because he has learned that this is the way to bring mother on the run to pick him up from his crib and give him the fondling and attention he craves. Such a baby is said to be "spoiled." However, opinion today tends to incline toward risking too much indulgence rather than the consequences of not giving the infant enough of the loving he wants. It is thought that the emotional tone of an individual is set during his first five years of life, and that the child who gets the proper amount of attention and affection has a better chance of maturing into a strong, stable person than the infant who suffers from emotional neglect.

Some babies, of course, may be spoiled from too much attention at the wrong time. Babies should be fondled and loved when they are *not* crying. If this attention is reserved for the infant when he cries, he soons learns to associate affection with his demand for it.

Babies who are spoiled tend to stop crying promptly when they are picked up and to start crying again when set down. Sick babies are apt to cry in or out of the mother's arms.

Parents who wish to develop a routine method for finding out why the baby is crying might follow a plan like this: First, examine the baby to see whether a wet diaper, pin or other condition may be a source of discomfort or pain; second, decide whether or not the baby is too hot or too cold; third, pick the baby up to see whether he is crying merely because he wants attention; fourth, feed the baby to see whether he will stop crying; fifth, take the temperature by rectum to see whether he has a fever; and, sixth, call a physician if the baby persists in his crying.

Why Babies Vomit

All babies normally drool, push out and,

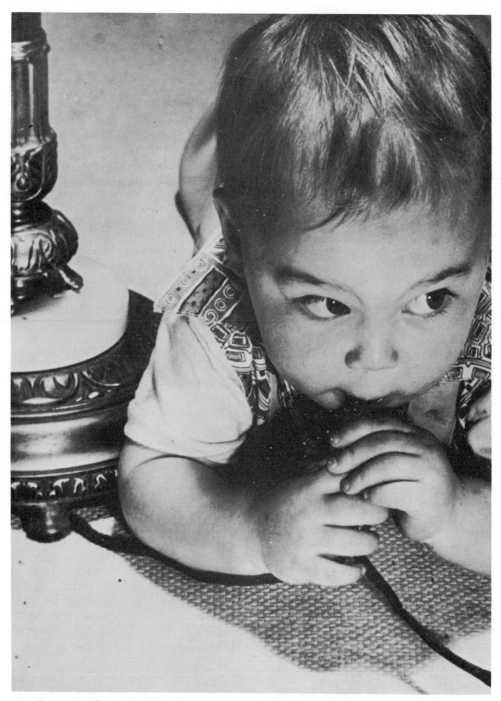

Figure 49.   Electrical outlets and worn extension cords can be as deadly as the electric chair itself.
Plug outlets and keep cords repaired. (Courtesy of Prudential Insurance Company of America.)

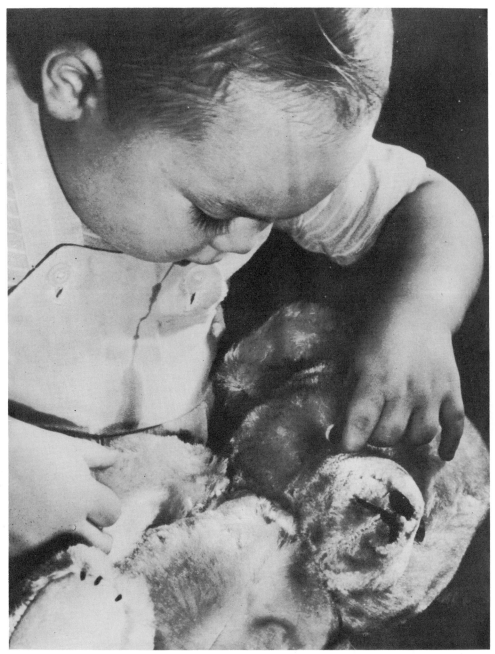

Figure 50.   Eyes and stuffing from toy animals and dolls can cause strangulation. Avoid nuts, carrot sticks, popcorn and similar foods with younger children. (Courtesy of Prudential Insurance Company of America.)

on occasion, vomit some of their food. Usually this is due to the fact that they have eaten too fast or too much. Eating too much, and thus overfilling the stomach is a common cause of vomiting. Ironically, the baby who does this may end up being hungry as a result of having got rid of his entire meal. Vomiting may be due to more serious causes, however, and this must be understood by the parents.

Vomiting may be induced by gastric indigestion, caused by too much fat in the milk. Giving the baby skimmed milk can ease this condition.

Respiratory infections, such as whooping cough, pneumonia or other infections of the upper respiratory tract, may cause vomiting.

An infection of the abdominal cavity, called acute peritonitis, and caused by a gangrenous hernia or the rupturing of an appendix, may cause vomiting.

Swallowing air by a child overeager in feeding may cause vomiting.

A baby may deliberately vomit to gain attention or revenge. This baby has been alert enough to discover from previous vomiting that this brings desired attention and excitement.

Vomiting which develops about three to five weeks after birth in a baby who has been healthy may be due to a narrowing of a portion of the digestive tract. This condition, known as pyloric stenosis, does not permit the passage of sufficient food. Surgery is required, for the disorder may cause death if it continues uncorrected.

If an obstruction occurs high in the digestive tract, vomiting is apt to result.

Vomiting is sometimes caused by a condition known as intussusception, occurring when one section of the intestine slides over another part, like a tube fitting over another tube. The circulation is impaired, and blood comes out in the stool. This is a serious problem, and the child must be placed in the doctor's care.

But, to repeat, all babies normally drool, push out food, and sometimes vomit. Mothers know this only too well, so usually a mother will notice when the baby's vomiting is excessive. Not until it is far more frequent than usual or is associated with some other sign of illness is there cause for real concern.

Bed-Wetting

A study of urinary control in 1,000 children has shown that bladder control is a self-learned skill which most children have developed by the age of four and one-half years. Under ordinary circumstances the child doubles his bladder capacity between the ages of two and four and one-half years. The larger the bladder capacity the greater the likelihood that the child will control bed-wetting.

According to Dr. S. Richard Muellner, most children can be taught to control bed-wetting. First, it must be explained to the child that his bladder is as yet too small and that he will have to make it larger in order to become cured of bed-wetting. When the child is instructed to force fluids during the day and to hold his urine as long as possible it may take three to six months before a satisfactory bladder capacity is reached. By forcing fluids it is meant that the child drinks as much as possible. By holding his urine he keeps from going to the toilet as long as he can. In this training period during which the child attempts to enlarge his capacity for holding urine, the wet bed is strictly ignored. Gradually the child should develop a capacity for holding larger and larger amounts of urine. Enlargement of the bladder gradually produces the capacity to retain the total output of night urine after which the child will no longer wet the bed.

Handicaps

Many children may have serious handicaps that appear early in life. It is impor-

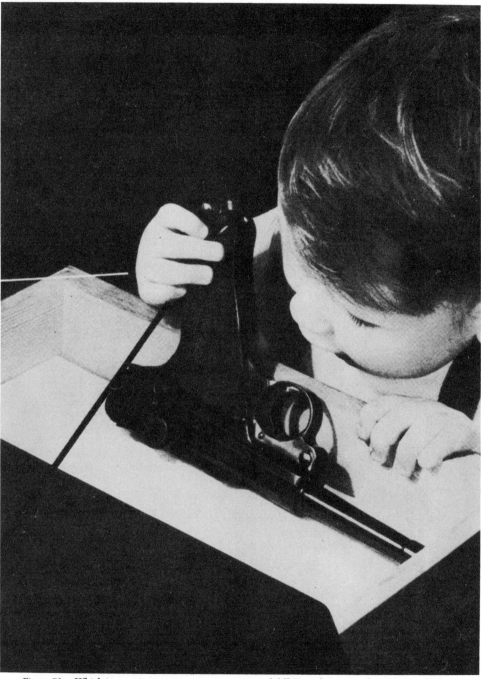

Figure 51. Which is more important—your gun or your child? Keep firearms and ammunition locked safely away from curious children. (Courtesy of Prudential Insurance Company of America.)

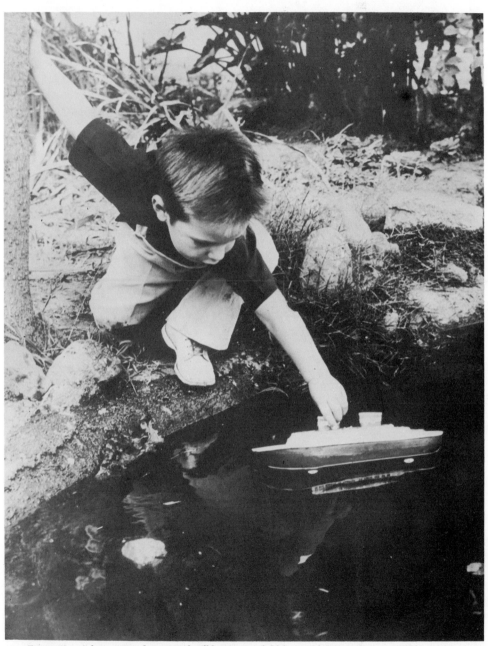

Figure 52.   A fence around your yard will keep your child from wandering into a neighbor's pool or fish pond. Teach children to swim early. (Courtesy of Prudential Insurance Company of America.)

tant for parents to be alert to these difficulties because early attention to them
may result in a permanent correction.
Often the psychologic impact of a handicap may be as great a problem as the physical defect itself. The ability to speak, see
and hear is especially important for the
normal growth and development of a
child. Any suspected deviations should be
carefully checked by the parents with the
pediatrician or family physician. The early
correction of some handicaps turn out to
be one of the greatest contributions that
parents can make to the present and future welfare and happiness of their children.

The Non-Speaking Child

The child who does not learn to speak
early is often a source of worry to his parents. The normal child knows at least 10 to
12 words at the age of 18 months and can
speak these words without hesitation.

When a child appears to be retarded in
his speech, parents should consult a physician or speech specialist. There are at least
four conditions that should be investigated
when a child is retarded in his speaking development. Perhaps the first thing that
should be suspected is an impairment of
hearing. The child who cannot hear well
cannot speak well. Of course, the child
may be mentally retarded, and if he is a
slow learner this will be reflected in his inability to speak at an early age. The child
who is emotionally disturbed may also fail
to speak at a normal age. This child may
have the capacity to speak but may stop
even after a normal beginning in his
speech. On the other hand, he may rarely
speak and this reticence may be interpreted as an inability to speak. A fourth
case for non-speaking at an early age is
damage to the brain. The brain-damaged
child may attempt to speak but his words
do not make sense. He may use words,
but they do not fit together in a pattern of
speech but appear indiscriminately.

The non-speaking, or inarticulate, child

should therefore be medically investigated
from the standpoint of his hearing, mental
retardation, emotional stability and brain
damage. Although there may be other
causes of non-speaking in a child, these are
four conditions that occur frequently
enough so that they should be investigated.

The Hard-of-Hearing Child

School surveys suggest that from 3 to 5
per cent of the children in the elementary
schools have a hearing impairment. Recent
studies by the United States Children's
Bureau indicate that between 3,500,000
and 7,000,000 persons under the age of 21
years have sufficient hearing impairment
to justify medical attention or treatment.

Although most of the hearing loss in
childhood comes from neglected infections of the middle ear there has been an
increase in recent years in hearing loss that
involves some impairment in the central
nervous system.

Pain in the ear should never be neglected. A child who says he has an earache
should be taken to a physician for careful
examination. This may be the only indication that a child has an infection of the
middle ear. To neglect such a condition is
to establish the possibility that the child's
hearing may be permanently impaired.
Research studies have shown that approximately 50 per cent of total deafness in
adult life is caused by neglected ear infections during childhood.

Accidents Are the Greatest Hazard

Serious thought should be given by all
parents to the safety of their children. In
early life the ages from one to four years
are especially hazardous. This is a time
when children can get away from their
parents, but it is also a period of inexperi-
ence and undeveloped judgment. The

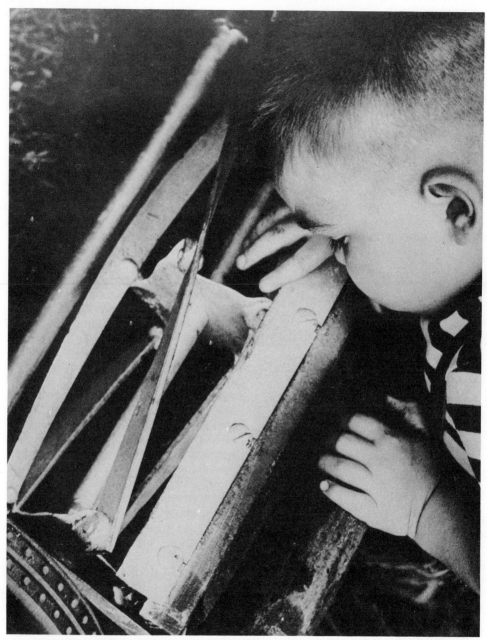

Figure 53.   Don't let useful machinery make useless children. Youngsters can be severely maimed if left alone with ordinary home appliances, garden and farm machinery. (Courtesy of Prudential Insurance Company of America.)

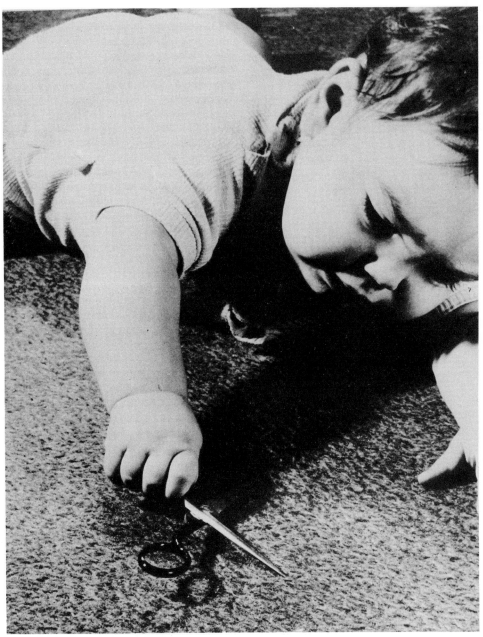

Figure 54. Scissors, ice picks and nail files are highly dangerous. Keep them from toddlers. Teach older children to walk—not run—when carrying sharp pointed objects. (Courtesy of Prudential Insurance Company of America.)

child of two, for example, can hardly be expected to exercise adult judgment in crossing a busy street.

THE EIGHT MOST DANGEROUS ACCIDENTS FOR BOYS AND GIRLS

Motor Vehicles
Other Transport
Poison
Falls
Fire and Explosion
Heat and Radiation
Fire-arms
Drowning
World Health Organization, June, 1960

Some parents attempt to insure the safety of their children by a rigid program of restrictions. This is not enough and is often not advisable. Parents might well put emphasis upon at least two other aspects in the prevention of childhood accidents. First, parents should be particularly diligent in the removal of hazardous conditions. If the handle of a pot containing hot water is never permitted to project over the edge of the stove then there is no need for the parent to make a great issue of leaving such handles alone. The hazard is obviated because it is never permitted to exist. A second emphasis that parents can employ is to educate the child within his capacity of comprehension of accident hazards. When the child understands why he should not do certain things he is more apt to be cooperative in the avoidance of hazards.

POISONING

"Some 95 per cent of poisoning cases occurred to children under five years of age. The rise . . . at the end of the first year is very pronounced . . . In the vast majority of cases the substances were within reach of the child."

Dr. R. M. Bissell and
Robert S. McInnes, M.P.H., 1960

What will work with one child, however, may not succeed with another. Par-

ents often overlook the basic and important problem of individual differences. One child responds instantly to a suggestion, while another resists and must be taught by different methods. Wisdom in the understanding of individual differences often comes to parents when there are many children in a family. Parents with only one child may never realize that every human being is distinctly different from all others even though there is basic physiologic and psychologic similarity.

Some of the leading causes of accidents involving children are indicated in the accompanying tabular and graphic materials. Whether or not the child survives depends mostly on his parents.

Children in Hospitals

When the sick child must be sent to the hospital it is likely that this may be an emotionally upsetting experience for the child.

Separation from parents and home in itself is a form of rejection and lack of affection on the part of the parents in the mind of the child. Parents who do a good job of explaining the situation to the child, who

---

ACCIDENTAL DEATHS IN CHILDREN AGED ONE TO FOUR YEARS

Rank	Accidental Cause of Death	Percentage of Deaths
1	Motor Vehicle	31
2	Fire and explosion	20
3	Drowning	14
4	All other causes	13
5	Poisoning	7
6	Falls	6
7	Choking from food and other objects	5
8	Burns and Scalds	4

From: Metropolitan Life Insurance Company. Accidents among pre-school children, Statistical Bulletin, *40*:6–8, August, 1959.

POISONINGS IN CHILDREN AGED FIVE
YEARS OR UNDER

	Type of Poison	Male	Female
1.	Aspirin	45	39
2.	Other drugs	30	24
3.	Household preparations	35	29
4.	Insect and rodent poisons	23	19
5.	Plants	2	7
6.	Unknown	1	0
	Totals	136	118

From: Bissell, Dwight M., and McInnes, Robert
S.: Epidemiology of accidental poisoning. California Medicine, 92:416–17, June, 1960.

prepare him in advance for hospitalization and who visit him frequently in the hospital can help to alleviate this problem.

For many children the hospital experience will be a frightening and lonely one. Some investigators of children's reactions to hospitals indicate that the child of three or four years of age is apt to be more sensitive than children of other ages to the absence of parents. Some children who appear to adapt well to the hospitalization are actually in a state of despair and self-repression.

The child should be told as much as possible about the hospital environment, why he is going to the hospital and why he should trust his doctor and other personnel while there. If the child cannot understand or cannot bring himself to trust others, it is much more likely that he will have emotional reactions to hospitalization. Selection of a physician or surgeon who understands children and knows how to contribute to their security and confidence should be arranged in advance, if this is possible.

Experience has shown that infants below the age of seven months accept the hospital environment without question. Crying that occurs in this age group is usually associated with hunger or discomfort rather than loneliness or fear. Older infants respond to separation from mother and family more vigorously.

On return from the hospital some children may become overly dependent on the mother, may cling to her and cry even when she leaves the room. In these children the appearance of strangers may also create emotional disturbances of insecurity and fear. After about two weeks, however, these reactions tend to disappear and the child becomes once more safely established in his own home.

Questions

1. What is sensible behavior on the part of a parent when a two-year-old child has a temper tantrum in a public place?
2. Should children be permitted to do almost anything they want to do on the theory that they will then learn by experience both "right" and "wrong"?
3. How can you tell whether or not an infant in a crying spell is sick, spoiled, uncomfortable or unhappy?
4. What is a normal temperature for a baby, when should the temperature be taken, and how should it be determined?
5. What should a girl or young woman know about children in order to make a superior baby sitter?
6. Should a child be punished for consistently wetting his bed?
7. What is the greatest hazard of infancy and childhood?
8. What hazards are there for children in hospitalization?

For Further Reading

1. Breckenridge, Marian E., and Vincent, E. Lee: *Child Development: Physical and Psychological Growth Through Adolescence.* Philadelphia, W. B. Saunders Company, 1960.
2. Byrd, Oliver E.: *Family Life Source Book.* Stanford, California, Stanford University Press, 1956.
3. Fraiberg, Selma H.: *The Magic Years.* New York, Charles Scribner's Sons, 1959.
4. Harris, I. D.: *Normal Children and Mothers.* Glencoe, Ill., Free Press, 1959.

5. Robertson, James: *Young Children in Hospitals.* New York, Basic Books, 1959.

6. Stuart, Harold C., and Prugh, Dane G.: *The Healthy Child.* Cambridge, Harvard University Press, 1960.

For Advanced Reading

1. Bakwin, Harry, and Bakwin, Ruth Morris: *Clinical Management of Behavior Disorders in Children.* Philadelphia, W. B. Saunders Company, 1960.

2. Martmer, Edgar E.: *The Child with a Handicap.* Springfield, Ill., Charles C Thomas, 1959.

Recommended Film

A New World for Peter. 16 mm., color, sound, 22 minutes, 1959. Ithaca, New York: Parent's Committee, Box 23. (Preparation of a child for hospitalization.)

27

THE PROBLEM OF MEDICAL CARE

DURING the last half century the American people and their representatives in Congress have become increasingly concerned about the problem of medical care.

This problem is not as simple as might appear on the surface. Most people, including physicians, are in favor of adequate, high quality medical care. Differences of opinion appear, however, as to how this high quality care is to be achieved. Some unthinking persons assume that if they get *more and cheaper* medical care they will automatically be assured of better quality. This is not necessarily so. It is a characteristic of business economy that quality declines with cheapness. Whether this applies to medical care is not certain, but people should think through the possible consequences of *cheap* medical care. *Quality* of medical care is probably more important than the amount of medical treatment that is received by any individual. As a matter of fact, *cheap* medical care on a national basis may turn out to be a costly service, because of administrative costs, if for no other reason.

In the United States it is possible to secure the best medical care in the world because American physicians now receive the finest training, and are produced in greater numbers than those of any other nation. This country has more highly trained physicians per capita than any other nation with the exception of Israel, which has an abnormally high ratio of physicians because of the influx of these professional people from abroad. On a national scale we have more and better medical care than other nations.

On an individual scale, however, many families have found it difficult to meet medical, hospital and nursing bills in the event of severe and sustained illness. In recent years this has been true partly because of the rise of the cost of living and to a lesser extent because of the rise in medical costs. The price of medical care, in fact, has risen less than the price of living in general.

Considerable attention has been given in the past thirty years to the possibility of a national health program based on compulsory health insurance. A careful analysis of the proposed programs has caused the medical profession to express sincere doubts that such an approach to the problem of medical care is best for the United States.

The Committee on
The Costs of Medical Care

Probably the earliest large study made in the United States on the cost of medical care was the one conducted by the Committee on the Costs of Medical Care.

This Committee was composed of professional people in the field of medicine and public health as well as nonprofessional members from other walks of life. They made a five-year study of the problem of medical care costs and made their report in November, 1932.

Even in this first report there was a clear-cut division of thinking on the amount and kind of governmental activity and control desirable in the health field.

The majority report was signed by thirty-five members, and their principal recommendations and conclusions were based on the belief that the costs of medical care had outrun the capacity of many people. They recommended expansion of public health services, more group medical practice by physicians, development of coordinating councils for better planning in the use of community medical facilities and services, improvement of medical education with greater emphasis on prevention, and distribution of the costs of medical care through group organization of individual members of the population.

The minority report was signed by nine members, with basic agreement on every point except the issue of governmental activity and control.

The National Health Survey

During the winter of 1935–36 the United States Public Health Service in conjunction with the Works Progress Administration and other cooperating agencies conducted a house-to-house survey of more than 700,000 homes to obtain data on the national health. This information was analyzed relative to underlying factors such as income, age, sex, marital condition, occupation, housing, sanitary facilities, and so on.

The survey gained information on such things as how many times a year the doctor was called, how much time was spent by members of the family in the hospital, how much nursing care was needed by the family, how much chronic disease existed in the group, how much gross physical impairment handicapped various members of the family, and how much time members had been ill for seven days or more during the year preceding the date of the survey. A record was also made as to the number of people who were ill on the day the study was conducted. It was concluded that illness is a great problem in the United States.

The American Foundation Report

The American Foundation Report of 1937 contained the opinions and recommendations of 2100 leaders in American medicine. Although this report did not end in a set of recommendations, certain conclusions were apparent from a careful study of the opinions of this representative group of American physicians.

The main conclusions of this investigation were that the physician is concerned with the health of the well person as well as that of the sick person, that the costs of medical service are too high, that health is a matter of national concern, and that a revision of medical practices was needed because of changing social and economic conditions.

The division of thought on the problem of medical care became more apparent when a committee of physicians (begun as the "Four-Thirty" and later expanded to more than 1000 members) approved the National Hospital Bill and urged that the Wagner Health Bill should be considered.

The National Health Conference

In July, 1938, a National Health Conference was held at Washington, D.C., to consider the need for a better national health program. Of the 171 persons invited to participate in this conference, only fifty-three held an M.D. degree. Other representatives come from the fields of public health, labor, journalism, education, industry, agriculture, and so on.

The recommendations adopted at this conference were based upon those made by a technical committee on medical care which had been set up to study this problem. They favored the expansion of public health, maternal and child health services, hospital facilities, insurance against loss of wages during sickness, and a general program of medical care to offset excessive cost to the individual.

The Wagner Health Bill

In February, 1939, Senator Wagner of New York introduced a National Health Bill in Congress. The Bill was a broad one intended to expand state and federal health activities by an annual expenditure of nearly one billion dollars when in full operation.

Although action on the Bill was postponed, parts of it were separated from the broader structure and subsequently passed by Congress. One segment became known as the National Hospital Act, which provided for federal grants to states, counties or districts for the construction or improvement of needed hospitals.

The National Resources Planning Board Report

In 1943 the National Resources Planning Board gave attention to the problem of health and emphasized the need for eliminating preventable diseases and disabilities, developing better national nutrition, obtaining better organization of health services, and assuring adequate health and medical care for all.

The Attitude of the American Public Health Association

On October 4, 1944, the American Public Health Association issued an official statement on its attitude toward the provision of medical care on a national scale. This statement was subsequently modified in various ways through the ensuing years.

The public health group favored comprehensive services for all people as well as social insurance and taxation for the support of health services. The group agreed with the American Medical Association in favoring construction of needed hospitals and other facilities as well as the creation of a single public health agency and expansion of research in health problems. The group also went on record as favoring financial assistance of medical students and those who were willing to practice in rural areas.

By 1950 the viewpoint of the American Public Health Association on the problem of medical care in a national health program was expressed in the following resolution, passed at the annual meeting of that year:

The Association urges all agencies, organizations, and individuals concerned with medical care problems to exchange views and experience and to pool their knowledge, their resources, and their efforts to the end that the best possible medical care for all the people may ultimately be developed under the conditions that now prevail in the United States.

By November 14, 1956, the recommendations of the American Public Health Association had taken on a more specific nature: *"Resolved,* That the . . . Association recognizes that the health of older people is a public health problem of national magnitude and concern, and thus warrants action by the Federal Government to stimulate the programs in the states designed to reduce the impact of chronic illness upon older people . . . and recognizes the need for financial support by the federal level of government . . ."

Ultimately this support was to be partially responsible for the passage in 1960 of federal legislation for greater financial support for the medical care of the aged.

President Truman's Proposed National Health Program

On November 19, 1945, President Harry S. Truman delivered a message to Congress on a proposed national health program and urged the adoption of a bill consisting of five main parts, as follows: (1) construction of hospitals and other needed facilities; (2) expansion of public health, maternal and child health services; (3) strengthening of medical education and research in health; (4) compulsory insurance for the prepayment of medical costs; and (5) payment of benefits to workers who incur wage losses because of sickness and disability.

This bill was essentially a modification of the original Wagner Health Bill, which Congress had not approved. President Truman's proposed bill brought conflicting viewpoints on governmental participation in medical care into the open on a greater scale than previously.

Parts of this bill were well supported by the medical profession and were adopted by Congress, which did not, however, pass the total bill.

In August, 1946, for example, the Hospital Survey and Construction Act became a law and laid the groundwork for expansion of hospital facilities throughout the country. A large share of the responsibility for this program was given to the individual states, and the latter participated in the provision of funds. Also passed in 1946 was the National Mental Health Act, which provided for increased research in mental disease, funds for the training of specialists in the field of mental health, and financial assistance to states for improvements in the field of mental health and disease.

The Brookings Institute Report

In 1948 the Brookings Institute report on compulsory health insurance was published.

In this report it was concluded that no great nation in the world had better health than the United States and that no *basic* defects existed in the voluntary American system for provision of medical care. This group also concluded that the great majority of American families have the resources to pay for adequate medical care through voluntary arrangements. The report opposed the establishment of compulsory health insurance and government participation in medical care.

The National Health Assembly

In 1948 a National Health Assembly was held which was attended by more than 800 delegates, including many physicians, labor union representatives, and others. A ten-year program of health goals for the nation was outlined. Although much agreement was achieved, the group was still split on the fundamental issue of compulsory health insurance and governmental control in medical care.

The President's Commission on the Health Needs of the Nation

On December 29, 1951, President Harry S. Truman created a commission of fifteen members who were instructed to make a careful evaluation of the health needs of the nation and to make a report of its findings and recommendations within one year.

This group, known among medical circles as the Magnuson Commission, after the name of its chairman, made its report available in five volumes in 1953 after examining statistical data, surveying health literature, and conducting hearings in various areas of the United States.

The Commission reported that during a single year the nation's total expenditures for civilian health services amounted to nearly $14 billion, a per capita cost of approximately $89 per year. *Only two-thirds of this health bill, however, was paid directly by the consumers.* Of each $100 spent by consumers on health, approximately $28 was paid to physicians and surgeons, $24 to hospitals, nearly $18 for drugs, and $11 to dentists. Of the remaining $19 approximately $6 went for eyeglasses, crutches or other appliances, $7 for insurance, and about $7 for nursing and miscellaneous items.

The Commission found that the average family was spending about $200 per year for health expenditures. It was concluded, however, that this average figure did not apply to many families in which excessive illness had occurred.

In one study it was found that one third of the families had paid medical bills of $100 to $400 a year *beyond the cost of health insurance.* Some families had paid more than $600 in excess of their health insurance coverage.

The Commission recommended that the principle of *prepaid health services be accepted as the most feasible method of financing the costs of medical care.* The group favored a cooperative federal-state program to assist in the financing of personal health services. This program, it was stated, should be administered by a single state agency, with an advisory council representing the public interest, and should provide services to all persons, as comprehensive as local resources would permit. Administration of the plan on a local or regional basis was favored. Federal assistance in the form of grants-in-aid should be made from general tax revenues, according to the Commission.

President Eisenhower's Message to Congress

On January 26, 1956, President Dwight D. Eisenhower sent a message to Congress in which he expressed the views of his administration regarding the health needs of the nation. The President stated that:

The Nation in recent years has made notable advances in the unending struggle against disease and disability. Human suffering has been relieved, the span of man's years has been extended. But in the light of the human and economic toll still taken by disease, in the light of the great opportunities open before us, the Nation still has not summoned the resources it properly and usefully could summon to the cause of better health.

Therefore, as a nation, we must now take further steps to improve the health of the people. . . . Such action should be taken in several general areas through:

1. A substantial increase in Federal funds for medical research.

2. A new program of grants for construction of medical research and training facilities.

3. Further steps to help alleviate health personnel shortages.

4. Measures which will help our people meet the costs of medical care.

5. Action to strengthen certain other basic health services throughout the Nation . . .

In respect to the cost of medical care President Eisenhower observed that "the need for more and better health insurance coverage can best be met by building on what many of our people have already provided for themselves—the voluntary health prepayment plans . . ."

President Eisenhower's Health Message to Congress received commendation from the American Medical Association shortly thereafter as "in general a sound approach to a solution of the problems in the health field."

Forand Bill

The Forand Bill was introduced in the 86th Congress by Representative A. J. For-

and of Rhode Island. The Bill proposed to amend the Social Security Act so that the Federal Government would provide health care for persons eligible for Social Security benefits, most of whom would be over the age of 65.

Under the proposed bill the government would enter into contracts to pay hospitals, nursing homes, physicians and dentists for the health services that they would provide to the 16 million eligible persons (estimated in 1960).

Financial support for the Forand proposal would come from an increase in social security taxes. The American Medical Association and physicians in general opposed the Forand Bill, believing that passage of the bill would put medical care on a political basis and would weaken the patient-physician relationship. In addition, opposition has stemmed from the fact that more and more of the older citizens are now protecting themselves by voluntary health insurance. As of 1960, the Health Insurance Institute reported that 65 per cent of the older citizens over the age of 65 had the protection of health insurance.

Early in 1960 the Eisenhower administration opposed any program of compulsory health insurance for the elderly and the proposed Forand Bill was not sufficiently supported in Congress to gain passage.

Medical Care for Older Persons

On September 13, 1960, President Dwight D. Eisenhower signed a bill into law that provides more adequate medical care for persons over the age of 65. This new law followed the deferment of the Forand Bill in Congress and provided for federal financial assistance to states developing programs for the improvement of medical care for persons over the age of 65.

Most states already had a program of medical care for needy, old persons who were on relief rolls. Under the new law the Federal government will assist the states in giving more and better medical care to these people. Part of the aid to the states will meet the medical bills of people over 65 who are not so destitute as to qualify for state relief for food, housing and clothing (in other words people who can support themselves except when health problems require medical cost beyond their financial capacity).

The bill does not provide for compulsory health insurance or for increased taxes under social security. It therefore differs greatly from the Forand Bill which would have provided medical care for all persons over 65 who are entitled to social security benefits. This new law is more consistent with the concept of voluntary health insurance coverage and minimal participation of the Federal government in health and medical affairs than the Forand Bill.

The Attitude of the American Medical Association

By 1939 the American Medical Association had formulated and published certain concepts that it believed to be fundamental in any relationship of government to medical care.

Since the A.M.A. had consistently worked for many years for the improvement of the national health, these concepts were primarily a reiteration and reorganization of views long held.

The American Medical Association went on record as favoring the establishment of a federal agency to coordinate and administer medical and health functions of the Federal Government, the provision of funds by Congress for the promotion of health and the care of the sick if states were in need of these funds. Also favored was local responsibility as a primary principle in the provision of medical or public health services and a local mechanism to

determine needs and administer programs. Approved also was extension of medical care for the indigent and the medically indigent, full utilization of established medical and hospital facilities, continued development of the private practice of medicine, and expansion of public health and medical services consistent with the American system of democracy.

The American Medical Association as a professional group has since been consistently against compulsory sickness insurance. This opposition has been based on the concept that government control would limit the freedom of the individual and result in a deterioration of the quality of medical care.

The medical profession has also challenged the validity of the health statistics which have been quoted by persons favoring federal compulsory health insurance. The point has been made by the medical profession that the draft rejection figures which have been quoted so frequently as evidence of the need for a better health program are not dependable because many persons who were first turned down by the armed forces were later accepted for military service; and that a tremendous number of those who were rejected could not be made healthier by any health program.

As a substitute for the National Health Bill, the Association has proposed a broad program featuring better housing, nutrition and sanitation; extension of public health services to prevent disease; voluntary health insurance; local voluntary hospital sickness insurance for the indigent; voluntary sickness insurance; federal aid to needy states; health surveys of each state to establish needs; education of the American people to ways of improving health programs without increasing taxes; continuous surveys of voluntary health plans; freeing of physicians from military services on a broader scale in order to provide better civilian medical care; an increase in the number of medical students; a slow and careful consideration of revolutionary changes; and a study of medical personnel needs.

Currently, the leadership of the American Medical Association has swung from mere opposition to compulsory health insurance to a broader program for the prevention and treatment of illness in the United States.

The medical profession is trying to achieve a better distribution of doctors throughout the country by rendering financial assistance, especially to young doctors, and providing other encouragement for physicians to practice medicine in rural areas or other places where more doctors are needed.

A serious attempt is being made to improve relations between hospital administrators and physicians to obtain better hospital service for patients. The medical profession has agreed on the principle of federal assistance for the construction, equipment and renovation of the physical plants of medical schools, although it feels that the operating deficits of medical schools can still be met on a voluntary basis. They are giving greater support to health insurance plans sponsored by various state medical societies. The Association is also cooperating with business organizations interested in simplifying and providing a better commercial health insurance program. The profession is also striving for greater cooperation with other professional groups such as the optometrists and others.

Dr. Iago Galdston of the New York Academy of Medicine has pointed out that many of the problems in medicine today are a result of great successes achieved. One hundred years ago there were few complaints about the cost of medical care or the difficulty of obtaining the services of a doctor; complaints were made about incompetence in medicine and the many disputes that split the medical profession. As late as 1870 the hospital was a place where only the critically ill person went to die. Today it is a refuge for the sick, a center

for teaching physicians and a research center for medical progress. Dr. Galdston also says that curative medicine, despite its marvelous ability to cure the ills of the individual, is relatively helpless when it comes to curing the social ills of a civilization. To meet new problems, medicine needs freedom and public support.

Can We Afford Medical Care?

One question that must be answered is whether the average American family can afford to pay for medical care at existing prices.

If we do not have the ability to pay for medical care, then the problem is definitely one of economics. On the other hand, if we have adequate income, but spend it foolishly, then the problem is one of re-education and restoration of a better sense of values. A family is hardly justified in complaining about the cost of preventing disease or treating illness if it spends a great share of the budget for relatively trivial things.

What is the case in respect to medical care?

HEALTH CARE SPENDING

"Americans are spending twice as much for recreation, alcohol, and tobacco as for medical care ... Two dollars out of every $18 the public spends on personal needs falls in the playing-drinking-smoking category, $1 in the medical bracket."

Health Insurance Institute, AMA News, April 4, 1960

During an average year people in the United States spend from 7 to 9 billion dollars on alcoholic beverages. The annual amount of money spent for medical care and death expenses combined is approximately the same, though in some years more is spent on alcohol. Although expenditures will normally fluctuate from year to year, it appears that we spend more for drinking alcohol than we do for the treatment of sickness.

In one year when we spent over nine billion dollars on health and death expenses, a figure that amounted to approximately 5 per cent of our total financial outlays, we also spent more than eleven billion dollars, or 6 per cent of our total expenditures, on recreation, and more than twenty-two billion dollars, or approximately 12 per cent, on automobiles and transportation. During this year, also, approximately three billion dollars was spent on tobacco.

From the foregoing data it can be seen that we are either so healthy or our medical bills are so small that we can afford to spend much more money for tobacco and alcohol, entertainment, automobiles and transportation than for medical care, or else our sense of values is so distorted that we find these other products and services of more value than the health of our families.

One interpretation that can be made of the foregoing figures is that we do have a national capacity to pay for medical care, but that we need a reorientation of our sense of values. We should learn to spend our money for the more important things.

One thing appears certain. If we are spending only 5 per cent of our per capita expenditures on the expenses of medical care and death, it seems clear that on a national scale we can afford to pay for medical care.

It should be noted that although physicians have been criticized by the public for the rising costs of medical care, their services have risen in price to a much smaller extent than has occurred in the general cost of living. *The physician has not been responsible for the great increase in the cost of medical care,* although he is in the mind of the public. There is need for greater reflection by the people of the United States on the complexity of the medical care problem.

A Question of Values

In a democracy that professes to place a high premium upon the development of individual initiative and personal responsibilities it would appear that every citizen should continue to accept at least a partial obligation for the protection of his own and his family's health.

Balance is needed between giving too much responsibility to others and accepting all responsibility oneself. It is likely that an extreme view in either direction may be unwholesome.

If a person cannot spend money wisely or make a sensible choice between paying for the illness of his family in contrast to supplying them with tobacco, alcohol, entertainment and automobiles, it is unlikely that protecting that person by compulsory health insurance will make him a person of stronger character or judgment. On the other hand, if it were possible to re-educate such a person to have a better sense of values, there would be a fundamental contribution to his character.

All the evidence indicates that there are extreme inequalities in the cost of medical care for individual families. Sickness and death do not strike all families with equal force. Some families may be economically distressed by illness, while others escape unscathed for years. The problem of providing high-quality medical care to all families in the United States in such a way that none become impoverished as a result of sickness has not yet been completely resolved. When an adequate solution is found, however, it should probably contain provisions for the continuation of individual responsibilities as well as for group or community sharing of the costs of excessive illness.

It will be up to the American public to decide whether compulsory health insurance will be the ideal solution to the problem of the costs of medical care. A decision on this question should not be made on an emotional basis, but on an analysis of the facts and moral issues involved.

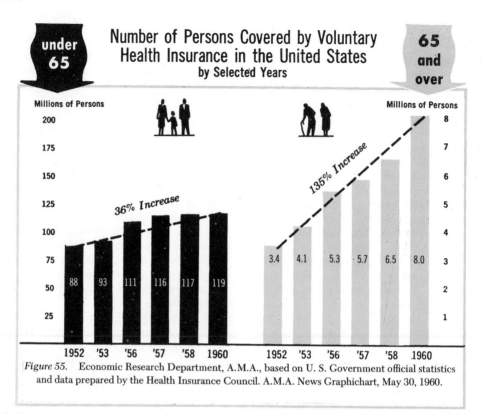

Figure 55.   Economic Research Department, A.M.A., based on U. S. Government official statistics and data prepared by the Health Insurance Council. A.M.A. News Graphichart, May 30, 1960.

Health Insurance

One solution to the cost of medical or surgical care is group insurance. It has been shown in the section on national expenditures that the country as a whole can afford to pay for medical care. There is always the problem of excessive costs due to long, sustained illness and surgical emergencies that may arise in any particular family, however. The national ability to pay for medical care is of little assistance to the individual family in such a case unless there is some means of sharing such additional costs.

Currently, a large number of individuals and families subscribe to health insurance. Insurance for hospitalization, accidents, medical and surgical care, and payment for time lost because of illness and absence from the job constitute the four main types of health insurance sold in this country.

In 1959 more than 123 million persons were covered with some form of prepayment sickness insurance on a voluntary basis.

In addition to the voluntary health insurance plans, most states now have workmen's compensation laws which require employers to carry insurance for their employees in case any are disabled because of the work in which they are engaged. A number of states have recently passed laws for sickness compensation consisting of cash benefits in case of illness or injury *that has no relation to the job.* Illness and disability benefits are also available in pension and retirement plans that now cover about five million people.

In 1955 President Eisenhower urged a reinsurance plan which he had put forth two years earlier, by which insurance companies might purchase insurance from the government to protect themselves against

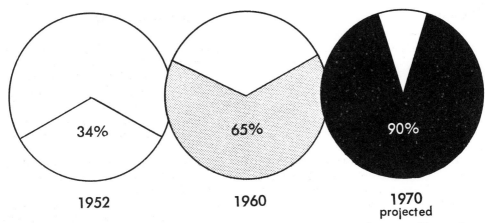

Figure 56. Percentage of health insurance coverage of United States population over 65 years of age who need and want this protection. (A.M.A. News Graphichart. Health Insurance Institute, March 7, 1960.)

heavy losses. The President believed that through such Federal support there would be a considerable expansion of health insurance plans that would give greater protection to more people for more illnesses. This plan was first beaten in the House, and in 1955 the bill never reached the floor of either the House or Senate. In his 1956 Message to Congress the President was no longer urging this type of reinsurance plan and acknowledged that the considerable growth of voluntary health insurance plans might meet existing needs, especially if the insurance companies could be permitted to share or pool their risks in offering broader benefits and extended coverage. Legislation that would permit such voluntary pooling of resources was being considered by the administration at the time of the President's message.

The number of persons covered by health insurance, especially the voluntary type, fluctuates widely from year to year. It is also likely that no individual health insurance plan can be found that will be perfect for everyone. Nevertheless, the more widespread the adoption of voluntary health insurance, the greater the likelihood that the medical, surgical and hospital needs of the average family will be met to a considerable extent. There is growing evidence that the people of the United States can provide themselves with adequate health insurance on the voluntary basis consistent with a democratic way of life.

Current Federal Legislation

Shortly after taking office in 1961, President John F. Kennedy and his administration made further legislative proposals in the field of medical care. Even the supporters of such legislation do not claim that its enactment would bring about a *final* solution to the many problems that have impelled similar legislation in the past. The adequacy of public health care and facilities, the level of public health, and the roles of the individual and federal, state, and local governments will be areas of discussion, change and progress for many years to come. It is of utmost importance that the college student familiarize himself with the issues involved.

Questions

1. How much medical care, if any, should a person expect without direct payment for services?
2. What value is there, if any, in paying for medical treatment through taxes and assessments, rather than in the traditional individual manner?
3. What suggestions do you have for spreading the cost of excessive illness in a family?
4. Should an individual ever be relieved entirely of the responsibility for maintaining his own health?
5. What is your opinion of deductible health insurance comparable to that in widespread use in the field of automobile insurance?

For Further Reading

1. Bachman, A. W., *et al.*: *Health Resources in the United States: Personnel Facilities and Services.* Washington, D.C., Brookings Institute, 1952.
2. Bauer, W. W.: *Santa Claus, M.D.* Indianapolis, Bobbs-Merrill Co., 1950.
3. Huntington, Emily H.: *Cost of Medical Care.* Berkeley, California, University of California Press, 1951.
4. Peterson, O. L.: *A Study of the National Health Service of Great Britain.* New York, Rockefeller Foundation, 1951.
5. Winslow, C. E. A.: *The Cost of Sickness and the Price of Health.* New York, Columbia University Press, 1951.

28

COMMUNITY HEALTH SERVICES

THE CONCEPT of needed community health services is changing. For many years medical and public health leaders have accepted the so-called Basic Six as an outline for the provision of public health services. The Basic Six consisted of the following: vital statistics, public health education, environmental sanitation, public health laboratories, communicable disease control and maternal and infant hygiene. Modern thinking calls for a much broader attack on the health problems of a community.

Some of the changes that are taking place in the field of public health that have significance for enlarged responsibilities and opportunities are as follows:

The increasing conquest of tuberculosis with successful treatment of many patients by private physicians is altering the quality and quantity of public health participation in this field.

379

Cooperation by schools, physicians, pharmaceutical organizations and many other groups in mass immunizations (such as for poliomyelitis) open new possibilities for extension of this service to the American public.

Scientific developments and the genesis of new techniques in the food industry calls for modification by public health authorities in the techniques of food and milk sanitation.

The great increase in the older population has given rise to a need for new approaches in the prevention and care of long term, chronic illnesses.

Psychiatric problems have become more of a concern of public health authorities in recent years. Programs for the rehabilitation of alcoholics and drug addicts are illustrations of changing practices in this zone of human relations.

Public health supervision of fluoridation programs has thrust public health authorities into the field of dental health on a broader scale than ever before.

The hazard of nuclear and other types of radiation exposure has given rise to completely new responsibilities for the mass protection of populations by public health and civil defense authorities.

The ascendancy of accidents as one of the major causes of death in this country has called for the development of a new kind of epidemiology.

In large cities the emergence of air polution as a serious public health problem gives rise to the need for new laws, new cooperative efforts, new scientific findings and the evolution of more effective public health weapons against this menace.

These and many other changes in the structure of our public health problems make adjustments imperative in our public health programs. The basic organization for the provision of public health services remains the same.

Community health organization exists in various forms and at many levels: from that of the village to international union.

There are at least six main categories in which organization for community health exists today. These are (1) the voluntary health agencies, (2) the professional health organizations, (3) the local departments of public health, (4) the state departments of public health, (5) federal public health activities and (6) the World Health Organization and other international bodies organized for the promotion and protection of human health.

The citizen can express himself in favor

of organization for community health in a number of ways. First, he can give voting support to measures on the ballot that foster protection of human health. Second, he can express himself in the community, by voice and written word, in favor of community health organization and activity. Third, he can take an active part in shaping the program for community health by participation in health projects, financial support of voluntary health agencies, and by serving on community health councils or health committees of other organizations.

In this chapter some of the multiple organizations that exist in our society for the improvement and maintenance of human health are described. The activities of these organizations are enumerated in part, so that a general understanding of the work of such public, voluntary and professional groups may be better understood. A more complete conception of these organizations must be obtained from an analysis of more detailed descriptions, although in some of the previous chapters many aspects of community health have been discussed.

The Voluntary Health Agencies

The voluntary health agencies are a unique development in the United States. These organizations exist for the promotion and protection of human health on a voluntary basis and receive their financial support by gifts and fund-raising campaigns, without governmental support of any kind.

The characteristic feature of the voluntary health agency is that it is composed of people with a common interest in a specific health problem. For example, the local Health and Tuberculosis Organizations are composed of people concerned principally with the prevention of tuberculosis and the protection of the public in general from this disease. Recently these organizations have begun to broaden their programs beyond that of the control of tuberculosis to other health problems. Members of the American Cancer Society are persons who have an especial interest in the promotion of research on cancer and education of the public regarding this disease. The National Foundation is composed of both professional and lay persons who have a special interest in the control of poliomyelitis, although this organization is also becoming more active in attempts to control other diseases.

An example of the health service provided by a voluntary health organization is found in the activities of the American Cancer Society. This organization, in a period of eleven years, devoted $41,213,-000 to research on cancer. This expenditure of funds reflected a basic philosophy that the organization could best serve humanity by specializing on the promotion and support of research.

During the years in question the society made 2439 grants-in-aid and supported 501 research fellows and scholars. More than 350 research grants were made to institutions for the investigation of problems relating to cancer. During one year financial support was being given in forty-four medical and scientific centers to 152 cancer-research projects in hospitals, universities and various laboratories.

All these activities are supported by funds raised voluntarily from the general public and by the time and energy contributed by thousands of members of the American Cancer Society.

An outstanding example of what a voluntary health organization can do for the promotion of human welfare is found in the relationship of the National Foundation to the Salk vaccine for the prevention of paralytic poliomyelitis. This vaccine, which has greatly reduced the deaths and paralysis from poliomyelitis, was produced by Dr. Jonas E. Salk on funds provided by the organization, which supported his basic research and subsequently made available large quantities of the vaccine for extensive field trials of its effectiveness.

One of the striking characteristics of recent years has been the sponsorship of new health services in cities and counties by the voluntary health organizations. About two thirds of the heart clinics and one half of the diabetes clinics in the United States have been operated by voluntary health organizations in recent years.

There has been some criticism of the voluntary health agencies because there is a tendency for such organizations to work independently of others because of their special interests, but such an inclination is not necessarily a total weakness, for often concentration of effort in a narrow field brings results that could not be obtained by a broader approach.

The Professional Health Organizations

An important and well organized force for the promotion of community health in the United States is the professional health society. The American Medical Association, for example, represents such a professional organization. The membership is composed of professionally trained and licensed physicians. Sometimes associate memberships in such organizations are available for persons in other categories, but the predominant feature of membership is that it represents professional qualification in a given field.

Other examples of professional organizations that have had an important influence upon the structure of public health in the United States are the American Public Health Association, the American Dental Association and the professional nursing groups.

It is safe to say that in the field of health the two organizations that have had the greatest professional influence are the American Medical Association and the American Public Health Association.

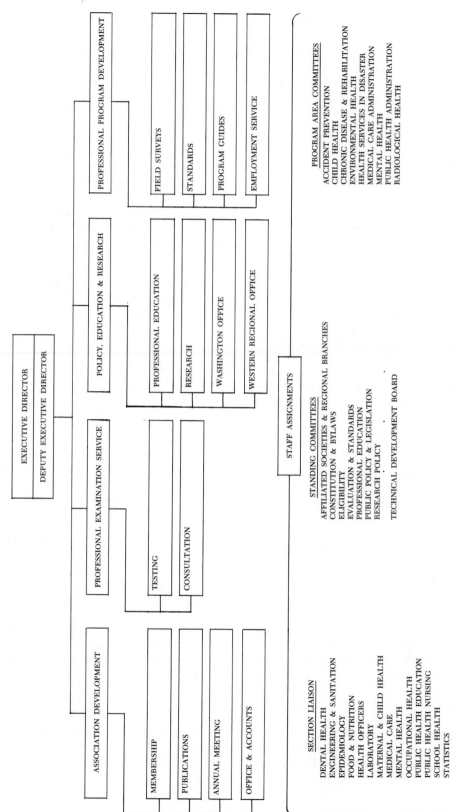

Figure 57. The organization and activities of the American Public Health Association. (Courtesy of American Public Health Association.)

The American Public Health Association

The American Public Health Association has taken a consistent lead in the fight for improved public health programs in this country. Being dissociated from any government structure or official agency, the public health group has been free to express its professional opinion on a multiplicity of health problems in the United States. A long and constructive influence on the development of public health has been apparent in the history of this organization. The1960 organization and activities of the American Public Health Association are shown in the accompanying chart.

The American Medical Association

Although predominantly occupied with the problems of medical treatment, the American Medical Association has exerted a powerful influence on the health of the American people in a variety of ways. One of the important influences of this group has been concerned with the improvement of medical education in the United States. Early in the twentieth century the American Medical Association fostered an examination of medical schools throughout the country that resulted in the establishment of certain high level standards for medical education. The application of high standards in the evaluation of medical schools has resulted in the dissolution of those schools with an inferior program. As a consequence of active leadership in this field, the medical schools in the United States now provide the highest quality of medical training that can be obtained in any country in the world.

An example of the numerous community relationships in which a professional society may be involved is offered in the chart on page 384, which is an organizational chart of the Santa Clara County Medical Society of California.

The American Medical Association has expressed itself on many aspects of health in this country. The organization has been especially concerned in recent years in safeguarding the basic relationship of the physician and his patient and the avoidance of state medicine.

The World Medical Association

The World Medical Association is an international organization of medical societies. It is not a part of the United Nations nor is it a part of the World Health Organization. This voluntary association was organized in 1947 for the purpose of exchanging medical knowledge, to protect the freedom of medicine, and to promote world peace. The association is supported both by dues from members and by contributions. More than 50 national medical associations from different countries of the world are now members of this group.

The American Dental Association

The American Dental Association has taken a leading role in the promotion of community programs for fluoridation of public water supplies. This may well represent the outstanding development in the field of dental health throughout the entire history of dentistry. The dental profession deserves great credit for its unselfish and untiring efforts to educate the American public to the values of fluoridation of the community water supplies. Research and experience both show that dental decay can be greatly reduced when fluoridation of the drinking water is adopted by communities, but in many areas ignorance and misinformation have caused public reluctance to adopt this important dental health measure. The American Dental Association has fought vigorously to dissipate this ignorance and to dissolve the prejudices that sometimes deprive communities of this desirable public health measure. The success of their efforts is illustrated by the fact that more than 1850 cities and towns in the United States have now adopted fluoridation.

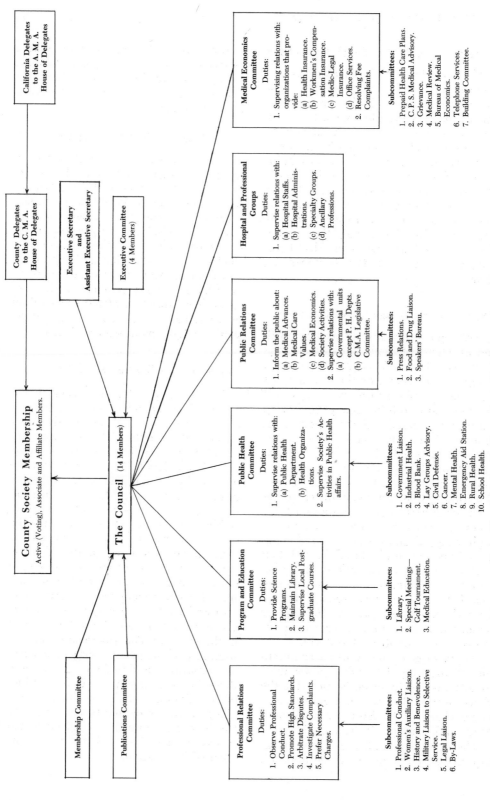

California Delegates to the A. M. A. House of Delegates

County Delegates to the C. M. A. House of Delegates

Executive Secretary and Assistant Executive Secretary

Executive Committee (4 Members)

County Society Membership
Active (Voting), Associate and Affiliate Members.

The Council (14 Members)

Membership Committee

Publications Committee

Medical Economics Committee
Duties:
1. Supervising relations with: organizations that provide:
   (a) Health Insurance.
   (b) Workmen's Compensation Insurance.
   (c) Medic-Legal Insurance.
   (d) Office Services.
2. Resolving Fee Complaints.
Subcommittees:
1. Prepaid Health Care Plans.
2. C.P.S. Medical Advisory.
3. Grievance.
4. Medical Review.
5. Bureau of Medical Economics.
6. Telephone Services.
7. Building Committee.

Hospital and Professional Groups
Duties:
1. Supervise relations with:
   (a) Hospital Staffs.
   (b) Hospital Administrations.
   (c) Specialty Groups.
   (d) Ancillary Professions.

Public Relations Committee
Duties:
1. Inform the public about:
   (a) Medical Advances.
   (b) Medical Care Values.
   (c) Medical Economics.
   (d) Society Activities.
2. Supervise relations with:
   (a) Governmental units except P. H. Depts.
   (b) C.M.A. Legislative Committee.
Subcommittees:
1. Press Relations.
2. Food and Drug Liaison.
3. Speakers' Bureau.

Public Health Committee
Duties:
1. Supervise relations with:
   (a) Public Health Department.
   (b) Health Organizations.
2. Supervise Society's Activities in Public Health affairs.
Subcommittees:
1. Government Liaison.
2. Industrial Health.
3. Blood Bank.
4. Lay Groups Advisory.
5. Civil Defense.
6. Cancer.
7. Mental Health.
8. Emergency Aid Station.
9. Rural Health.
10. School Health.

Program and Education Committee
Duties:
1. Provide Science Programs.
2. Maintain Library.
3. Supervise Local Postgraduate Courses.
Subcommittees:
1. Library.
2. Special Meetings—Golf Tournament.
3. Medical Education.

Professional Relations Committee
Duties:
1. Observe Professional Conduct.
2. Promote High Standards.
3. Arbitrate Disputes.
4. Investigate Complaints.
5. Prefer Necessary Charges.
Subcommittees:
1. Professional Conduct.
2. Women's Auxiliary Liaison.
3. History and Benevolence.
4. Military Liaison to Selective Service.
5. Legal Liaison.
6. By-Laws.

Figure 58. Organization chart—Santa Clara County Medical Society.

The Local Public Health Department

From the preventive viewpoint it is the local public health department that the average person may encounter in his daily life. Local public health departments may exist on the individual community or town basis or may be on a somewhat broader scale, such as a county department of public health.

The local public health departments are sustained by public funds, most of which are obtained by taxation at the local level; however, substantial financial amounts are received from the state department of public health in most states. In addition, the local public health department may profit by funds from special federal programs. These federal monies are usually obtained through the state department of public health.

The functions of the local public health department vary considerably from area to area in the United States. This should be expected, since local public health problems may be quite different in one community from those in another community. It should be obvious that an effective local public health program can exist only if the activities of this department are based upon the needs of the community.

One way to understand the functions of the local public health departments in the United States is to study how the employees of health departments spend their time on the job. Dr. Edward M. Cohart and Dr. William R. Willard, co-directors of the Yale Public Health Personnel Research Project, reported a study in which 92 per cent of the employees of eight local health departments in Michigan kept a time log of their activities for one week.

This study found that the percentage of total working time devoted to various aspects of the local health department program was as follows:

From the foregoing table it can be seen that the activities of the local public health department are concerned with many

Rank	Program Activity	Time Percentage*
1.	School health..............	27
2.	Environmental sanitation.....	23
3.	Maternal and child health.....	16
4.	Tuberculosis...............	13
5.	Acute communicable disease..	10
6.	Crippled children...........	3
7.	Mental hygiene.............	3
8.	Venereal disease	2
9.	Chronic disease.............	1
10.	All other aspects of the program	2
	Total...................	100

* Rounded to the nearest whole number.

health problems other than the sanitation of water supplies, sewage disposal, registration of deaths and other vital statistics, milk sanitation and the control of communicable diseases. Such functions are usually assumed to represent the total health concern of the local public health department. Actually, depending upon the locality, the functions of a particular health department at the local level may be strikingly different from one community to another. In one area, such as in Los Angeles, there may be a vital concern about smog control, whereas in another community this may be no problem at all. Perhaps the fundamental thing to remember is that the functions of the local public health department will differ according to needs of the local community.

Ferguson, Graning, and Cheney reported a study of the activities of 186 local public health officers in thirty-five different states.

This study showed that the local health officer spends in a typical work week about 2538 minutes on seventy-four activities in twelve different health programs. Seventy-five per cent of this average, or 1896 minutes, involves the expression of medical judgment.

The types of activities in which local health officers engage and the percentage of time spent in each of these activities are indicated in the accompanying table.

Rank	Activity	Per Cent of Time
1.	Individual conferences	10.3
2.	Clinic participation	10.2
3.	Correspondence	8.6
4.	Group conferences	8.5
5.	Travel	7.6
6.	Program planning	6.4
7.	Direction and supervision	6.0
8.	Records and reports	4.3
9.	Meetings attended	4.2
10.	Telephone	3.8
11.	Field investigation	3.2
12.	Board participation	3.2
13.	Community activity	2.6
14.	Self-improvement—reading, etc.	2.5
15.	Budget and fiscal	2.2
16.	Preparation of educational material	2.0
17.	Personnel	1.8
18.	Enforcement of ordinances	1.8
19.	Licensing and permits	1.6
20.	Professional consultation services	1.4
21.	Evaluations and surveys	1.4
22.	Talks given	1.2
23.	Teaching	1.1
24.	Education-in-service	1.1
25.	Housekeeping and errands	0.8
26.	Purchasing	0.7
27.	Personal and unidentified	1.5

An example of the many activities of the local health department is given in the chart, on page 387, of the organization of the health department of the City of Newark, New Jersey.

The State Department of Public Health

In each state there are certain legal requirements approved by the state legislature for the promotion and protection of the public health. The structural organization with the responsibility for supervising state regulations and providing a statewide program for the promotion of health is, of course, the state department of public health.

This public health organization receives its principal financial support from taxation on a state level plus rather substantial income from the federal government for statewide development of special programs, including the development of the state public health organization itself.

A rather clear-cut indication of the activities of the state public health department can be gained from a study of the way in which the budget is expended. This financial accounting gives a precise indication of the state health activities of a department.

It should be expected that the programs of state departments of public health will differ according to the health needs within that state. Nevertheless there is a general structure in most states. An example of activity analysis by financial cost accounting is offered in the following table, in which the Florida State Board of Health gives an itemized account of the public health dollar for a particular year.

Rank	Activity or Unit	Cents
1.	County health units	52.92
2.	Preventable diseases, exclusive of tuberculosis control	7.58
3.	Laboratories	6.79
4.	Entomology and mosquito control	6.78
5.	Chronic diseases	5.84
6.	General administration	5.07
7.	Sanitary engineering	3.00
8.	Vital statistics	2.49
9.	Tuberculosis control	2.16
10.	Maternal and child health	1.95
11.	Training	1.82
12.	Bureau of local health service	1.55
13.	Health information	1.15
14.	Narcotic enforcement	0.90

The scope of the state department of public health is also revealed by study of the personnel employed in this branch of government. In the typical state department there is a state health officer, various medical personnel, dental directors, sanitary engineers, laboratory directors,

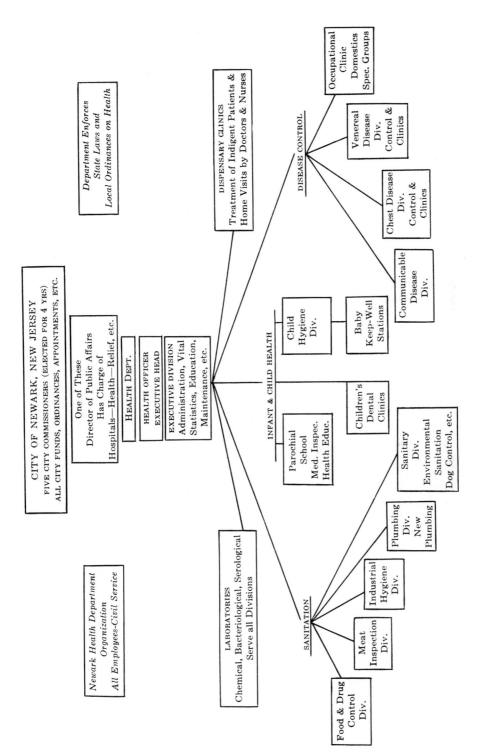

Figure 59.

*Department Enforces
State Laws and
Local Ordinances on Health*

*Newark Health Department
Organization
All Employees–Civil Service*

CITY OF NEWARK, NEW JERSEY
FIVE CITY COMMISSIONERS (ELECTED FOR 4 YRS)
ALL CITY FUNDS, ORDINANCES, APPOINTMENTS, ETC.

One of These
Director of Public Affairs
Has Charge of
Hospitals—Health—Relief, etc.

HEALTH DEPT.

HEALTH OFFICER
EXECUTIVE HEAD

EXECUTIVE DIVISION
Administration, Vital
Statistics, Education,
Maintenance, etc.

DISPENSARY CLINICS
Treatment of Indigent Patients &
Home Visits by Doctors & Nurses

DISEASE CONTROL

Occupational
Clinic
Domestics
Spec. Groups

Venereal
Disease
Div.
Control &
Clinics

Chest Disease
Div.
Control &
Clinics

Communicable
Disease
Div.

INFANT & CHILD HEALTH

Child
Hygiene
Div.

Baby
Keep-Well
Stations

Children's
Dental
Clinics

Parochial
School
Med. Inspec.
Health Educ.

Sanitary
Div.
Environmental
Sanitation
Dog Control, etc.

Plumbing
Div.
New
Plumbing

Industrial
Hygiene
Div.

SANITATION

Meat
Inspection
Div.

Food & Drug
Control
Div.

LABORATORIES
Chemical, Bacteriological, Serological
Serve all Divisions

vital statisticians, nurses and associated personnel such as laboratory assistants, stenographers, clerks and so on.

The multiple bureaus and divisions of a state department of public health are illustrated in an analysis of the California State Department of Public Health, in which there are twenty-eight divisions and bureaus which reflect different kinds of public health services. These are (1) the Bureau of Business Management, (2) the Bureau of Health Education, (3) the Bureau of Records and Statistics, (4) the Training Office, (5) the Division of Dental Health, (6) the Bureau of Food and Drug Inspections, (7) the Bureau of Sanitary Engineering, (8) the Bureau of Vector Control, (9) the Bacteriology Laboratory, (10) the Branch Laboratory of Los Angeles, (11) the Food and Drug Laboratory, (12) the Laboratory Field Services, (13) the Sanitation Laboratory, (14) the Viral and Rickettsial Laboratory, (15) the Division of Local Health Services, (16) the Bureau of Acute Communicable Diseases, (17) the Bureau of Adult Health, (18) the Bureau of Chronic Diseases, (19) the Bureau of Crippled Children Services, (20) the Bureau of Hospitals, (21) the Bureau of Maternal and Child Health, (22) the Bureau of Public Health Nursing, (23) the Bureau of Tuberculosis, (24) the Bureau of Venereal Diseases, (25) the Medical Social Service, (26) the Nutrition Service, (27) the Mental Health Service and (28) the Division of Medical and Health Services (under the office of civilian defense).

An official statement of the American Public Health Association indicates that, in general, the responsibilities for assurance of proper public health services at the state level may be grouped into seven divisions, as follows: (1) administration, (2) promulgation of health rules and regulations, (3) enforcement of state health laws and regulations, (4) state program planning and policy determination, (5) evalua tion of existing programs, (6) assistance to local health units and (7) health education.

It must be remembered that the state department of public health is a legally constituted unit of state government which usually operates independently of other units and is responsible directly to the governor.

Each state of the union is likely to have many different kinds of health problems as compared to other states. Because of this it would be an error to have state departments of public health that were exactly like those in all other states. Uniformity of organization should not be expected. The pattern of the department should reflect the needs and resources of each state, and should be flexible enough to permit change and adaptation to new health problems.

Federal Public Health Activities

At the national level in the United States there exists a considerable structure for the promotion and protection of human health. The financial support for this structural organization comes entirely from federal funds, which, of course, come in turn from the people of the United States.

In terms of organization, federal health activities have been historically centered in the Public Health Service, although many other branches or divisions of federal administrative units have had responsibilities directly concerned with the health of our people.

The Public Health Service Act, which was signed by President Roosevelt on July 3, 1944, was hailed by health authorities as a milestone in the 146-year history of the United States Public Health Service. This new law brought together in a more orderly arrangement all the laws affecting the Service, but retained the important duties that had been delegated to the latter over a period of more than fifty years. These duties included responsibilities for scientific research in the field of health, the control of biologic products (drugs and antibiotics), the medical care of lepers and narcotic drug addicts, the medical and hospital care of merchant marine seamen, members of the United States Coast Guard and other Federal beneficiaries, and direction of the National Quarantine Service.

Under the new law the Public Health Service was organized into four main administrative units: the Office of the Surgeon General, the National Institutes of Health, the Bureau of State Services, and the Bureau of Medical Services.

In 1953, under President Eisenhower, another great change in organization with respect to the administration of federal health services occurred. At that time the Federal Security Agency was elevated to the rank of a department and became known as the Department of Health, Education and Welfare. This new department consisted of four main subdivisions: the Public Health Service, the Social Security Administration, the Office of Education, and the Office of Vocational Rehabilitation.

Under this new administrative arrangement Public Health Service activities were accentuated and broadened, especially along the lines of social welfare as related to health problems. It can be said, in fact, that federal legislation pertaining to health in the United States during the current century has been predominantly concerned with, and dominated by, a broad social approach.

The World Health Organization

At the international level the outstanding organization for the promotion of human health is the World Health Organization.

The World Health Organization is mostly concerned with the control of communicable diseases on an international scale and in building up the public health organization in various foreign countries with backward programs. The organization is also much concerned with the edu-cation and training of medical and auxiliary personnel as well as with the training of public health personnel. There are many other activities which this organization carries on, such as the provision of professional leadership in the establishment of sound statistical services on health, the dispensing of medical information throughout the world, the encouragement of the construction in various countries of the necessary factories for the production of essential drugs and in practical assistance to individual countries in the control of particular diseases.

The assistance given to various countries by the World Health Organization in the organization of their public health departments may be the most important work of this group over a long period of time, since such encouragement develops individual capacities for the control of disease on a lasting basis. Currently, however, the most spectacular activities of the World Health Organization have been those concerned with the attempted conquest of specific diseases, such as malaria, tuberculosis and the venereal diseases.

The constitution of the World Health Organization should be studied in full for a full understanding of the scope and intent of this international body. Article 1 of Chapter I and Article 2 of Chapter II, which express the objective and the functions of the World Health Organization, are reproduced here in order to give a swift over-view of the work of this international body.

CHAPTER I. OBJECTIVE
Article 1—The objective of the World Health Organization (hereinafter called Organization) shall be the attainment by all peoples of the highest possible level of health.

CHAPTER II. FUNCTIONS
Article 2—In order to achieve its objective, the functions of the Organization shall be:
(a) to act as the directing and coordinating authority on international health work;
(b) to establish and maintain effective collaboration with the United Nations, specialized agencies,

governmental health administrations, professional groups and such other organizations as may be deemed appropriate;

(c) to assist governments, upon request, in strengthening health services;

(d) to furnish appropriate technical assistance and, in emergencies, necessary aid upon the request or acceptance of governments;

(e) to provide or assist in providing, upon the request of the United Nations, health services and facilities to special groups, such as the peoples of trust territories;

(f) to establish and maintain such administrative and technical services as may be required, including epidemiological and statistical services;

(g) to stimulate and advance work to eradicate epidemic, endemic and other diseases;

(h) to promote, in cooperation with other specialized agencies where necessary, the prevention of accidental injuries;

(i) to promote, in cooperation with other specialized agencies where necessary, the improvement of nutrition, housing, sanitation, recreation, economic or working conditions and other aspects of environmental hygiene;

(j) to promote cooperation among scientific and professional groups which contribute to the advancement of health;

(k) to propose conventions, agreements and regulations, and make recommendations with respect to international health matters and to perform such duties as may be assigned thereby to the Organization and are consistent with its objective;

(l) to promote maternal and child health and welfare and to foster the ability to live harmoniously in a changing total environment;

(m) to foster activities in the field of mental health, especially those affecting the harmony of human relations;

(n) to promote and conduct research in the field of health;

(o) to promote improved standards of teaching and training in the health, medical and related professions;

(p) to study and report on, in cooperation with other specialized agencies where necessary, administrative and social techniques affecting public health and medical care from the preventive and curative points of view;

(q) to provide information, counsel and assistance in the field of health;

(r) to assist in developing an informed public opinion among all peoples on matters of health;

(s) to establish and revise as necessary international nomenclatures of diseases, of causes of death and of public health practices;

(t) to standardize diagnostic procedures as necessary;

(u) to develop, establish and promote international standards with respect to food, biological, pharmaceutical and similar products;

(v) generally to take all necessary action to attain the objective of the Organization.

Questions

1. How many voluntary health agencies are there in your community, and what are their purposes?

2. What support has the local medical profession given to health measures in your community?

3. If there is a health council in your community, what activities has it been engaged in during the past year?

4. What services to your community does the public health department provide?

5. How would you go about organizing a health council in your community if none exists?

6. Are there any special health problems in your community that are more important than in other towns and cities?

7. If you were the public health officer in your home town what ten health problems would you give the greatest emphasis?

For Further Reading

1. Burn, J. L.: *Recent Advances in Public Health.* Boston, Little, Brown and Company, 1959.

2. Hanlon, John J.: *Principles of Public Health Administration.* St. Louis, C. V. Mosby Company, 1960.

3. Hilleboe, Herman E., and Larimore, Granville W.: *Preventive Medicine.* Philadelphia, W. B. Saunders Company, 1959.

4. Mustard, Harry S. and Stebbins, E. L.: *An Introduction to Public Health.* New York, Macmillan Company, 1959.

5. School of Public Health: *Legal Aspects of Public Health.* Ann Arbor, Michigan, University of Michigan Continued Education Service, 1959.

For Advanced Reading

Apple, Dorrian: *Sociological Studies of Health and Sickness: A Source Book for the Health Physicians.* New York, Blakiston-McGraw-Hill Book Company, 1960.

Recommended Films

1. *For the Nation's Health.* 16 mm., color, sound, showing time 16 minutes, 1957 (History of the Public Health Service), United World Films, Inc., 1445 Park Avenue, New York 29, N.Y. or Communicable Disease Center, attention Audio Visual, Atlanta 22, Ga.

2. *The National Institutes of Health.* 16 mm., color, sound, showing time 24 minutes, 1960 (Medical Research and Related Activities) United World Films, Inc., 1445 Park Avenue, New York 29, N. Y. or Communicable Disease Center, attention Audio Visual, Atlanta 22, Ga.

3. National Health Council. *Community Health in Action.* 16 mm., color, sound, showing time 23 minutes, 1955. Rental or purchase from Sam Orleans and Associates, Inc., 211 W. Cumberland Ave., Knoxville 15, Tenn.

29

RADIATION AND HEALTH

EVERYTHING in life is composed of atoms of various elements. Some of these atoms are not fixed and stable. Unstable elements give off parts of their atoms which fly off into space at tremendous speed, with great penetrating power. These particles are called rays and the giving off of the parts of the unstable atoms is known as radiation.

The particles given off in ionizing radiation have been given specific names as follows: *alpha, beta, gamma* and *x-rays.* These rays come from different parts of the atom. The *gamma* rays and the *x-rays* have the greatest penetrating power and it is primarily from these that we need the greatest protection, but they are also very useful to humanity in the diagnosis of disease, medical research and the treatment of certain kinds of illnesses.

The discovery of nuclear fission has greatly stimulated interest in, and investigation of, the effects of radiation on human life. The effects of radiation from pre-existing sources are being re-examined. Possible damage from radioactive fall-out associated with nuclear fission bombs is in part a matter of speculation at this time, but considerable thought is being given to this problem.

Measurement of Radiation

Scientists have developed certain terms for the measurement of radiation. These are technical terms but the important thing to remember is that they measure the *amount* of radiation that is involved. The three commonest terms are roentgens, rads, and rems.

The *roentgen* is a measure of the amount of radiation *exposure* and consists of the amount of radiation that will produce a certain amount of ionization in a specified volume of air. The important thing to remember about a roentgen is that it measures the amount of exposure to radiation that a person may experience.

The *rad* is a measurement of *dosage*. It measures the amount of energy from radiation that is absorbed by a material, such as human tissue. One rad represents the absorption of 100 ergs (units of energy) that is absorbed per gram of material (such as human tissue). An exposure of one roentgen from x-rays will usually result in about

one rad of radiation absorption in soft tissue.

The *rem* is a unit of absorbed radiation dosage which takes into account the relative biological effectiveness of different types of radiation. For x-rays, one rem is equivalent to one rad and this degree of absorption may be thought of as a "rad-equivalent-man." Since one rad is equivalent to about one roentgen of exposure with x-rays, some persons prefer to identify the rem as a "roentgen-equivalent-man." In either case, the initials come out the same: rem.

Sources of Radiation

Current exposure to radiation in the United States comes from three main sources: (1) the natural background of cosmic rays from outer space and other natural sources that have always been present in our environment, (2) medical and dental x-rays and (3) radioactive fall-out from the testing of atomic weapons.

A number of states have now passed laws that require the registration of all sources of ionizing radiation, including x-ray machines and radioactive substances used in the practice of medicine and other professions.

The primary purpose of such registration has been that of providing satisfactory protection to patients and the technical experts who use this kind of equipment.

Exposure to radiation occurs at a steady pace regardless of any efforts to protect ourselves. This steady exposure comes from what is known as the "natural background" of radiation. The natural background consists of radiation from cosmic rays of outer space, radioactive soils, atmospheric radiation and certain small amounts of internal radioactivity. The total radiation dosage for a year from this source is about 0.1 rems.

Other sources of radiation may come from dental, medical, occupational and

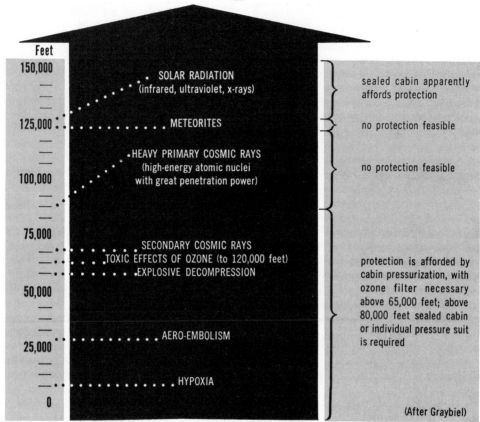

Figure 60. Health and radiation hazards at high altitudes. (Therapeutics Notes, October, 1957.)

miscellaneous sources including radioactive fallout from the testing of nuclear weapons.

When radiation from the natural background is combined with all other radiation dosages that we are currently receiving, the average person receives about 0.3 to 0.4 rems per year over the whole body.

If the current exposure to radiation from all sources continues at the same level of exposure and absorption, then in the first 30 years of life the average person would be exposed to approximately 5 to 8 rems. The reasonable limit of exposure and absorption that scientists believe is permissible without damage is thought to be about 13 to 15 rems.

It thus appears that the average person could be safely exposed to approximately twice as much or more radiation than he is currently receiving without harmful effects upon human health or future generations.

The hazards of radiation appear to be exaggerated in the popular mind. Nevertheless, various sources of radiation will be discussed more fully in later portions of this chapter.

Health Hazards from Excessive Radiation

It is true that unwise and excessive exposure to radiation may produce harmful effects upon human beings. Uncontrolled radiation of an excessive amount has been shown to produce genetic changes, birth defects, cancer, leukemia, skin disorders, ulceration, loss of hair, tissue destruction, sterility, a decreased life expectancy and even death.

The answer to these harmful effects from the unwise use of radiation is relatively simple. Only professional persons, such as a radiologist, should be permitted to expose a person to radiation. The x-ray can be safely used by radiologists, physicians and surgeons, dentists, veterinarians and other professionally qualified persons. Patients should learn not to insist upon needless x-rays, but should be guided to the constructive use of radiation in both diagnosis and treatment by the professional advice of their qualified medical advisors.

Particular attention should be paid to the protection of the developing embryo during the time of pregnancy. At this stage of development human cells are most sensitive to radiation. The reproductive tissues, in general, should be protected against radiation because genetic research has indicated that there are long range hazards to the human race in needless exposure of the germinal tissue. Undesirable changes or mutations may appear generations hence if the reproductive tissues of persons now living are exposed to excessive radiation.

This hazard involves only a part of the population, notably children, young people, and women during pregnancy. The genetic hazard does not exist for women after menopause, for those who will not have children or for the older part of the population. Another important point regarding genetic hazards is that they may be expected to be of significance in future generations only if a large or total part of the population has received damaging radiation to the germinal tissue. Damage to the individual would have little or no impact in future populations.

On June 12, 1956, the National Academy of Sciences of the United States and the National Research Council of England released official information on their investigations of the effects of radiation on humans. Although these studies were conducted independently, the findings were basically identical.

It was concluded from these investigations that over a period of thirty years (most children are born before their parents are of this age) the reproductive tissues of humans receive an average radiation dosage between 4.3 and 5.5 roentgens, depending upon the altitude at which a person lives. The average exposure from x-rays during this same span of years is about 3 roentgens. Radioactive fall-out from the testing of atomic weapons over a period of thirty years, if conducted at the current experimental rate, would be about 0.1 roentgen. This is relatively low exposure.

From the genetic (reproductive) viewpoint radiation can do damage over a very long time through mutations. These mutations, or changes, are significant only if they occur in the reproductive tissues. To control possible effects upon future generations it is recommended that the accumulated exposure of reproductive tissues over a period of thirty years be kept to 15 roentgens or less. This suggests that a record should be kept of each person's exposure to radiation on a cumulative basis, that the use of diagnostic x-rays should be kept to a minimum, and that greater effort should be made to protect the reproductive tissues when there is exposure to radiation.

Chest X-rays

From the genetic point of view, it is not important how much radiation may be involved over the whole body. The important thing is how much of this radiation reaches the reproductive tissue. One cannot calculate the amount of radiation that reaches these tissues on the basis of the amount of radiation reaching the chest in a chest x-ray, for example. Although a person who has a large chest x-ray taken may be exposed to 0.1 roentgen, such a person would be exposed to only 0.00025 roentgen so far as the reproductive tissue is concerned. It must be remembered that when other parts of the body are subjected to radiation, that only about 1/200th or less of this radiation will reach the reproductive tissues. As one radiologist has expressed it, "We are way on the safe side."

MOBILE X-RAY SURVEYS

"It has been determined that the amount of exposure . . . for one x-ray picture is 0.0015 Rem. Since we only receive that amount of radiation during one chest x-ray of this type, it is clear that we could have 750 of them made and only receive one Rem . . . remember we are allowed ten Rems of such exposure during our lives. To get your permissible limit of such radiation, you would have to have 7,500 such chest x-rays. This is not very likely to happen."

Florida Health Notes, April, 1960

The possibly harmful effects of diagnostic x-rays have been greatly over-rated according to a research team headed by Dr. Reynold F. Brown, radiation safety officer at the University of California Medical Center in San Francisco.

A research team, headed by this physician, made a study of a large representative sample of the population. They found that the average person would receive only 1.2 to 1.5 roentgens of radiation in the first 30 years of life from x-ray examinations. This is less than 1/3 to 1/2 of the amount of radiation that a person gets from the natural background of the cosmic rays, soil and so on.

The findings were based on the medical records of 100,000 members of the Kaiser Foundation Health Plan.

Cosmic Rays

The air contains minute concentrations of radioactive materials, and the amount of radiation to which a person is naturally exposed varies a great deal. Denver has about three times as much radiation in its environment as San Francisco. This is probably due to the fact that Denver lies at a greater altitude than San Francisco, and, in consequence, receives a more intense concentration of cosmic rays from space. Cosmic rays, which emit gamma rays, are increasingly absorbed as they pass through our atmosphere.

Radioactive Soils

Natural radioactive materials are widely present in the earth's soil. Most are found in uranium and thorium, which occur, on the average, in these amounts:

Uranium . . . . 6 parts per million by weight
Thorium . . . . 12 parts per million by weight

Much smaller amounts of radium and actinium are also found in nature. These are the only four naturally occurring elements known to be spontaneously radioactive.

Many areas of the earth contain naturally radioactive soil. In 1958 three investigators reported that natural radioactivity of the soil was contributing about eleven times as much radioactivity as fallout from nuclear fission products.

There are many difficulties associated with the measurement of the radioactivity of surface soils, but investigations all over the world do indicate that fission products in fallout from bomb tests may be less significant than the radioactivity that already exists in the soil.

A study of congenital defects among children born in areas of greater radioactivity suggests that there is a definite association between malformations at birth and increased levels of radioactivity in bedrock.

A public health investigation of congenital defects reported on birth and death

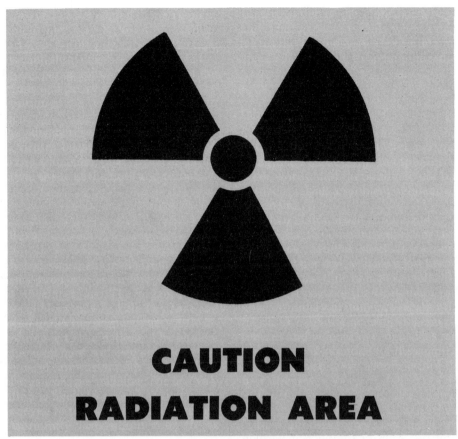

Figure 61. Each area using radioactive material is required by the Atomic Energy Commission to post conspicuously a sign bearing the above symbol and wording. On a background of yellow the above symbol is printed in magenta or purple. (Florida Health Notes, April, 1960.)

certificates in areas with radioactive soils was reported in 1959. This investigation indicates an association between the rate of birth defects and higher levels of radioactivity in bedrock. The United States Congress appropriated $50,000 for the fiscal year 1960 to investigate further the problem of radioactivity in areas of rock outcroppings.

It is reported that a population of about 80,000 persons has lived in India on the Travencor Monazite sands for generations. This area provides a soil that is several times more hazardous in radiation than soil at sea level. The Indian Government, with assistance from the World Health Organi-zation, is planning to make a special study of this population to see if there is evidence of undue hazard from living in this region of high natural radioactivity. Special attention will be paid to the possibility of a greater prevalence of leukemia, birth defects, and shorter length of life.

Radioactive Fallout

Dr. Willard F. Libby, Commissioner of the U. S. Atomic Energy Commission, reported on January 19, 1956, that the long-term affects of radioactive fallout are not as great as has been generally supposed. Strontium 90 is commonly recognized as the greatest long-term danger, but worldwide evidence from the recent testing of weapons provides the conclusion that the hazard from this source is insignificant.

In the ordinary atom bomb, for each 20,000 tons of TNT-equivalent explosive energy, about 2 pounds of radioactive materials are produced. In these 2 pounds are about ninety different radioactive substances or species which will last from only a few seconds to many years. This mixture decreases in radioactivity tenfold for every sevenfold increase in age. Seven hours after a nuclear explosion the radioactivity has decreased to one tenth of what it was at one hour. In forty-nine hours the radioactivity is only one hundredth of what it was at one hour. In two weeks the radioactivity is only one thousandth and in three months only one ten thousandth of its initial level.

Fading Radiation Hazard

According to Dr. Simon Kinsman, Ph.D., "In estimating the probable decrease of the radiation hazard with time, the decay rate of the ashes of the nuclear weapon can be approximated by considering that for every seven-fold increase in the age of fission products, there will be a ten-fold reduction in the radioactivity or intensity of radiation as illustrated below:"

Contamination in Curies of Radioactive Material	Time After Formation of Fission Products	Radiation Intensity from Fission Products (Roentgens per Hour)
1,000 ..	1 hour	10,000
100 ..	7 hours	1,000
10 ..	49 hours (2 days)	100
1 ..	14 days (2 weeks)	10
0.1 ..	14 weeks (3 months)	1

Many people do not understand that there is a substantial difference in the radiation hazard from fallout materials between different kinds of nuclear explosions. Scientists agree that the fallout from a reasonably high level air detonation gives little or no hazard from radioactive materials. The same is true if a nuclear bomb penetrates the surface of the ground and detonates below it. It is thought that the radiation hazard from a sub-surface explosion would be restricted almost to the point of ground impact.

The most substantial radiation hazard from fallout materials will occur when a nuclear weapon is detonated close to the surface of the earth. In such an explosion the fireball which is formed and starts to ascend would become diluted with dust and dirt from the ground and from pollution materials in the air close to the surface. As the vaporized parts of the fireball cool, they condense into solid materials on the dusts and other materials that have been sucked into the nuclear cloud. These solid particles thus become radioactive and begin to fall out of the nuclear cloud as rapidly as they are swept out of it by air currents. The settling of these radioactive particles is known as the fallout.

The amount of territory that would be affected by this radioactive fallout depends, as indicated, on the type of nuclear explosion. It would also depend upon weather conditions and the direction of prevailing winds. The small radioactive dust particles would fall out at the slowest pace and might be spread for a considerable distance if the explosion had been a surface burst.

Studies of the H-bomb tests in the Pacific indicate that from a 15-megaton weapon, within one hour after the burst about 250 square miles of territory would be contaminated by an average intensity of 2,500 roentgens of *gamma* radiation per hour. Six hours after this same burst approximately 4,000 square miles would be contaminated but to a much lower average intensity of only 30 roentgens of *gamma* radiation per hour.

Strontium 90

Strontium 90 is one of the radioactive substances produced by nuclear fission that is considered a hazard to human health. The reason for this is its persistent radioactivity over a number of years. This substance has a ½ life of approximately 28 years and an average life of about 40 years.

Strontium, like calcium, on gaining entrance to the body tends to be deposited in the bones, thus it could be expected that strontium might remain in the body for a long time, with possible damaging effects. However, no evidence to date suggests that the fallout of strontium 90 has been sufficient to produce harmful effects in human beings.

Rivers have been found to be virtually free of radio strontium and studies indicate that the top two or three inches of soil hold the substance tenaciously. On plowing, the farmer buries radio strontium deeper and it may not move for two or three years.

The Atomic Energy Commission has made extensive studies on this problem. Findings suggest that most of the radioactivity from nuclear weapons is dissipated in the stratosphere but that radio strontium is apt to be the greatest hazard from nuclear fallout.

During 1959 the Public Health Service took samples of water supplies at 51 different points throughout the United States. These samples were tested for radioactivity. Seventeen major rivers were included in the study.

Although the levels of radioactivity fluctuated, they were well below the level set by the National Committee on Radiation Protection and Measurements as being permissible throughout the entire lifetime of the population.

Radioactivity in milk collected from eleven stations around the country was also found to be below the safe levels advocated by the national committee.

The Public Health Service is currently expanding the number of stations throughout the United States that check regularly on the radioactivity of water and food. Plans call for the establishment of 250 of these public health stations.

Strontium 90 is brought to earth and contaminates surface soils and water primarily by rainfall. Studies of surface runoff and rainfall have shown that only a small part of the strontium 90 that falls on cultivated soils is carried away by the runoff.

Studies in Wisconsin and Georgia have been made in which the amount of strontium 90 falling in the rain was sampled by collecting the water in wash tubs three feet in diameter which were left in the open near the soil to be tested. Samples of run-off water from soil were also taken for a radioactive analysis. It was found that about one per cent of the fallout usually appeared in the run-off, although there were exceptions to this. In Wisconsin as much as 25 per cent of the fallout was carried away in the run-off. This higher percentage of the removal of strontium 90 was associated with greater amounts of erosion or soil loss. Since erosion is not a major problem in most agricultural areas, the investigators concluded that the majority of the strontium 90 that is brought to earth by rainfall will remain in cultivated soils.

Treatment for Radiation Sickness

Treatment for radiation sickness varies according to the degree of injury. In general, there are three groups of patients so far as the effects of radiation are concerned.

In group 1 it is unlikely that any person will survive; there has been such intensity of injury from radiation that no matter what is done for the patient he probably will not recover. These patients begin heavy vomiting soon after they have been injured by the radiation. They have fever, diarrhea and loss of appetite, and suffer profound damage to the circulatory system. These symptoms coming immediately after an atomic bombing probably indicate that the person will die within several weeks. Even if this patient is treated with antibiotics, blood transfusions, penicillin or other measures, recovery cannot be assured.

Unfortunately, the only medical treatment for patients in this group should be that which is intended to alleviate pain and to make the patient comfortable until death occurs.

In group 2, patients can be expected to survive. In this category are those who start vomiting on the day of exposure to radiation, but whose symptoms then disappear and who seem to be in good health for one to three weeks. During this time, however, certain blood changes may be taking place, such as a decrease in the white blood cell count. This decrease in the body's ability to fight disease is followed by infections, bleeding gums, oozing of blood through the skin or the body cavities, and other symptoms. Injury to the bone marrow may cause an anemia, and the same condition may result from an excessive loss of blood because of hemorrhage. Weakness may result from both bleeding and infection.

The primary medical treatment for this group of patients is that of blood transfusion. The tranfusion should be of whole blood. Infections may be countered with the antibiotics.

With proper medical care based mainly on blood transfusion and antibiotics, a great many of these patients may survive.

In group 3, persons suffering from radiation will most likely survive. Treatment is based upon transfusions and the use of antibiotics just as in group 2. This category of patients has definitely had a smaller dosage of radiation and therefore the effects are less severe. These patients suffer no vomiting on the day of exposure, although they may have mild symptoms the day after being injured by radiation.

The Atomic Bomb Casualty Commission of the United States Government has been making extensive studies of the effect of atomic radiation on survivors of the Hiroshima and Nagasaki bombings.

This Commission has found a definite increase in the number of cases of leukemia among those survivors who were within 6,000 feet of the atomic explosion. New cases of this disease are still developing, and it is not yet known exactly how many will occur in future years, although it is already obvious that leukemia is occurring among atomic bomb victims at several times the rate in a normal population.

It has also been found that survivors who were within two-thirds of a mile of the atomic explosion have unusual numbers of cataracts of the eye. About one in ten have shown some changes in the lens of the eye. Some estimates have indicated that at least 500 persons who survived the atomic bombings have become partially or totally blind as a result of damage to the eyes.

In the Japanese bombings it must be remembered that the great majority of victims died from burns. Only 15 per cent of the deaths were due to radiation.

In general, the Japanese survivors who were injured by radiation have shown a variety of signs and symptoms such as bleeding gums, bloody stools, anemia, fever, loss of appetite, loss of hair, bleeding through the skin, general weakness, cataracts, leukemia and still other disorders. Only a small minority of babies born of parents injured by radiation appear to show any genetic deformities. A slight trend in this direction is apparent, however.

If a nuclear bomb should be exploded under water off a nearby coast, a great cloud of radioactive water vapor would be a dangerous hazard to the surrounding area. Radioactive dust from a land explosion would also create a hazard and, if inhaled, would undoubtedly cause death.

If radioactive dusts or water vapor should contaminate foods or water supplies, they could cause severe illness and death to many people. However, the problem of sterilizing or cleaning certain food and drink is not as complicated as one might think.

Protection against and decontamination of radioactive substances are discussed in the next chapter.

Peaceful Uses of Radiation

Public preoccupation with the potentially damaging effects of radiation has caused most persons to overlook the constructive uses to which it may be put.

The benefits of radiation as used in research, medicine, dentistry and other scientific fields far outweighs the hazards that are involved. Greatest benefits have probably come to human health through X-rays and radioactive isotopes in medicine. Industry also has many constructive uses for properly controlled radiation, both in research and in many phases of industrial production.

The additions to human knowledge from the research use of radioactive isotopes is very great. These substances are discussed in the next few paragraphs.

Radioactive Isotopes in Medicine

Although only radium, uranium, thorium and actinium are known to be radioactive as found in nature, many other elements can be made radioactive artificially.

This is done by placing a portion of an element within an atomic reactor, to be bombarded by showers of neutrons. Some of the neutrons are then absorbed into the nuclei of the iodine, carbon, cobalt, phosphorus, iron or whatever element is being treated. When this occurs, the previously nonradiating element becomes radioactive.

Some artificially radioactive elements are called isotopes of their original form. These isotopes retain all their former chemical and electrical properties; but, in addition, they have the property of radiation. This newly acquired characteristic makes radioactive isotopes of very great importance in science and medicine.

Even before the development of the atomic bomb, scientists in medicine and biology had been using radioactive isotopes as tracers, in order to study the processes of life. The radiations emitted by the atoms of radioactive carbon, phosphorus or iodine, for example, serve as tags to signal the presence of such atoms wherever they go in a person's body. With an instrument like a Geiger counter, the location of the "tagged" substance can be readily detected. Experimenters realized for some time the value of such tagged atoms both for research and for developing new methods of treating disease.

The Stanford Research Institute reported in 1960 that about 400,000 administrations of radioisotopes to human beings are given each year by physicians in the United States.

Most of the isotopes are used for diagnostic purposes and more than 40 per cent are given to people over the age of 50.

It was calculated by the Institute investigators that three out of every one thousand persons who go to clinics and hospitals undergo some sort of diagnostic procedure involving the use of radioisotopes. The use of radioactive materials is expected to nearly double by 1965.

According to a report by the Atomic Energy Commission, there were nearly 5,500 licensed users of radioisotopes in the United States by 1960. Most of these licenses have been granted in the fields of medicine, industry and federal and state laboratories.

Ten radioactive substances are in use at present. New radioisotopes made available to medicine during 1959 were cadmium[109] with a half life of 1.3 years and iodine[130] with a half life of 12.5 years.

Today, as by-products of our great industrial plants manufacturing nuclear materials for defense purposes, we have an

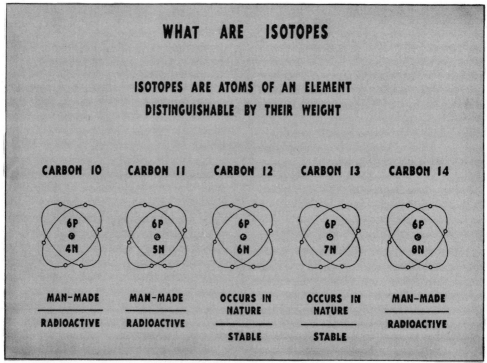

Figure 62. Isotope is a word of Greek derivation meaning "same place." An isotope is therefore one of two or more atoms occupying the same place in the table of the elements, but differing slightly in composition of protons, neutrons and electrons. When the atom contains an unbalanced number of these components it is considered unstable, and it emits or releases the unbalancing parts and is therefore "radioactive." (Florida Health Notes, April, 1960.)

abundance of radioactive isotopes available. The result is that a vast program of tagged atom research has been launched.

Public Health Controls

The Executive Board of the American Public Health Association expressed the view in March, 1960, that: "Ionizing radiation, if properly utilized, is instrumental in improving the health and welfare of the people. Exposure to radiation, however, results in damage which may not be apparent immediately. Therefore, consistent with good medical practice, expo-

sure to radiation from all controllable sources must be minimized."

Extracts from the supporting statement of the Association follow:

1. All Ionizing Radiation Injurious —

The effect of ionizing radiation on living tissue is to injure or to destroy cells . . .

2. The effects of small doses of radiation may be imperceptible and slow to appear. Once the injury has occurred, however, there is no known means of repairing the damage . . .

3. Public Health Responsibility —

It is a responsibility of government to safeguard its people against potentially harmful exposures, when the exposures cause significant health hazards against which individuals are unable to protect themselves by their own efforts . . .

4. Prevent Unnecessary Radiation Exposure —

It is sound radiological health policy to prevent all unnecessary human exposures to radiation . . .

5. For the total population the recommended limits of maximum permissible exposure are well below those currently accepted for persons occupationally exposed to radiation . . . The actual radiation exposure of large populations that is likely to have significant consequences is yet to be determined . . .

6. Evaluation of Radiation Hazards —

The cumulative exposure of individuals and the total public exposure to radiation results from various and often unrelated sources . . .

7. Protective Approaches —

The technics for protecting the public are of two kinds—those limiting the creation of radiation sources and those controlling the environment . . .

8. Where elimination of radiation sources is impracticable, the alternative is to control the environment . . .

9. Urgent Need for Action —

. . . The potentialities of radiation exposure of individuals and the population are steadily increasing. In many places present demands and hazards require immediate action . . .

Questions

1. How much of a radiation hazard are chest x-rays?

2. Do the diagnostic benefits outweight the hazards from the use of x-rays?

3. Why can people over the age of 30 years be exposed safely to more radiation than younger persons when they must have already absorbed more radiation?

4. How can a person defend himself against the hazards of radiation from the fallout from nuclear explosions?

5. What is the natural background of radiation?

6. What persons in our population are most liable to suffer ill health because of radiation damage?

For Further Reading

1. Schubert, Jack, and Lapp, Ralph E.: *Radiation: What It Is and How It Affects You.* New York, Viking Press, 1957.

2. United Nations: *Peaceful Uses of Atomic Energy.* Vols. *10* and *11*. New York, Columbia University Press, 1956.

For Advanced Reading

1. Blatz, Hanson: *Radiation Hygiene Handbook.* New York, McGraw-Hill Book Company, 1959.

2. Brucer, Marshall: *The Acute Radiation Syndrome.* Washington, D.C., Office of Technical Services, Department of Commerce, 1959.

3. Brues, A. M.: *Low-level Irradiation.* Washington, D.C., American Association for the Advancement of Science, 1960.

4. Dunham, Charles L.: *Radioactive Fallout.* Washington, D.C., Office of Technical Services, Department of Commerce, 1959.

5. Halnan, K. E.: *Atomic Energy in Medicine.* New York, Philosophical Library, 1957.

6. Oughterson, Asley W., and Warren, Shields: *Medical Effects of the Atomic Bomb in Japan.* New York, McGraw-Hill Book Company, 1956.

Recommended Films

Off-site Monitoring of Fallout From Nuclear Tests. 16 mm., colored, sound, showing time 29 minutes, 1958. Atlanta 22, Georgia, Communicable Disease Center, Attention Audiovisual.

30

CIVIL DEFENSE

IN THE EVENT of nuclear war the problem of civilian defense will represent a challenge to national survival.

The development of nuclear warheads and guided missiles as well as many other efficient means for the delivery of the most destructive bombs the world has ever known makes the problem of national survival acute in the event of a modern war.

Psychologic, chemical and bacteriologic warfare add grave potentials to that of nuclear bombing. In the face of such devastating possibilities for mass extermination the individual may surrender all hope of survival in a fit of despair, or he may face the problem squarely and do what he can to survive. Personal attitudes can make the difference between extinction and survival.

The danger of nuclear attack lies in four directions: heat, blast, radiation and panic.

The production of heat is instantaneous when a nuclear bomb explodes. The area of destruction by heat from such a bomb will depend upon the size of the bomb and other factors. The heat is of the instantaneous or flash type; therefore, any damage that occurs from this source takes place within a split second. In the Japanese explosion, burns occurred more than two miles from the center of the blast. In a modern thermonuclear explosion they would occur at a greater distance.

Radiation, like heat, is produced instantaneously at the time of the bomb explosion. In fact, radiation is produced only for a few seconds. Within even a few minutes much of the radiation will be dissipated, but some will persist and may spread over a large area.

A great shock or blast wave caused by expansion of gases from the nuclear explosion surges outward immediately after the heat blast. This shock wave may do extensive damage mechanically by destruction of buildings from rushing winds.

Fear and panic may aggravate the situation during a nuclear attack and may result in much greater loss of life because of people not acting intelligently.

Burns

The heat from a nuclear explosion, although of tremendous intensity, is of very short duration. People in homes or beyond barriers will be reasonably well protected against flash burns unless they are close to the center of the explosion.

The type of clothing that a person happens to be wearing at the time he receives a nuclear burn may make a considerable difference in the intensity of his injury. Light-colored clothing tends to reflect heat, whereas dark clothing tends to absorb the heat. People wearing white or light-colored materials may be reasonably well protected by them if they are far enough way from the center of intense heat, but those with dark clothing may be burned not only by the heat of the explosion, but also because the dark clothing may catch fire from the retention of heat and cause additional burns on the skin beneath.

Large numbers of burns may be expected from buildings that may be set afire by the heat and blast of the nuclear explosion.

Almost any type of protection at the time of explosion will give an excellent chance to escape a serious flash burn. The transmission of heat in a nuclear explosion appears to be in a line-of-sight direction.

The medical treatment for burns has been revolutionized in the past few years. The main problems appear to be those of the treatment of pain and shock, the prevention of infection and the replacement of protein and body fluids.

A major objective in any type of first aid rendered for burns should be the relieving of pain and the prevention of shock and infection. The application of ointments and salves to burns is no longer advised, since this merely complicates the problem for the physician or surgeon who treats the case later. The application of a sterile bandage, however, is advisable. In general, the less an amateur attempts to treat a burn, the better the opportunity for the physician or surgeon to prevent infection and secure recovery of the patient.

One of the latest treatments for the emergency relief of pain and shock in the treatment of burns is the thrusting of the burned part of the body into ice water. The application of ice packs to the burn might achieve somewhat the same effect in the relief of pain and shock, but the ice water solution is better for the prevention of infection since antibacterial substances can be added to the ice water.

Shock from burns seldom occurs unless at least 15 per cent of the total body surface is damaged. It is probably advisable, however, to start shock treatment if more than 10 per cent of the body surface is burned. The best treatment for shock is the giving of blood plasma or whole blood. In a mass emergency in which there might be a severe shortage of such supplies, however, the giving of water and salt by mouth for the first twenty-four to thirty-six hours might be lifesaving. After this time, however, the amount of salt should be sharply reduced in order to prevent swelling and accumulation of fluid in the lung tissues. Only a physiologic salt solution (one containing approximately the same concentration of salts as is normally found in body fluids) will be helpful, since if there is an excessive amount of salt in any fluid, the person taking this solution by mouth may become nauseated and vomit, and other complications may occur.

Recent research at the Massachusetts General Hospital in Boston has indicated that damage to the respiratory system is a major factor in death from severe burns. Research by two Boston surgeons that involved 1,141 cases of burns indicated that damage to the lungs and respiratory system caused a much higher percentage of deaths than did shock. It was found that over a period of years, only one per cent of the deaths from severe burns were caused by shock, but that respiratory conditions were a cause for 33 per cent of the deaths. In another study of 54 burn deaths, respiratory damage was responsible for 50 per cent of the deaths and only one person died from shock.

These investigators also found that if the face is not burned there is much less likelihood that respiratory damage will occur. This suggests that special protection should be given to the face in the presence of severe heat or flame if this can be done.

Burns should be covered with dressings, since this tends to reduce pain as well as prevent contamination.

In general, the emergency care of a person who had been badly burned should center around (1) evaluation of the extent of the injury, (2) relief of pain, (3) application of an emergency dressing, (4) treatment of shock, (5) giving of fluids to insure an adequate urinary output, and (6) prevention of infections.

In the event of mass burn casualties from a nuclear bombing there would also be a tremendous need for skin grafting. Advance planning for the use of plastic surgeons or other physicians skilled in such techniques is essential if such care is to be readily available in event of need.

Some authorities estimate that 90 per cent of the injured who survive a nuclear bombing will suffer from burns. Probably most of these burns will have occurred from the nuclear heat itself, but some will result from the burning of homes and public buildings that have become ignited after the blast.

Plans should be made in advance by the officials of any community to see that sufficient fire-fighting apparatus is available from areas outside of that which is likely to be damaged by an atomic explosion. Such fire-fighting equipment, if quickly available, could do much to prevent the wholesale destruction of large parts of a community as well as to prevent many individual burns.

Blood transfusions are of great importance in the treatment of burns. Because of the relatively short time that blood may be stored, it is impossible to stockpile a huge reservoir of human blood for use in the event of a nuclear bombing. There is always the possibility, too, that if blood banks were not strategically located, they might be destroyed by the bombing which they were intended to counteract. Advance organization of a huge "walking blood bank" appears to be the only possible solution to the problem of handling the thousands and thousands of burn cases that might exist after a nuclear assault on a large city. In other words, a large-scale organization for on-the-spot blood transfusions from human donors is needed. Under this plan the donors keep their own blood until they are called upon to participate in transfusion.

It has been found that injections of gamma globulin may reduce infections after burns by about 50 per cent. The use of this substance in combination with antibiotics has been found to be highly effective in the prevention of infections following burns. Infections constitute a serious threat to life and may cause death several days after severe burns.

Tremendous quantities of medical supplies would be needed for the proper treatment of burns on a mass scale. Adequate supplies of oxygen, blood plasma, fluid, bandages, antibiotics and various pain-killing medicines would be needed in order to control shock, reduce infection, and ease the suffering of the burned patients. In addition, a large staff of nurses and physicians would be required.

By careful advance planning it is estimated that at least 50 per cent of the burn casualties from a nuclear bombing could be saved.

Nuclear Blast

The radius of blast damage from a nuclear explosion depends upon the strength of the detonation, which is measured in TNT equivalents, one megaton representing one million tons of TNT. Thus, the blast from a 1-megaton nuclear weapon explosion would virtually demolish structures within a range of about four miles and would seriously damage buildings within a range of about six miles. However, the effects of blast damage would be greatly reduced by proper shelter within this range of effects. Strongly built structures, or underground structures, would give substan-

tial protection against blast injuries from falling or flying debris.

Blast injuries to the human are especially associated with the lungs, eardrum, sinuses and parts of the body in which there is the greatest variation in tissue density. The most dangerous injury, and one which results in death within a few minutes, involves the lungs and the emergence of air bubbles in the blood which may reach the heart or brain. Because blast may cause hemorrhage or swelling of the lung tissues there is also the immediate danger of suffocation and heart failure due to the lack of oxygen because of the nonfunctioning lungs. If the person survives the immediate lung injury from blast he may soon develop pneumonia or other lung infections, because of impaired lung function due to bruising or hemorrhage. The heart, liver, spleen and abdominal organs may be damaged by blast also and this may result in internal hemorrhage or rupture of specific organs of the body.

Blast injuries would be superimposed upon the burn or heat injuries from nuclear explosion since both physical forces would be involved within immediate range of the nuclear explosion. It is estimated that on a national scale a nuclear attack on the United States would result in a combined blast and heat casualty list of nearly 20,000,000 fatalities on the first day, with subsequent fatal injury to approximately 12,000,000 more persons. Deaths from radioactive fallout would follow and be superimposed upon this staggering loss of human lives.

Blast from a nuclear explosion first results in a tremendous shock or *outward* exertion of physical force, followed by winds of terrific velocity moving *inward* to fill a vacuum. This combination of physical forces involving primary shock, tornado-like winds, and a vacuum or collapsing type of force can be expected to cause the collapse of buildings on a massive scale for miles around the point of nuclear explosion. Injuries to persons within blast range would result from all of these forces, and would involve direct blast injury as well as secondary, and perhaps fatal, results from falling buildings, flying debris and other effects.

People caught in the open without time to seek shelter would have their best chance to escape fatal or serious injury from blast by lying on the ground and covering the face and head with their arms, and curling up to protect the chest as much as possible. Any space below the surface of the ground is better.

Psychological Warfare

In the event of modern warfare, citizens must be prepared for psychologic assaults upon their will to resist. Efforts to create fear, panic, and general confusion may be expected to arise from conscious efforts of internal enemies as well as from the general reactions of the population to nuclear bombings.

Civilian defense leaders have called attention to three widely held fallacies among the American people. These three misconceptions are: (1) that the military forces will take over in the case of an attack on civilians, (2) that the Soviet Union will not use the hydrogen bomb and (3) that no one can survive hydrogen bomb warfare. The three fallacies might well have their origin in misconceptions deliberately planted by internal enemies. Civilian communities would find it necessary to depend upon themselves in case of casualties from a nuclear attack. Strong evidence suggests that an enemy in possession of the nuclear bomb would not hesitate to use this weapon. Evidence also indicates that the survival rate in any community would depend mostly on its civil defense preparations. People could and would survive in the event of nuclear warfare. Intelligent preparation for protection of self and family would make substantial differences in any community in the number of people who survive.

Psychiatrists have pointed out that the loss of life in case of nuclear bombing might be greater because of panic than as a result of the disaster itself.

Panic, which is a sudden and groundless fright or terror accompanied by unreasoning or frantic efforts to secure safety, involves temporary disorganization of thinking and control of fear.

Factors that contribute to panic are tension and insecurity, imitative behavior, suggestibility, rumor, fear of the unknown, lack of preparation, and strong sensory stimuli such as loud noises, burning objects and the sight of people running.

Good organization, able leadership and adequate motivation for maintaining emotional balance in the face of disaster, as well as a basic understanding of fear and how people react in fear situations, are important factors in the prevention of panic.

Protection from Radiation

In the event of the radioactive fallout that might follow a nuclear attack, there would be plenty of time for survivors to seek protective shelter. In most cases radioactive materials would not begin to reach the ground until about one-half hour after the nuclear explosion. A longer time would be involved at greater distances from the detonation.

The greater the space between the individual and the fallout materials, the greater the protection. Ordinarily, three feet of dirt is sufficient to stop the penetration of radiation; underground shelters that provide this much protection enable survivors to escape damaging effects from radiation.

A simple one-story wooden building can reduce the hazard from radiation by about one-half. Large reinforced concrete buildings can greatly reduce the radiation hazard especially if people withdraw to the inner portions of the building. In the basement of such a large building, the radiation hazard may be reduced to as little as one-thousandth. In fact, anything that catches the radioactive dust and keeps it away from a person gives a certain degree of protection.

Hazards from radiation decrease rapidly. Even without protection, the intensity of the hazard decreases to about one-hundredth after about two days and to as little as one-thousandth after about two weeks, because most radioactive materials decompose rapidly. Even on the day of a nuclear explosion the intensity of radiation after about seven hours would be only about one-tenth of what it was one hour after the explosion. It can be seen that even if a person stayed underground or in a sheltered area for as little as twenty-four hours the chances of escaping damage from radioactive materials would be greatly enhanced. If windows have not been broken by blast or other damage, they should be closed or substitutes for the glass should be found. Remember, anything that keeps radioactive dust at a distance reduces the hazard of injury.

Decontamination

It is possible to achieve radiologic decontamination. It is not possible to judge how much radioactive contamination takes place except by the use of some electronic device such as the Geiger-Mueller counter. However, it can be assumed that if there is a radioactive fallout that there will be contamination of shoes, outer clothing, tools, grounds, buildings, and so on. In general, people and small objects can be decontaminated by the removal of clothes and by thorough washing and bathing, if water is available. Washing with damp rags is advisable if a shower bath cannot be taken. The use of a detergent or other cleansing substance is advisable if the skin has been contaminated. It is very important to

change clothes if the individual has been personally contaminated with radioactive fallout.

It must be remembered that when radioactive materials are removed by washing and bathing, the radioactivity will then be in the bath or wash water. Decontamination, therefore, involves the removal of this water to a safe distance from human beings. In washing or bathing, the individual must also take pains to do a thorough job and to remove dirt and dust from the hair, ears, nose, fingernails and every other part of the body.

Incoming water can be decontaminated quite successfully if it runs through the common ion-exchange water softener, which is effective in removing radioactive particles that have fallen into the water. If the household has water softener equipment and it is necessary to use water after fallout has occurred, then it would be best to use only the water that has been drawn through such equipment.

For decontamination of the area outside the home, the most effective procedure is to use garden hose for washing off the dust from roofs, walls, sidewalks, driveways, lawns, trees or other objects. The decontamination of outside objects should not be attempted immediately after the fallout. It is best to wait until some decomposition of radioactive materials has taken place. When outside decontamination is begun, the roof and nearby concrete surfaces, such as walks and driveways, should be washed down first.

Warning Signals

A knowledge of the warning signals will save human lives in the event of nuclear attack.

There are two warning signals for the general public. The first of these is the "alert" signal and the second is the "take cover" warning.

The alert signal consists of a continuous,

steady blast on a siren, or other appropriate instrument, for a period of three to five minutes. Remember, this signal is a *continuous* steady blast.

The "take cover" signal has two variations. It may occur as a continuous wailing tone or as a series of short blasts of three minutes duration. Fire stations will be the ones most apt to give these signals.

In the event of either of the foregoing warning signals, all members of the family should start at once to put into operation their survival plans in keeping with the responsibilities that they may have.

A third source of warning about an impending nuclear attack may come over the radio. Wave lengths at 640 kc or 1240 kc have been designated by civilian defense authorities for communication with the population in the case of emergency. These wave lengths are known as CONELRAD, but it takes about 20 minutes to convert from a standard broadcast to a CONELRAD cast and during this time it is possible that all radio stations may be silenced. If this extensive silence occurs and you become aware of it then the previously agreed-upon survival plan should be put into operation.

Flight or Shelter?

In the event of nuclear attack a person has three choices in his attempt to survive.

A first choice is to get out of hazardous areas into a safer region. Evacuation may or may not be possible because of congested highways, limitation of available means of transportation, the remoteness of safe areas and so on. Nevertheless, this is one choice that is available to the individual in the event of nuclear attack.

Each individual or family should become thoroughly familiar with the areas of least hazard and should plan a sensible means of reaching these areas if judgment indicates that this is the soundest thing to do. Because families may be separated at

the time of nuclear attack, but may have separate transportation facilities available, a family plan should be made so that a meeting on a particular day and at a particular hour may be arranged in the event of the separation or disorganization of the family.

A second chance for survival is available if the family has its own individual shelter. A family basement that has been prepared in advance for maximum protection against blast and radiation hazard may give the most immediate and best chance of survival. This shelter ought to be prepared in keeping with recommendations of the Office of Civilian and Defense Mobilization and should be stockpiled with water, food, disinfectants, battery, radio, various tools, clothing and bedding, cooking and serving equipment, recreational and religious supplies, first-aid and medical supplies, an instrument for the evaluation of radioactivity and other items.

> **PLANNING**
> "If disaster strikes today can I say tomorrow that lives were saved because I planned well?"
> *William M. Lamers*

There should be enough supplies in such a shelter to last for two weeks, although it may not be necessary to remain underground for this period of time.

A third chance for survival lies in the use of an industrial or community shelter. Such shelters are apt to be better constructed and to give greater protection against blast and radiation. They may be difficult to reach for some members of the family because of the distance involved and because of transportation problems. Knowledge of such shelters should be possessed by each individual and his family. Whether or not such shelters are to be used in preference to home shelters remain a matter of judgment. Industrial or community shelters that permit the advance storage of survival supplies are highly desirable for those who have no provisions for such measures.

Germ Warfare

Germ warfare is nothing new. It has been used many times in history.

Bacteriological warfare may be hazardous even for the side that uses it, for the simple reason that nowadays mass epidemics of serious diseases are seldom confined to one part of the world. Epidemics generated by an enemy may return to the originators with the production of mass casualties on both sides.

Defense against bacteriological warfare rests upon precisely the same medical and public health activities that protect us against communicable disease in peacetime. The widespread use of immunizing substances can protect against many infections. The prompt use of antibiotics may prevent many deaths from diseases. Despite these defenses, however, it is always possible that the research laboratories of the enemy may evolve a more dangerous strain of some virus or other microscopic organism that can cause extensive illness and mass casualties.

Active immunization represents the best and most effective protection against bacteriological warfare. Unfortunately, we can only be immunized against those diseases for which we have immunizing substances. Both children and adults should be immunized against as many diseases as possible. When new immunizing substances become available, they should also be used for the establishment of personal and family protection against the contingencies of bacteriological warfare.

This protection should be achieved as soon as possible and should be sustained by periodic booster immunizations. To wait until there is a mass need for such protection is to run the risk that the supplies of protective materials will be exhausted by unprecedented demands.

It can be anticipated that biological warfare will be used against civilian populations, because the incubation period of most communicable diseases is of such duration that time is needed to produce ef-fects. This limits their usefulness in military operations although over a period of time military forces may be devitalized through germ warfare. The importance of health and vitality in industrial production also implies that enemy efforts will be made against civilians in order to reduce the production of military supplies.

The United States Public Health Service maintains an epidemic intelligence service where trained investigators act promptly to give notice of significant outbreaks of communicable diseases. This intelligence service network is constantly on the alert for the first signs of a bacteriological warfare attack.

In the event of biological warfare, it must be remembered that enemy agents may contaminate the public water supplies, may use infectious vapors and mists in air conditioning and ventilating systems and may contaminate food, milk and other supplies. Bacteriological warfare may also be directed against edible plants and animals.

It is now possible to spread bacteria viruses and toxins by spraying them into the air as a fine mist which quickly becomes invisible. Heavy concentrations of disease-producing substances or their toxins can be sprayed over large areas through the use of guided missiles and other objects. Research has shown that invisible clouds of infectious materials can diffuse through buildings and homes in much the same manner as a gas.

Some of the diseases apt to be spread through bacteriological warfare are anthrax, plague, glanders, brucellosis, tularemia, bacillary dysentery, Q-fever, Rocky Mountain spotted fever, psittacosis, encephalitis and influenza. Efforts to foster other diseases may be anticipated.

Chemical Warfare

According to reports from the Office of the Surgeon General of the United States

Army, there are at least two groups of important chemical warfare agents. These are the incendiaries and the nerve gases.

The nerve gases appear to be far more hazardous than the former. They may gain access to the body through the respiratory system or may be absorbed through the eyes or skin as well as through the digestive system.

The nerve gases were first developed by the German military forces during World War I. They were liquids, nearly colorless and odorless, which turned to gas on evaporation.

Although the Germans were the first to use war gases, the Allies retaliated with the use of chlorine, phosgene, chloropicrin, mustard and other gases. These gases caused well over one million casualties, but they are now obsolete.

During World War II both sides had such effective chemical weapons that they were afraid to use them. German research teams produced new and even more toxic chemicals now known as the nerve gases Tabun, Sarin, and Soman, which are about twenty times more toxic than hydrogen cyanide. They could cause casualties before they could be detected. When the Russians captured the German Tabun plant intact, they moved it to Russia with top ranking German chemists and technicians. Tabun is now the main chemical warfare weapon of the Soviets and by 1960 it was reported that they had stockpiled more than 50,000 tons of this chemical. The United States military forces have concentrated on the production of Sarin and stockpiles of this chemical are available for retaliation in the event of chemical warfare.

War gases of much greater hazard are now being produced, although some gases are intended to incapacitate rather than kill. They can produce temporary physical disability through blindness, paralysis and deafness. Other chemicals in this new category can cause temporary mental disorder. The great advantage of these gases is that they can be used in the liberation of captive cities without heavy loss of life among subjugated peoples. Friendly civilian populations under military control of an enemy may be spared while being liberated by military attack.

Whether the temporarily disabling or more toxic and lethal gases are used, the nerve gases are apt to be effective in concentrations of as little as one part of gas per million or more parts of air.

Fortunately the lethal effects of the nerve gases can be blocked by certain chemical compounds. It may be possible to secure civilian and military protection by the use of such antidotes and by the production and use of special gas masks that are now being devised.

Disaster Medical Care

In the event of mass casualties from nuclear, bacteriological or chemical warfare there would be need for a vast emergency medical program in every community.

The MEND program, more properly called Medical Education for National Defense, is currently operating in a majority of the medical schools of the United States. In this program medical students, medical faculties, and medical graduates are being trained in field operations that simulate civilian catastrophes from various causes, including those that may be expected in the event of modern warfare.

The program acts as a bridge between the military forces and the medical schools. Faculties of the latter are exposed to disaster and survival problems as expected by the military forces. The physicians themselves do the planning as to how the problems are to be met through medical training, organization, and experimental trials. All phases of nuclear, germ, and chemical warfare expectancies and possibilities are being covered in the training.

The organization of local and county medical societies for disaster medical care has been much stimulated by the foregoing MEND program and it can be anticipated that in most communities an organized plan now exists for the care of mass casualties in the event of wartime disasters. The details of this program need not be discussed. It is to be hoped that there will be no occasion in any community for the provision of such services because of modern warfare.

Questions

1. What is the greatest hazard of a nuclear explosion: heat, blast or radiation?
2. If you heard the "alert" warning signal for an impending nuclear attack at this very moment, what would you do?
3. What kind of a sensible family plan should be made in advance of a nuclear attack?
4. How can you defend yourself now against bacteriological warfare?

5. How can your own home or residence be prepared to give maximum protection against the hazard of radiation from nuclear attack?
6. What can you do to decontaminate a person who has been exposed to radioactive fallout?
7. Which of the three survival plans would be best for you and your family?

For Further Reading

1. Office of Civilian and Defense Mobilization: *The Family Fallout Shelter.* Battle Creek, Michigan, 1959.
2. Office of Civilian and Defense Mobilization: *Handbook for Emergencies.* Battle Creek, Michigan, 1958.
3. Office of Civilian and Defense Mobilization: *What Your Should Know About Radioactive Fallout.* Battle Creek, Michigan, 1958.
4. Stanford Research Institute: *Live.* Menlo Park, California, 1960.

Index